*To my parents
and to Héctor*

CONTENTS

ACKNOWLEDGMENTS

Researching a book about scientists, laypeople, and the nature of expertise could not help but spur me to reflect self-consciously on what it means to present myself as an "authority." To whatever extent I can offer a credible analysis of the politics of AIDS research, there is no mystery or magic behind my own expertise: I have benefited at every step from the labor of others who have helped me understand this material or whose work I have learned from over the years. I should therefore begin by acknowledging the researchers, activists, and government officials who fit me into overcrowded schedules and allowed me to interview them about their work and their ideas. They deserve my deepest thanks.

I am indebted to my dissertation adviser, Jerry Karabel, who, at the University of California at Berkeley, supervised the dissertation on which this book is based. His thoughtful and judicious comments have challenged me and moved my work in fruitful directions. I am grateful, as well, for the efforts of my other dissertation committee members, Michael Burawoy, Troy Duster, and David Kirp, whose incisive observations often forced me to rethink my assumptions. Barry Adam, Héctor Carrillo, Adele Clarke, Louis Corrigan, Mark Jones, Brian Martin, Steve Murray, Ken Plummer, Leslie Salzinger, and Steve Shapin all took the time to provide me with substantial comments on drafts of the manuscript or portions of it at various stages along the way. Steve Shapin also dropped any number of useful hints over coffee and in the hallways. The final product would be of far poorer quality without the efforts of these individuals.

I have also benefited from the insights of many other friends and colleagues with whom I have discussed this work, including Dennis Altman, Olga Amsterdamska, Marc Berg, Charles Bosk, Jane Camerini, Larry Casalino, Monica Casper, Nancy Chodorow, Jon Cohen, Susan Cozzens, Melinda Cuthbert, Marcy Darnovsky, Anni Dugdale, Ellie Ely, Ivan Emke, Barbara Epstein, Jeffrey Escoffier, Andy Feenberg, Melia Franklin, Joan Fujimura, Josh Gamson, Ty Geltmaker, Deborah Gerson, Tom Gieryn, Joe Gusfield, David Halperin, the late Carol Hatch, Karen Hossfeld, Leslie Kauffman, Philip Kitcher, Rebecca Klatch, Elizabeth Knoll, Cathy Kudlick, Kristin Luker, Harry Marks, Marcia Meldrum, Mary-Rose Mueller, Chandra Mukerji, Kevin Mumford, Sarah Murray, Cindy Patton, Trevor Pinch, Brian Powers, Jonathan Rabinovitz, Roddey Reid, Evelleen Richards, Alan Richardson, David Rier, Billy Robinson, Aron Rodrigue, Charles Rosenberg, Michael Rosenthal, Pam Rosenthal, Debra Satz, Beth Schneider, Andy Scull, Steven Seidman, Leigh Star, Arlene Stein, Nancy Stoller, Verta Taylor, Francine Twine, Chris Waters, Jeff Weintraub, Bob Westman, Andrea Williams, Ara Wilson, Alan Yoshioka, Yuval Yunay, the audiences at many conferences and talks where I have presented my work, and the anonymous reviewers of work I have submitted for publication.

Barbara Marin and Linda Derksen provided invaluable assistance on statistical matters. Alex Boese, Linda Derksen, and Josh Dunsby painstakingly transcribed interviews. Sarah Groisser scoured the manuscript for typographical errors. Bill Walker of the San Francisco Lesbian & Gay Historical Society archives and Michael Flanagan of the D.A.I.R. archives in San Francisco assisted me in finding AIDS-related materials. Reference librarian Elliot Kanter of the University of California at San Diego applied his expertise to database searches. Peter Duesberg graciously permitted me free access to his personal archives. Mark Harrington, Jon Cohen, and Mary-Rose Mueller also provided access to materials.

I am grateful to colleagues and students in the Sociology Department and the Science Studies Program at UCSD for furthering my education; to the administrative staff members in the department and the program for their technical assistance; and to my department chair, Tim McDaniel, for his support. For advice on publishing matters, I am indebted to Andy Scull and William Abrahams. My editor, Stanley Holwitz, has guided me through the publication process with a steady hand, and I have benefited from his good sense and accumulated wisdom. Others affiliated with the University of California Press, including production editor Scott Norton and copy editor Bonita Hurd, contributed greatly to the final product.

The dissertation on which this book is based was made possible by a Doreen B. Townsend Center for the Humanities Fellowship and a Spencer Dissertation Year Fellowship. Additional research and fundamental rethinking was accomplished under the auspices of a postdoctoral fellowship in the UCSD Science Studies Program, sponsored by a National Science Foundation grant. My capacity to bring this project to closure was then greatly enhanced by a UCSD Academic Senate Research Grant and a Chancellor's Summer Faculty Fellowship.

Close friends in the San Francisco Bay Area, San Diego, and elsewhere provided their encouragement over the years. My parents and my sister gave their love and support. And my partner, Héctor, helped in innumerable and unforgettable ways.

INTRODUCTION

CONTROVERSY, CREDIBILITY, AND THE PUBLIC CHARACTER OF AIDS RESEARCH

It was the first day of classes at Harvard Medical School in fall 1988. As students arrived for the new semester, members of the Boston chapter of ACT UP (the AIDS Coalition to Unleash Power) took positions in front of the building. Equipped with hospital gowns, blindfolds, and chains, the activists broke into a chant: "We're here to show defiance / for what Harvard calls 'good science'!" While some of the demonstrators poured fake blood on the sidewalk, others presented the medical students with a mock "course outline" for an "AIDS 101" class. The outline listed discussion topics like:

PWA's [People with AIDS]—Human beings or laboratory rats?

AZT—Why does it consume 90 percent of all research when it's highly toxic and is not a cure?

Harvard-run clinical trials—Are subjects genuine volunteers, or are they coerced?

Medical elitism—Is the pursuit of elegant science leading to the destruction of our community?[1]

This wasn't a large demonstration; indeed, it was a lesser episode in the annals of AIDS activism. But it suggested the contours of a

I

distinctive terrain. The concepts embedded in the "course outline" were relatively opaque, especially in contrast with the graphic symbolism of the protest—the blood and the chains. These were no simple slogans of the "Up with *this,* down with *that*" variety; each cryptic item hinted at arguments of some depth and complexity. In fact, the activist agenda reflected critical engagement with the nuts and bolts of clinical research into the Acquired Immunodeficiency Syndrome and a desire to take the science of AIDS as seriously as a deadly illness demanded.

These protesters were not rejecting medical science. They were, however, denouncing some *variety* of scientific practice—"elegant" science, "what Harvard calls 'good science'"—as not conducive to medical progress and the health and welfare of their constituency. To the uninitiated, such a challenge might well be baffling: What would "inelegant" science look like, and why should anyone desire it? What would be the alternative to the "good science" that the medical students were absorbing in their lecture halls? What precisely were the activists claiming, both about the nature of AIDS and the nature of biomedical research? And from where did they derive the authority to make their allegations and proposals?

This book is a study of how varied classes of AIDS experts, diverse conceptions of scientific practice, and distinct claims of knowledge about AIDS have all been generated out of relationships of conflict and cooperation in the United States since the early 1980s. Inside a large and often floodlit arena with a diffuse and porous perimeter, an eclectic assortment of actors has sought to assert and assess credible knowledge about AIDS: biomedical researchers and health care professionals of different stripes; activists, advocacy groups, and people with AIDS or HIV infection; health educators and social scientists; politicians and public health officials; government agencies and advisory committees; pharmaceutical and biotechnology companies; writers, journalists, and the institutions of the mainstream and alternative media. "What we know about AIDS" is the product of this elaborate, often heated, and in some ways quite peculiar complex of interactions.

I seek to identify the pathways by which specific beliefs and spokespersons have become accredited as authoritative: How is certainty constructed—or deconstructed? How are scientific controversies adjudicated? How are debates closed, and what is the character of that closure? Who becomes an "AIDS expert" and by what means? In short, how is the linkage of power, knowledge, and order forged in the United States in the context of the AIDS epidemic? My analysis shows how knowledge emerges out of *credibility struggles*—and how the unusual politicization of AIDS in the United States has altered the conduct and resolution of such struggles.

By scientific "credibility," I mean to refer to the believability of claims and claims-makers. More specifically, credibility describes the capacity of claims-makers to enroll supporters behind their arguments, legitimate those arguments as authoritative knowledge, and present themselves as the sort of people who can voice the truth.[2] Credibility is, of course, a quality that can be established in many different ways in different arenas. The credibility of a speaker can rest on academic degrees, "anointment" by the media, or the speaker's access to esoteric forms of communication; the credibility of any knowledge claim can depend on who advances it, how plausible it seems, or what sort of experimental evidence is invoked to support it. In the case of AIDS, credibility struggles have had distinctive characteristics, and the involvement of such a large cast of characters in the controversies has important implications for the study of credibility and knowledge-making.

From a scientific standpoint, the sheer complexity of AIDS has ensured the participation of scientists from a range of disciplines, all of them bringing their particular, often competing, claims to credibility. But AIDS has also been a politicized epidemic, and that political character has had consequences: it has resulted in *multiplication of the successful pathways* to the establishment of credibility and *diversification of the personnel* beyond the highly credentialed. The construction of facts in AIDS controversies has therefore been more complicated and the routes to closure more convoluted. Credibility struggles in the AIDS arena have been multilateral: they have involved an unusually wide range of players. And the interventions of laypeople in the proclamation and evaluation of scientific claims have helped shape what is believed to be known about AIDS—just as they have made problematic our understanding of who is a "layperson" and who is an "expert." At stake at every moment has been whether specific knowledge claims or spokespersons are credible. But at a deeper level, the stakes have involved the very mechanisms for the assessment of credibility: how are scientific claims adjudicated, and who gets to decide? As this study shows, debates *within* science are simultaneously debates *about* science and how it should be done—or who should be doing it.

The science of AIDS, therefore, cannot be analyzed "from the top down." Rather, it demands attention to what Michel Foucault calls the "microphysics of power" in contemporary Western societies: the dispersal of fluxes of power throughout all the cracks and crevices of the social system; the omnipresence of resistance at every site; and the propagation of knowledge, practices, meanings, and identities out of the deployment of power.[3] At the same time, my analysis suggests that—as Foucault would have it—the attempt to master specialized forms of knowledge can make people "objects" of that knowledge as well as "subjects." This is no romantic tale of resistance that privileges the "purity" of knowledge-seeking from below; rather, I argue that the cultures of experts significantly encroach upon and transform those of the laypeople who would engage with them. Nor am I interested in cheerleading, despite my strong sympathies for AIDS activism. What make the story of this engagement with biomedical expertise interesting and important are the ironies and tensions embedded in the process of forging novel scientific, political, and moral identities. This is a complicated history in which no party has had all the answers. All players have revised their claims and shifted their positions over time; all have had to wrestle with the unintended consequences of their own actions.

The immediate goal of my analysis is to shed light on the scientific and political dynamics of a health crisis of immense social import. With so many lives at stake, it behooves us to understand the configuration of interests, beliefs, and practices that determine how we come to believe what we think we know about the epidemic. However, I intend this analysis to do more. By emphasizing the role of laypeople in the production of biomedical knowledge, this study challenges approaches to the social study of science that tend to assume that knowledge-making is the province of a narrow circle of credentialed experts. And by exploring the vicissitudes of lay interventions in AIDS research, particularly on the part of grassroots activists, this study addresses some important and intractable questions about the politics of expertise and the place of science in the larger culture: What is the nature of the power wielded by experts? How does a society reconcile competing commitments to scientific autonomy and participatory democracy? What possibilities are there for laypeople to involve themselves meaningfully in the processes of "doing science," and what are the consequences of such incursions?

In the broadest sense, the analysis that follows reflects a historical and institutional approach to the study of controversies about knowledge. It is concerned with the minute details of the construction of facts, but it assumes that the dynamics of fact-making become apparent only through a more thoroughgoing examination of power, meaning, and social organization. It focuses on the institutions of biomedicine and their particular organizational features and interests, but it argues that these institutions are constrained, and in some sense constituted, by their relations to other institutions and actors, notably forms of popular resistance. Because the pattern of these interrelationships in the case of AIDS has taken shape only gradually over the course of the epidemic, the body of my analysis assumes the form of narrative history. And because the actors and institutions in the story are so diverse, I have been deliberately eclectic in my selection of the theories and concepts that give the narrative its structure. Specifically, this book unites approaches from social studies of science, the sociology of medicine and the professions, and the sociology of social movements. In so doing, the book suggests directions for the development of a more comprehensive inquiry into the politics of knowledge in modern Western societies.

The Crisis of Credibility and the Rise of the AIDS Movement

THE POLITICS OF TRUST AND DISTRUST

Why is AIDS research so fraught with conflict and controversy? Why is this arena of fact-making so unusually public and porous? It has been suggested that a line of scientific research is likely to be controversial when any of a number of characteristics are present: if the research has direct applications, if it challenges or threatens the "natural order," if it is relevant to some politicized social issue, if sentiment has mobilized a related social movement, or if the research is in competition for scarce resources.[4] Since AIDS research is marked by all five characteristics, one need not search hard for explanations of the volatility of the encounters surrounding it.

At the same time, both the controversies enveloping AIDS research and the invasion of the domain of science by outsiders presuppose a specific historical moment—one in which the authority of experts has extraordinary cultural centrality yet seems possessed of a curious fragility. Certainly there is no avoiding reliance on experts who are crucial transmitters and translators of technical knowledge to the lay public.[5] Increasingly, science is the resource called on to promote consensus, and experts are brought in to "settle" political and social controversies. Yet this "scientization of politics"[6] simultaneously brings about a "politicization of science": the fact that political disputes tend to become technical disputes means that different parties rally their own experts to support them in a controversy, much like lawyers offering to the jury a parade of expert witnesses. Ironically, the outcome is that the very reliance on experts to adjudicate disputes tends to undercut the authority of expertise in general, "[highlighting] their fallibility [and demystifying] their special expertise."[7]

Growing distrust of established experts is magnified by our culture's ambivalent attitude toward the institutions of science and their technological products. To be sure, science remains in relatively high esteem, especially considering the overall decline in confidence in many social institutions in the United States in recent decades.[8] Yet science has been subject to attack from a range of points on the political spectrum, and the powers and prerogatives of the expert technocracy have been called into question.[9] Postmodernist perspectives have unseated an Enlightenment confidence in the forward march of history, raising troubling questions about the role of science in a world stripped of the old warrants of reason, truth, and progress.[10] And in a post-Hiroshima world, each passing technological disaster—DES, asbestos, Three Mile Island, Chernobyl, the space shuttle *Challenger*, the *Exxon Valdez*—heightens the perception that the fruits of scientific discoveries may be bitter as often as they are sweet. Overpromising by scientific experts, and claims of certainty that must later be watered down or retracted, are other instigators of "flip-flop thinking" on the part of the public—a tendency to alternate between mythologizing and demonizing scientists.[11]

Medicine, as the most visible—and indeed most popular—form of applied science, has been a particularly important target of recent critiques of science.[12] Doctors, in the words of Paul Starr, "serve as intermediaries between science and private experience."[13] More profoundly than the abstract sciences, medicine seems to entrap its consumers in a fierce love-hate relationship, a tight nexus of need and fear. Over the course of the nineteenth and early twentieth centuries, doctors rose to positions of privilege in the United States, able to reap substantial social rewards on the basis of their authority. This authority, according to Starr, rested on the twin pillars of legitimacy and dependence: people believed that medical knowledge could help them, and they felt that only doctors possessed that special knowledge and the skill to use it. The victory of medical authority therefore required the popular abandonment of an earlier, Jacksonian belief that the healing arts were accessible to "common sense" and the acknowledgment, on the contrary, of medicine's "legitimate complexity": no longer could everyone be his or her own physician.[14]

In the 1950s, as Starr notes, "medical science epitomized the postwar vision of progress without conflict"—but this vision faltered in the 1960s and 1970s.[15] Leftists advanced a thoroughgoing critique of the "medical-industrial complex": lurking behind the white coats and the reassuring smiles were profit lust and the dominance of large corporations.[16] While conservatives and liberals argued that medical costs were out of control, feminists strove to take back control over their own bodies, criticizing medical science as a patriarchal institution. Revelations of past abuses in medical experimentation on human subjects led to an expanded emphasis on "informed consent," premised on the notion that the patient's trust in a physician is not automatically granted but "must be earned through conversation."[17] At the same time, these revelations prompted the emergence of new institutions and bureaucratic structures designed to safeguard the interests of patients and research subjects vis-à-vis their own doctors.[18]

The AIDS epidemic has magnified these various misgivings about doctors and researchers. Indeed, in the face of death and disease, popular ambivalence about biomedicine has undergone a peculiar amplification: distrust has been accentuated, but so has dependence. Despite their suspicion of expertise, people in advanced industrial societies typically expect doctors and scientists to protect them from illness and death. Yet, a decade and a half into the epidemic, researchers have not found an effective cure or vaccine. Scientists insist this is not surprising, given the complexity of AIDS and the "normal" rate of progress in biomedical investigations. Nevertheless, the failure of experts to solve the problem of AIDS quickly, as they were "supposed to," has heightened popular resentment and sparked a "credibility crisis."[19] This in turn has opened up more space for dissident positions, both among scientists and doctors and within the lay public.

In theory, science is a quintessentially public enterprise. As Yaron Ezrahi notes, every scientific finding is legitimated by the notion that it is "grounded in impersonal non-private reproducible procedures through which it can be certified by anyone who cares to do so, provided he has the competence and the patience."[20] In fact, as Steven

Shapin and Simon Schaffer have described it, the evolution of modern science is an ironic story of the construction of "a public space with restricted access." The consequence is that "a form of knowledge that is the most open in principle has become the most closed in practice."[21] Scientists themselves are often anxious to police the boundaries of their professional domain and keep out unqualified interlopers or traffickers in "pseudoscience."[22]

Yet the experts themselves ruefully acknowledge that the traditional conception of scientific autonomy is little in evidence in the case of AIDS. "We are no longer in that period of splendid isolation in science," the director of the National Institutes of Health (NIH), Dr. James B. Wyngaarden, remarked in 1989. "AIDS has politicized research, brought scientists face to face with many social issues and disaffected individuals, and gotten the attention of an activist community."[23] If, as some have sought to argue, the "purity" of science is guaranteed by its insulation from external pressures,[24] then AIDS research is a clear-cut case of impure science.

THE DISTINCTIVE CHARACTER
OF THE AIDS MOVEMENT

Perhaps the most striking feature on the landscape of AIDS politics is the development of an "AIDS movement" that is more than just a "disease constituency" pressuring the government for more funding, but is in fact an alternative basis of expertise. The members of this movement are not the first laypeople to put forward claims to speak credibly on biomedical matters. But this is indeed the first social movement in the United States to accomplish the large-scale conversion of disease "victims" into activist-experts. In this sense, the AIDS movement stands alone, even as it begins to serve as a model for others.[25]

The movement is broad based and diverse, ranging from grassroots activists and advocacy organizations to health educators, journalists, writers, and service providers; it cuts across the various communities and constituencies affected by the AIDS epidemic, and includes gays and lesbians, people with hemophilia, injection drug users, and members of many hard-hit African-American and Latino communities. Over the course of the epidemic, members of the AIDS movement have taught themselves the details of virology, immunology, and epidemiology. They have criticized scientific research that seemed to be fueled by antigay assumptions, defended speculation about alternative theories of AIDS causation, asserted that community-based AIDS organizations have the expertise to define public health constructs such as "safe sex," demanded scientific investigation of potentially useful treatments, established a grassroots base of knowledge about treatments, conducted their own "underground" drug trials, and criticized the methodologies employed in AIDS clinical research. They have established their credibility as people who might legitimately speak in the language of medical science, in particular with regard to the design, conduct, and interpretation of clinical trials used to test the safety and efficacy of AIDS drugs.

Medicine is, to be sure, a more likely target of lay intervention than other, more private and remote domains of scientific practice. On a national level, biomedical politics constitute "one arena of science-government relations" where interest groups flourish and "where ordinary people get some of what they want."[26] On a more intimate scale, the health of one's body is an issue of considerable salience to most people in a way that, say, astrophysics or oceanography typically is not. And individuals have much easier access to at least the frontline institutions of biomedicine—hospitals, clinics, and so on—than to the inner sanctums of science. Indeed, there is a substantial, if recent, history of political challenges to the doctor-patient relationship and of the emergence of the "educated patient"—a history that prefigures the claims-making projects of the AIDS movement. Patients with chronic illnesses such as diabetes, multiple sclerosis, and arthritis may be particularly inclined to become expert in therapeutic options and even the theories about underlying disease mechanisms.[27]

Of course, the expertise of the individual educated patient is not likely to "travel" far beyond a restricted domain. But as patients begin to organize and exchange information, the breadth and durability of their lay expertise is enhanced. Such organization can take a variety of forms. Creation of patient self-help groups—a rapidly proliferating phenomenon particularly in the United States—is an important step in the development of an organized base of alternative expertise.[28] A different kind of example is the attempt made by groups of cancer patients in the 1970s to promote access to unapproved therapies, such as use of laetrile; their efforts resulted in public hearings and Supreme Court rulings.[29] Perhaps most consequential for the cultural redefinition of relations between medical experts and lay consumers was the emergence in the 1970s of the feminist health movement. Linking a systematic critique of patriarchal institutions to a concrete praxis of self-help, the feminist health movement sought, in Sheryl Ruzek's words, to "[reduce] the knowledge differential between patient and practitioner, [challenge] the license and mandate of physicians to provide certain services, [reduce] professionals' control and monopoly over related necessary goods and services, . . . and [transform] the clientele from an aggregate into a collectivity." [30]

However, neither self-help groups nor cancer activists nor even the feminist health movement has had much success in extending its critique of medical *practice* into an engagement with the methodologies of biomedical *research*. Examples of this sort of lay intervention are few and far between, although analysts have described some intriguing parallel cases. For example, in the late 1980s the RSI (Repetitive Strain Injury) Association in the United Kingdom not only produced patients who were "better informed about the disorder than their treating physician" but also played a role in the very conceptualization of this new illness within the biomedical establishment. [31] The German Retinitis Pigmentosa Society, founded in 1977, encouraged scientists to pursue specific lines of research that otherwise might not have been investigated, judging from the absence of such research in other European countries. [32] Yet even these examples pale when compared to the breadth, depth, and, certainly, the *militance* of the AIDS movement.

What gives AIDS activism its distinctive character? To some extent, the unique features of the clinical picture of AIDS have shaped the development of an activist response. First, AIDS has affected many young people in their twenties and thirties who are little inclined simply to lie down and wait to die. Second, those who test positive on HIV antibody tests (available since 1985) are likely to be told by medical authorities to expect some number of years of outwardly normal health before the onset of symptoms—years in which activism is not only feasible from a physical standpoint but may seem eminently practical from a political and psychological standpoint. Indeed, AIDS activism, as opposed to many other activist projects, holds out the promise of some profoundly tangible immediate rewards, most notably access to potentially life-prolonging medications.

Even more fundamental, the distinctive social epidemiology of AIDS has shaped the character of the public engagement with science. Unlike many other diseases, which affect the population in a relatively random fashion, AIDS has had a strikingly uneven impact, being disproportionately prevalent within specific groups, subcultures, and communities. This may seem an obvious point, yet its significance cannot be overemphasized. From the start—and up to the present day—AIDS has been understood both in epidemiological and lay parlance as a disease of certain already-constituted social groups distinguished by their "lifestyle," their social location, or both.[33] The result is that the very meaning of AIDS has been bound up with the cultural understanding of what such groups are like, while the very identity of the groups has been shaped by the perception of them as "the sort of people who get this illness." If AIDS were not deadly, if it were not associated with taboo topics such as sex and drug use, and if the groups affected were not already stigmatized on other counts, such linkages between identity and illness might be of little consequence. As it is, the AIDS epidemic has engendered fear and prejudice and has sparked the necessity, on a massive scale, for what Erving Goffman has called "the management of spoiled identity."[34]

Gay men, the group whose identity has been most thoroughly shaped by the confrontation and association with the epidemic, entered the era of AIDS equipped with a whole set of resources crucial for engagement in the struggle over social goods and social meanings.[35] In the recent past, gays and lesbians in the United States had achieved a singular (if incomplete) redefinition of social status, challenging the dominant conceptions of homosexuality as illness or immorality, and reconstituting themselves as a legitimate "interest group" pursuing civil rights and civil liberties. With the limited successes of the "homophile" movement of the 1950s and 1960s and the more substantial impact of the gay liberation and gay rights movements of the 1970s, gay men and lesbians challenged social norms, constructed organizations and institutions, and established substantial and internally differentiated subcultures in urban centers throughout the United States.[36] By the time the AIDS epidemic was recognized in 1981, the gay movement was deeply engaged in projects of "identity politics"—the linkage of tangible political goals to the elaboration and assertion of an affirmative group identity.[37] A threat to identity, therefore, was a threat that the movement could easily understand and one against which it was quick to mobilize.

An engagement with the medical profession was not entirely foreign to this movement either, since a specific accomplishment of gay liberation had been to "demedicalize" homosexuality by removing it from the official list of psychiatric illnesses. Indeed, while gay activists on the margins of U.S. society had developed an oppositional stance regarding many social institutions, they had for some time been particularly inclined to view medical authorities with suspicion.[38] And many lesbians (and heterosexual women) who would become active in the AIDS movement were schooled in the tenets of the feminist health movement of the 1970s, which likewise advocated skepticism toward medical claims and an insistence upon the patient's decision-making autonomy.[39]

Thus, in its emergence and mobilization, the AIDS movement was a beneficiary of "social movement spillover":[40] it was built on the foundations of other movements and borrowed from their particular strengths and inclinations. Most consequential was the link to the lesbian and gay movement of the 1970s and early 1980s: It mattered that gay communities had preexisting organizations that could mobilize to meet a new threat; these community organizations and institutions also provided settings for the face-to-face interactions that are so important in drawing individuals into activism.[41] It mattered, too, that these communities included (and in fact were dominated by) white, middle-class men with a degree of political clout and fund-raising capacity unusual for an oppressed group. And it was crucial that gay communities possessed a relatively high degree of "cultural capital"— that they had cultivated a disposition for appropriating knowledge and culture.[42] Within these communities are many people who are professionals, artists, and intellectuals of one sort or another—not to mention many doctors, scientists, educators, nurses, and other health professionals. On one hand, this has provided the AIDS movement with an unusual capacity to develop its own "organic intellectuals"[43] and contest the mainstream experts on their own ground. On the other hand, it has afforded important sources of intermediation and communication between "experts" and "the public."

This particular historical conjuncture has given birth to a movement that is uniquely inclined and empowered to challenge the scientific and medical establishments. In some respects, the AIDS movement resembles other social movements that have challenged scientific authorities in the recent past—movements that have focused on issues as diverse as evolutionary theory, IQ testing, nuclear power, fetal tissue research, and recombinant DNA research. However, while there often are similarities among these oppositional groups, even across the political spectrum,[44] the differences in how they approach science are striking.[45] Some movements are essentially negative, confining themselves to the politics of distrust: "We don't believe you when you claim that fluoridation is harmless." Others ultimately just want to show that science and truth are on their side. They seek to acquire for themselves the cachet of scientific authority by finding the expert who will validate their given political stance: "Low level radiation is dangerous"; "the greenhouse effect isn't a serious threat." Members of a third category, typified by some advocates of mysticism and "New Age" philosophies, reject outright the scientific way of knowing and advance their own claims to expertise from some wholly different epistemological standpoint.

Perhaps the most interesting of the social movements that position themselves in relation to science are those which try to stake out some ground on the scientists' own terrain. These activists wrangle with scientists on issues of truth and method. They seek not only to reform science by exerting pressure from the outside but also to perform science by locating themselves on the inside. They question not just the *uses* of science, not just the *control over* science, but sometimes even the very *contents* of science and the *processes* by which it is produced. Most fundamentally, they claim to speak credibly as experts in their own right—as people who know about things scientific and who can partake of this special and powerful discourse of truth. Most intriguingly, they seek to change the ground rules about how the game of science is played.

The AIDS movement can best be compared with the relatively short list of movements that neither simply enlist experts nor attack them but, rather, undergo the process of "expertification." A participant in such a movement learns the relevant knowledge base so as to become a sort of expert; more broadly, such participants transform the very mechanisms by which expertise is socially constituted and recognized. Phil Brown, for example, has studied the engagement of citizens of Woburn, Massachusetts, in the determination of health risks from toxic waste. Brown characterizes their efforts as "popular epidemiology," in which "laypersons gather scientific data and other information and also direct and marshal the knowledge and resources of experts in order to understand the epidemiology of disease." [46] Such movements, as Susan Cozzens and Edward Woodhouse note, are not "anti-science" but "pro-knowledge": they seek "to re-value forms of knowledge that professional science has excluded, rather than to devalue scientific knowledge itself." [47]

AIDS activism is distinctive, however, in the duration of intense working relationships between the movement and the research community. And AIDS activism is unusual in the extent to which activists necessarily depend on the energy and goodwill of their own interlocutors. Antinuclear activists who master the technical jargon of nuclear engineers have the luxury of treating those experts as the enemy. AIDS activists, by contrast, have no illusions about their ultimate dependence on the biomedical enterprise for the discovery and testing of treatments. Although some community spokespeople endorse New Age therapeutic methods ranging from "creative visualization" to healing crystals, most activists accept that a solution to the deadly AIDS epidemic will arrive via some variety of scientific process, if it arrives at all. They are caught, as Ronald Bayer puts it, "between the specter and the promise of medicine."[48]

Analyzing AIDS Controversies

CREDIBILITY AND TRUST IN SCIENTIFIC FACT-MAKING

The sociology of scientific knowledge is particularly well suited to shedding light on such phenomena as scientific controversy, credibility crises, and the public trust and distrust of experts: this body of work identifies credibility and trust as the very underpinnings of scientific knowledge-production. Not just relations between laypeople and experts, but also relations among scientists themselves are enabled by the social organization of trust and the construction of credibility.

Since its inception in the 1970s, the sociology of scientific knowledge has argued that scientific fact-making is a collective process amenable to sociological investigation.[49] As Steven Shapin explains, "no scientific claim 'shines with its own light'—carries its credibility with it. . . ." Analysts of science have therefore "become intensely interested in the specific processes of argumentation and political action whereby claims come to be accepted as true or rejected as false."[50] In practice, a range of theories has been offered as to how the credibility of knowledge claims is secured.[51] For Bruno Latour and his colleagues and collaborators, credibility is the stake in an agonistic struggle. In this approach, science is "politics by other means," and the credibility of a knowledge claim depends on the play of power: the scientist who can appear to make nature "behave" in the laboratory, whose rhetoric is more persuasive, who is able to summon up the more compelling citations, and who is able to enlist more allies, patrons, and supporters by "translating" their interests so that they correspond with the scientist's own is the one who constructs credible knowledge and gains access to further resources as a result. The most effective claims are those which become "obligatory passage points": the journal article that all must cite to justify their own work, the technology that all must employ to accomplish their own research—in general, the way stations through which other scientists, patrons, or members of the public necessarily must pass in order to satisfy their interests or achieve their goals. The more well traveled such passage points, the more fully institutionalized the knowledge claims become.[52]

Alternatively, analysts such as Barry Barnes, Harry Collins, and Steven Shapin, while emphasizing the role of conflict, also understand scientific credibility as emerging from the nexus of cooperative relationships that constitute scientific communities.[53] Since no one can "know" all or even a fraction of the corpus of scientific knowledge through direct experience, science is made possible through the allocation of trust. "Trust and authority," writes Barnes, "are the wires of a great system of communication which makes the specialized knowledge of society widely credible and widely usable."[54] Clearly, laypeople are almost always in the position of having to trust what experts tell them is true. But trust is crucial even to the relationships among scientists, as Collins demonstrates in his arguments concerning the phenomenon of "experimenters' regress": "The competence of experimenters and the integrity of experiments can only be ascertained by examining *results,* but the appropriate results can only be known from competently performed experiments."[55] Independent replication of a finding does not resolve the dilemma of whether to believe, because no two experiments are ever exactly the same in all details, and so the status of an experiment as a replication must also be socially negotiated. In order, then, for any finding to be accepted, scientists cannot be utter skeptics. Either they must trust that the experiment was competently performed (thus granting credibility to the result) or they must trust the result (thereby conceding that the experiment was competently performed). At any given moment, *some* knowledge must be taken on faith, if science is to proceed as a social institution. Even expressions of distrust are "predicated upon a background of trust," explains Shapin: a scientist cannot distrust a particular finding or person except against the background of other shared knowledge which is unproblematically trusted.[56]

These conceptions of the social relations that govern scientific knowledge-production have several implications for understanding cases such as AIDS research. First, these analyses suggest that scientists, other professionals, and laypeople alike find themselves frequently in the business of assessing the credibility of knowledge claims and claimants, and asking who or what they should trust and believe. The difficulty is that—for laypeople and to a considerable extent for experts as well—such assessments can usually be made only indirectly, through the scrutiny of external markers of credibility. Who conducted the study? Where was it published? What does the *New York Times* have to say about it? What does my doctor think? Even such everyday iconography as the diploma on the wall serves an important signaling function within a social system stitched together by assertions and assessments of credibility.[57]

Second, this understanding of credibility implies a special role for certain face-to-face interactions, such as those between doctors and patients. In a world significantly organized by impersonal bureaucracies, doctors serve as "'access points' . . . at which 'faceless institutions' present a particular human face to those who encounter and pass through them."[58] Doctors are among the experts that laypeople are most likely to encounter firsthand; their credibility can be read in their words, body language, and "bedside manner." This social location gives practicing physicians a distinctive function in controversies involving doctors, patients, and scientists.

Third, since trust and credibility may be fragile resources, scientists, doctors, and other experts are keenly attuned to potential disruptions in the social circulation of credibility. In effect, scientists barter their credibility for the extension of resources by patrons and the public, who typically stand back and respect the autonomy of scientists, allowing them to determine the specific division and allocation of research funds, judge one another's work, and police abuses.[59] One consequence of this arrangement for the expert claims-maker is that maintaining legitimacy (both one's own and that of science in general) becomes of paramount importance: when legitimacy is threatened, the credibility of one's claims is in jeopardy, and with it, the availability of resources and the maintenance of professional autonomy.[60] Like other professional groups, scientists frequently participate in shoring up their legitimacy,[61] including engaging in public relations work and attempts to manage the presentation of scientific findings in the mass media.[62] This labor is made difficult by the number of factors that can diminish the public's perception of the legitimacy of science, including instances of scientific fraud, malpractice, and incompetence; technological disasters; the failure to solve problems considered socially significant; the perception that scientists are "crossing the line" into politics or advocacy; admissions of uncertainty on the part of experts; and dogmatic professions of overcertainty.[63] The very existence of disputes between experts can cause legitimacy problems for science, given the "belief that science 'naturally' produces consensus by the collective pursuit of 'the scientific method.'"[64]

The AIDS crisis is a case in which the normal flow of trust and credibility between experts and laypeople has been disrupted. The autonomy of science has therefore been challenged; outsiders have rushed into the breach. But something else has happened as well: some of those outsiders, particularly groups of AIDS activists, have constituted themselves as a new class of "lay experts" and put forward their own claims to speak credibly about the epidemic.

SCIENCE STUDIES AND THE PROBLEM
OF KNOWLEDGE-MAKING FROM BELOW

How do we analyze moves on the part of AIDS activists to assert and assess scientific credibility? In a recent summary of credibility studies in the sociology of scientific knowledge, Shapin takes it as a point of methodological principle that "there is no limit to the considerations that might be relevant to securing credibility, and, therefore, no limit to the considerations to which the analyst of science might give attention."[65] Nevertheless, analysts of science have paid little attention to the specific and novel mechanisms by which lay outsiders establish beachheads of credibility on the terrain of modern scientific institutions.

In Collins's influential formulation, knowledge in scientific controversies is made by a relatively small "core set" of researchers.[66] Collins notes that members of the public may rely on other experts to challenge the claims of the core set. But he offers no discussion of the processes by which laypeople can construct alternative ways of knowing or new varieties of expertise that—sometimes—alter the pathways of knowledge construction.[67] Restricting analysis to a core set of experts makes little sense in controversies where part of what is "up for grabs" is who gets to count as an expert and which set of characteristics qualify one as such. Collins's own studies of parapsychology

demonstrate precisely this point.[68] But most appropriations of his notion of the "core set" use the term as synonymous with a small circle
of insiders. Similarly, Latour's "actor-network" theory assumes in
principle that, just as scientists may enroll laypeople in support of scientific facts and approaches, so laypeople may attempt to enroll scientists. But in practice, as a number of critics have pointed out, Latour
and his collaborators "have not developed the implications" of this
assumption[69] and have opted for what Susan Leigh Star criticizes as
the "executive approach," in which it is assumed that the powerful
scientist does the claims-making and seeks to recruit others, including
laypeople, behind his or her banner.[70]

How can science be studied without assuming in a priori fashion
which groups at which social locations create scientific knowledge? It
would be wise to take seriously Latour's injunction simply to "follow
the actors" wherever that may lead the analyst and not to worry about
what is really "inside" and "outside" of science.[71] Indeed, social studies of science have stressed that the boundaries between what is internal and what is external to science are themselves constructed in the
course of scientific practice—that scientists perform "boundary work"
to circumscribe a domain they can then call their own.[72] Another
school of science studies, which draws on the interactionist tradition
in sociology, is also helpful in thinking about a case such as this one.
These analysts study the "negotiation of order" in the encounter between different "social worlds"—"groups with shared commitments
to certain activities sharing resources of many kinds to achieve their
goals."[73] From this frame of reference, the scientific study of AIDS
can be viewed precisely as the product of the encounter—or clash—
between members of many different social worlds. Phenomena such
as a virus, a medication, or a clinical experiment, in this view, may
have the status of "boundary objects": each one has an identity that
cuts across social worlds, but understandings of the phenomenon may
vary in subtle yet significant ways depending on the social standpoint
from which it is viewed.[74]

Each participating social world can be treated as distinct, at least
for analytical purposes, yet somehow out of their intersection there
emerges a *field* that generates knowledge about AIDS. The borders of
this field may be relatively porous, its parameters may be evolving over
time, but it has an emergent logic—itself the product of negotiation
and cooperation—that conditions the practices of the diverse actors
within it. In my conception of the "field" of AIDS research and knowledge production, I am influenced by the work of Pierre Bourdieu, who

describes fields as specific, relatively autonomous, domains of social action—domains of social production and reproduction—that both reflect and constrain the interests, positions, strategies, and investments of the actors within them.[75] Inside each field, players compete with one another subject to the current rules of the game, but in so doing they seek to reshape the rules to suit the means at their disposal.

This is precisely what emerges in credibility struggles related to AIDS—the constant attempt by different players to rephrase the definition of "science" so that their particular "capital"—their forms of credibility—have efficacy within the field. Or as the AIDS activists in Boston put it: "We're here to show defiance / for what Harvard calls 'good science.'"[76] To understand the dynamics of such negotiations, however, it is useful to look beyond the domain of science studies. Studies of social movements, the media, and the professions all offer important resources for analyzing the politics of knowledge in AIDS research.

SCIENCE STUDIES AND
SOCIAL MOVEMENT RESEARCH

The relation between activism and science has been considered from a variety of directions by scholars working within the sociology of social movements, the sociology of science, and other fields. Analysts have investigated such topics as the reliance of some activist movements on outside, credentialed expertise,[77] the antipathy of groups such as the animal rights movement toward the scientific enterprise,[78] the formation of activist groups or advocacy movements by scientists or professionals themselves,[79] and even the tendency of delegitimated clusters of scientists to work in ways that resemble social movements.[80]

Few studies, however, have explored the role of movements in the construction of credible knowledge, and few sociologists of scientific knowledge have engaged significantly with the sociological literature on social movements.[81] To understand the complex dynamics of the field of AIDS research and in particular to conceptualize the interventions of organized groups of laypeople in scientific practice, it makes sense to borrow generously from this literature. On one hand, attention to the means by which social movements engage in claims-making—how they mobilize,[82] how they construct collective identities,[83] how they "frame" social issues and represent reality[84]—can shed light on their capacity to engage with medical and scientific expertise. On the other hand, it is worth asking how the encounter with science affects the social movement in turn: in what ways does this engagement transform the movement's collective identity, mobilization potential, framing practices, and representational strategies?

James Petersen and Gerald Markle apply the "resource mobilization" perspective (a dominant approach within the study of social movements) to the cancer treatment movement, analyzing how activists "try to form coalitions, seek sponsorship, and appeal to a wider audience . . . as a means of increasing their movement resources."[85] And Debbie Indyk and David Rier likewise emphasize resource mobilization in their useful analysis of the particular case of alternative knowledge-production in the AIDS epidemic.[86] But analysts of science have paid little attention to the extensive theoretical and empirical literature on "new social movements"—works describing the ecology movement, the women's movement, the antinuclear movement, racial and ethnic movements, the gay and lesbian movement, and so on—a literature with obvious relevance to the study of the AIDS movement.[87]

Theorists of new social movements differ greatly in their approaches to the topic, though most tend to agree that the actors within the new movements are drawn primarily from the "new middle class" or "new class" of culture producers, particularly that strand of it that Alvin Gouldner calls the humanistic intelligentsia.[88] But unlike in working class politics, the class character of these movements is not emphasized by the activists. They are involved not (or at least not only) in a distributive struggle, where a quantity of resources is being parceled out to competing groups, but in a struggle over cultural forms—what Jürgen Habermas calls the "grammar of forms of life."[89] Their emphases tend to be on "personal and intimate aspects of human life," their organizations tend to be "segmented, diffuse, and decentralized," and their theatrical protest tactics emphasize civil disobedience and a politics of representation.[90]

An epidemic whose social definition lies at the intersection of cultural discourses about sexuality, the body, and identity is, arguably, the ideal staging ground for the emergence of a new social movement. Perhaps most significantly, the politics of AIDS are interwoven at the deepest level with the explosive politics of sexuality in contemporary Western societies. "It would be difficult to imagine a more powerful or urgent demonstration than the AIDS crisis of the need to conceptualize sexuality, after the manner of Foucault, as 'an especially concentrated point of transversal . . . for relations of power,'" writes David Halperin.[91] AIDS activists have sought to challenge the ideological linkages between sex and death and put forward "sex-positive" programs of AIDS prevention that assert the right to sexual pleasure and sexual freedom.

The body, another key site for the elaboration of AIDS activism, is "the tangible form of selfhood," the "symbolic frame through which [the] paradoxes of existence are most powerfully mediated."[92] But as Alberto Melucci notes, in the contemporary period the body has also "become a field of action on which social and cultural contradictions are delineated."[93] This is perhaps most obviously true when the body is confronted by the physical threat of annihilation through disease: it can itself become the most potent signifier of crisis and resistance.[94] "We in the communities most touched by AIDS have learned that the ultimate site of this struggle is the body," commented ACT UP/New York activist Jim Eigo in a presentation at a scientific conference: "So here I am, my own and my only audiovisual aid. There will be no 'next slide.'"[95]

Central to the self-understanding of new social movements is the focus on the values of autonomy and identity. Yet the salient feature of the new social movements is not so much that they assert identities as the fact that the actors within them are *conscious* of their own active involvement in a public and contested process of identity construction.[96] While the constitution of identity may sometimes become an end in itself, William Gamson argues that it also serves an instrumental function in the mobilization process, influencing not only people's willingness to "invest emotionally" in the fate of the movement and "take personal risks on its behalf" but also their choices of strategies and organizational forms.[97]

These are exactly the characteristics one finds in ACT UP, which was, in the late 1980s and early 1990s, the premier social movement organization within the broader AIDS movement. ACT UP "operates largely by staging events and by carefully constructing and publicizing symbols"; its theatrics "are part of a continuing process of actively forging a gay identity while challenging the process through which it is formed *for* gay people at a time when the stigma of disease has been linked with the stigma of deviant sexuality."[98] This emphasis on identity politics has, in certain crucial respects, facilitated AIDS activists in their capacity to engage with scientific knowledge-production. Because identity politics are preoccupied with nonmaterial issues— with questions of representation and meaning—these activists are inclined to wage struggles over the definition of reality. And because identity politics stand in opposition to what Foucault calls "normalization," these defenders of identity are highly sensitive to the imposition of norms, categories, and labels by outside authorities.[99] Drawn often from the ranks of those with significant cultural capital, AIDS activists have both a greater inclination and capacity to participate in the construction of social meanings and challenge the purveyors of "symbolic violence."[100]

THE MEDIA AND THE
CONSTRUCTION OF CREDIBILITY

The AIDS movement's possession of cultural capital and its facility with manipulating symbols are manifested in another way that is central to the story I tell—the movement's possession of its own media institutions. A large number of studies have emphasized the important role of the media in establishing the public dimensions of scientific and medical controversies. Such studies reveal how the media filter and translate scientific information, construct public images of scientific certainty and uncertainty, shape the ways in which people understand the "sides" and "boundaries" of a debate, certify scientific and medical celebrities, affect perceptions of risk, and reinforce popular stereotypes of scientists and doctors as both heroes and villains.[101] David Phillips and his collaborators have shown that even professional scientists rely on prominent mass media organs, such as the *New York Times,* to provide them with a sense of which scientific findings are most important, and that "the direct transmission of information in the medical literature . . . is enhanced or amplified by secondary transmission in the lay press. . . ."[102] By the same token, the mass media can bring the perspectives of delegitimated actors into the public eye. As Bert Klandermans explains in a study of social movements, the media "are able to diffuse beliefs the organization itself would never had been able to diffuse," with the result that "the movement organization itself gains greater credibility. . . ."[103]

The analysis in this book reinforces the notion that the institutions of the mass media can play a critical role in shaping how scientific controversies are interpreted and adjudicated. But in addition, I emphasize the impact of alternative media institutions, including the lesbian and gay press, movement publications, and grassroots literature about AIDS treatments.[104] The extensive coverage of medical and scientific issues in these publications has been a significant factor in the construction of knowledge-empowered communities, and the particular analytical frames employed by writers and editors have helped shape the orientations of the AIDS movement. Indeed, some media organs of the AIDS movement, such as the publication *AIDS Treatment News,* are widely recognized as agenda-setting vehicles for the circulation of scientific knowledge, and are read by activists, doctors, and researchers alike.[105] Such developments pose an important challenge to the conventional "top-down" models of how expert knowledge is disseminated.[106] As Indyk and Rier suggest, the spread of knowledge about AIDS is best conceived as "a multisite process, involving not *hierarchies* of diffusion but *webs* of exchange."[107]

MEDICINE AND THE PROFESSIONS

The sociology of the professions is also of particular relevance to the study of credibility and expertise, since professionalism, as Andrew Abbott notes, is precisely "the main way of institutionalizing expertise in industrialized countries."[108] A crucial focus of my study is the relations between professional groups and lay clients, and I take seriously Foucault's suggestion that this is a pivotal arena of struggle in modern societies—that power is manifested in the ability of professionals to label, classify, and condemn, as well as in the capacity of clients to resist the imposition of such meanings.[109] However, my analysis also seeks to avoid reifying the categories "professional" and "layperson" as if they were invariant or monolithic entities. I therefore analyze tendencies toward professionalization *within* social movements that engage with expert knowledge.

Furthermore, my analysis assumes that the interests of the various researchers and doctors who figure in the AIDS controversies are shaped by their specific relations to organizations, institutions, and social groups. For example, I analyze the fundamental differences in interest and orientation between biomedical researchers, whose primary commitment is to science, and practicing physicians, whose immediate commitment is to patients. As Eliot Freidson notes, medicine is an "impure" social form—a profession with a lay clientele, coexisting with a scientific community of peers.[110] In debates over how to interpret research findings, practitioners of the healing "arts" who are in direct contact with patients may produce different readings than researchers who are invested in a conception of biomedicine as "science"—and, of course, some individuals occupy both roles simultaneously.[111] In analyzing such debates, this study seeks to reinforce the emerging links between studies of medical practice that have been central to the sociology of medicine and analyses of knowledge production that have been developed by the sociology of science.[112]

CONSTRUCTING SOCIAL REALITY

Although an understanding of the AIDS controversies demands broad attention to science, medicine, the professions, social movements, and the media, my employment of the various theories and concepts from these literatures does reflect an underlying commonality. In each case, I am concerned with theoretical perspectives that emphasize the active, collective, and competitive construction of the social world: how do individuals and groups diagnose social problems and propose solutions?[113]

The notion of "framing" is used commonly as a metaphor to describe the constructive dimension in different arenas of social practice—a metaphor that resonates clearly with conceptions of claims-making and translation in science studies. Frames are "principles of selection, emphasis, and presentation composed of little tacit theories about what exists, what happens, and what matters."[114] Frames impose order upon experience—but never arbitrarily or neutrally. Todd Gitlin provides the telling example of reporters' use of the crime story as a frame for understanding political protest.[115] Charles Rosenberg has analyzed how diseases come to be framed, in particular through attributions of causality and blame, and he describes how diseases, once framed, can then serve as frames for the organization of other social phenomena (as when for example we speak of "social lepers" or "computer viruses").[116] And somewhat similarly, analysts of "social problems" describe the role of claims-making in the genesis of "typifications"—the identification by an actor of the true "nature" of some problem and its "typical" manifestations—and in the assertion of group "ownership" over various social issues and how these issues are defined and conceived.[117]

Analogously, as the promoters of a "dramaturgical" model of social movement activism have usefully contended, social movements are not simply "carriers" or "transmitters" of ideology but are fundamentally and necessarily engaged in the framing of reality.[118] Social movements seek to "frame, or assign meaning to and interpret, relevant events and conditions in ways that are intended to mobilize potential adherents and constituents, to garner bystander support, and to demobilize antagonists."[119] Frames serve as "accenting devices" that underscore the seriousness of movement claims, they promote the attribution of blame and causality, and they help activists to "align" events and experiences into digestible "packages."[120]

Each of these perspectives is useful in understanding the varied contributions of the key players in the construction of credible knowledge about AIDS. To engage in the politics of knowledge, individuals and groups must be able to present themselves as credible representatives of social interests and engage in the framing of reality through techniques of representation. They must be able to mobilize a constituency by framing or translating issues and interests in ways that attract adherents. And they must succeed in constructing enabling identities with relatively well-defined boundaries.[121] Different actors will seek to frame AIDS, or construct knowledge, or assert their claims to expertise in quite different ways depending in part on their interests, their social locations, and the organizations to which they belong. By means of these framings, credible knowledge is both assembled and taken apart.

This review of the claims-making practices of scientists, professionals, activists, and the mainstream and alternative media confirms that, indeed, "there is no limit to the considerations that might be relevant to securing credibility. . . ."[122] Credibility, as I use the term, rests on the dual supports of power and trust.[123] On one hand, credibility is both a stake and a weapon in the skirmishes between all those who are in competition to say what the world is like. On the other hand, credibility is the mechanism for forging durable relationships within which knowledge can reliably be exchanged. The construction of credibility is thus simultaneously an outcome of the competing forces brought to bear in struggles and a marker of the thickening of social ties.

The achievement of credibility can be demonstrated by its real-world consequences: Are claims accepted or rejected in different fields? What language is used to qualify or characterize scientific claims (there is a huge difference between "Many scientists believe that AIDS is caused by a virus called HIV" and "HIV, the AIDS virus, . . .")?[124] Are the evaluative capacities of different actors acknowledged or disputed? Who is successful in bringing controversies to closure, and who has the capacity to reopen them? Do the rules of credibility assessment remain fixed, or do they shift in response to struggle?

And crucially, what actions are taken or policies implemented on the basis of credibility granted to claims or to claims-makers?

The Plan of the Book

Two sets of controversies demonstrate with particular force the centrality of credibility struggles in the constitution of scientific knowledge about AIDS: debates about the *causes* of the syndrome and debates about *treatments*. The analyses of these two controversies occupy the first and second halves of this book, respectively. These debates strike at some of the central questions that confront biomedical science: What is AIDS and what causes it? How can its effects be curtailed?

PART ONE: THE POLITICS OF CAUSATION

Who could doubt that HIV, the human immunodeficiency virus, causes AIDS? That proposition has been the accepted scientific wisdom since the mid-1980s, after several groups of researchers reported finding a previously unknown virus in the blood of AIDS patients.[125] It is a conclusion endorsed by preeminent virologists, immunologists, epidemiologists, and clinicians; by the World Health Organization and the Centers for Disease Control and Prevention (CDC); and by prominent AIDS service and advocacy organizations. In the mainstream media, HIV is casually referred to as the "AIDS virus"; among insiders, AIDS is increasingly understood as simply the end stage of "HIV disease." The claim that HIV is the etiological agent in the Acquired Immunodeficiency Syndrome is the guiding assumption behind billion-dollar programs for HIV antibody testing, antiviral drug development and treatment, and vaccine research around the world. It is the cornerstone of "what science knows about AIDS."[126]

Yet the search for the cause of AIDS took many twists and turns before settling on HIV. Indeed, the notion that AIDS might be caused by a previously unknown virus was initially a relatively *unpopular* one. Beginning from a zero point of near-total uncertainty, competing groups of scientific claims-makers, under the watchful gaze of interested segments of the public who sought to establish "ownership" over the epidemic, advanced various hypotheses. Then, between 1984 and 1986, a bandwagon formed behind the proposal that a particular virus, eventually named HIV, was the causal agent.

Nevertheless, in the late 1980s and early 1990s, some years after the discovery of HIV and the large-scale implementation of social policy based on it, the markers of controversy abounded. Symptomatic were debates about "cofactors" needed to cause disease, investigations into the mysteries of "pathogenesis" (Just *how* does HIV cause disease?), and scares about cases of an "AIDS-like" illness in HIV-negative people. Most astounding of all have been the claims of Peter Duesberg, a molecular biologist at the University of California at Berkeley and a member of the elite National Academy of Sciences. Beginning in 1987 in an article in *Cancer Research* and subsequently in articles in publications such as *Science* and the *Proceedings of the National Academy of Sciences,* Duesberg has maintained that HIV is a harmless passenger in the AIDS epidemic, "just the most common among the occupational viral infections of AIDS patients and those at risk for AIDS, rather than the cause of AIDS." [127] He argues that there is no solid evidence establishing a causal role for the virus and, furthermore, that a retrovirus such as HIV simply cannot cause a syndrome like AIDS. Instead, Duesberg's current alternative hypothesis is that "the American AIDS epidemic is a subset of the drug epidemic," [128] attributable primarily to long-term consumption of recreational drugs and secondarily to what Duesberg calls "AIDS by prescription"—the toxic effects of the medication azidothymidine (AZT), widely prescribed to fight HIV infection.

Duesberg is only one of a number of researchers, doctors, and activists who have cast doubt on the "HIV hypothesis," but he has attracted by far the most attention. Duesberg's claims have prompted dozens of articles and communications in scientific journals and several hundred articles and letters in the mainstream English-language press. In 1994, *Science,* one of the most important general science journals in the world, devoted eight pages to the "Duesberg phenomenon." [129] The story has found its way into *Naturwissenschaften* and the *Gaceta Médica de México;* [130] the *Los Angeles Times,* the *New York Times,* and the *Times* of London; [131] National Public Radio and *Penthouse;* [132] the position papers of an AIDS advocacy organization and the columns of a pop music magazine; [133] and perhaps every gay and lesbian news source in the United States. [134] Reporters are quick to stress Duesberg's impressive credentials. He is frequently cast as a "heretic" who, like Galileo, has been excommunicated by dogmatic proponents of "orthodoxy" less interested in truth than in their hold on the faithful. [135] And reporters are often quick to mention that Duesberg has declared himself in principle "quite happy to [be] publicly injected with HIV." [136] Many scientists who think Duesberg is dead wrong are made apoplectic by the mention of his name. "I'm so tired of hearing the Peter Duesberg crap about HIV," said Donald Francis, a prominent AIDS researcher formerly with the CDC, to an audience of one thousand at a 1992 public forum on AIDS in San Francisco. "News reporters looking for an AIDS angle should look for another story. . . . The disease is caused by the virus, dammit, and the press should understand that." [137]

To describe the construction of facts such as "HIV causes AIDS," sociologists of scientific knowledge have adopted the phrase "black box." [138] As Bruno Latour explains, the concept is borrowed from cybernetics, where black boxes are used in diagrams as a quick way of alluding to some complex process or piece of machinery: if it's not necessary to get into the details, one just draws the box and shows the input and the output. Then no one has to worry about what goes on inside the box itself, and the nonexpert may never even realize just how messy the inside really is. Scientific facts are similar: masked beneath their hard exterior is an entire social history of actions and decisions, experiments and arguments, claims and counterclaims—often enough, a *disorderly* history of contingency, controversy, and uncertainty.

Scientists strive to "close" black boxes: they take *observations* ("The radioactive isotope count that indicates the presence of reverse transcriptase, an enzyme associated with retroviruses, rises over time in specially prepared lymph tissue from a person with an illness believed to be AIDS-related"), present them as *discoveries* ("A novel human retrovirus has been grown in T-lymphocytes of AIDS patients"), and turn them into *claims* ("The probable cause of AIDS has been found") which are accepted by others ("HIV, the putative cause of AIDS, . . .") and may eventually become *facts* ("HIV, the virus that causes AIDS, . . .") and, finally, *common knowledge,* too obvious even to merit a footnote. Fact-making—the process of closing a black box—is successful when contingency is forgotten, controversy is smoothed over, and uncertainty is bracketed. Before a black box has been closed, it remains possible to glimpse human actors performing various kinds of work—examining and interpreting, inventing and guessing, persuading and debating. Once the fact-making process is complete and the relevant controversies are closed, human agency fades from view; and the farther one is from the research front, the harder it is to catch glimpses of underlying uncertainties. [139] It then becomes difficult to ask, Was the examination accurate? Was the interpretation defensible? Was the persuasion logical? Those who want to challenge a claim that has been accepted as fact must effectively "re-open" the black box.

What are the dynamics of fact making when science is closely scrutinized by attentive spectators? What are the processes by which black boxes are closed and reopened when scientific arguments become the stuff of news reports and street conversations? There are examples of important controversies in science—the debate over continental drift is one[140]—that barely get any airplay in the "outside" world. AIDS is something else again. With millions of people around the world believed to be infected with HIV, the human stake in the causation controversy is gigantic, immediate, and inescapable. It should therefore come as no surprise that the cast of characters in AIDS debates is diverse. A full-fledged inquiry into the controversy immediately bursts us out of the "scientific field" narrowly construed. It forces an examination of the ensemble of social actors, with varying and conflicting social interests, who at different points have struggled to assert credible knowledge about the epidemic or to assert their capability to weigh and evaluate such knowledge.

At a different level, the causation controversy reflects a struggle for "ownership of" and "democracy within" science. An agenda has emerged, well expressed in the words of writer Jad Adams, one of the "HIV dissidents" and author of *AIDS: The HIV Myth*: "Ultimately, expert advice must be evaluated by the people who are not experts—politicians, journalists, and the public. This is part of democratic life and a scientist has no more right to exclusion from public scrutiny than a treasury official."[141] In the intervention of laypeople in debates about the causes of AIDS, claims about causes are interwoven with claims about the very right to intervene. It makes sense that the opponents of the orthodox position on causation so frequently take aim at what they call the premature "rush to judgment" in 1984 on the question of causation: from their perspective, this moment represented the stifling of democratic openness of opinion and the authoritarian imposition of closure. In many ways the debate has become a *debate about closure*—that is, a debate about when and how scientific controversies end.[142] But concerns about closure in this case break down into a number of important dimensions: *epistemological* (When is causation proven?), *methodological* (How should rival theories be weighed and compared?), *empirical* (Was closure arrived at too early? What conclusions did the evidence permit in 1984 and what conclusions are reasonable today?), and most notably, *political* (Who decides? Which social actors are qualified or entitled to participate in the process of establishing the scientific knowledge about AIDS?). In other words, the controversies about what causes AIDS are simultaneously *controversies about scientific controversies* and how they should be adjudicated—controversies about power and responsibility, about expertise and the right to speak. As frames of knowledge and belief about AIDS have become fixed in place, a range of social actors have engaged in credibility struggles to defend, refine, subvert, overturn, or reconstruct those frames.

Conceived as a series of multilateral credibility struggles, the controversy surrounding the causation of AIDS raises a number of important questions that I consider in the chapters that make up part one:

> How did the hypothesis that was initially considered relatively unlikely—that AIDS is caused by a previously unknown virus—come to supplant more popular alternatives?

> What were the processes by which the HIV hypothesis, once formulated, became "black-boxed" and achieved the status of fact— among doctors and scientists, in the mass media, in gay communities, and in the AIDS movement? To what extent was there dissent, and how was it manifested?

> How is it that Duesberg, initially presenting views that had minimal credibility among established AIDS researchers and mainstream AIDS organizations, has been able to attract allies and adherents not just among sectors of the AIDS movement but, eventually, within legitimate scientific circles as well?

> How has Duesberg been able to accomplish this when others with somewhat similar views have been marginalized?

My reconstruction of the history of claims-making necessarily ranges widely. It is not just that the controversy extends across a range of scientific disciplines—virology, epidemiology, immunology, molecular biology, pharmacology, toxicology, and clinical medicine. The controversy also spins off into a series of more general debates about the nature of disease and the methods of scientific reasoning: Do diseases typically have a single cause or multiple causes? Are established rules of scientific proof inviolable, or are they subject to revision as scientific knowledge changes and technologies improve? When anomalies are found that appear to falsify an existing hypothesis, when should the hypothesis be scrapped and when is it proper scientific procedure to work with the hypothesis, tinkering with it so that it can account for the anomalies? Does normal, peer-reviewed "establishment science" produce the best results in the end, or do the truly revolutionary findings come from the mavericks and iconoclasts who challenge, or work outside of, the system?

And finally, as the controversy has expanded from one social arena to the next, it has never been articulated in a vacuum, separate from other social concerns. On the contrary, a variety of apparently tangential beliefs and values have spilled over into (indeed, partially constitute) the AIDS etiology debates. These beliefs and values include divergent attitudes toward homosexuality, promiscuity, and drug use; inferences that link the causes or origins of a disease with theories of social blame; and assumptions about whether illnesses are attributable primarily to microbes, lifestyles, or societies. In short, the AIDS causation controversy is inexplicable outside of the larger context of how AIDS has been constructed as a social problem against the backdrop of contested attitudes about scientific medicine.

PART TWO: THE POLITICS OF TREATMENT

Find the cause, then find the cure: this is the mission of biomedicine in a nutshell. But how does it work in practice? What are the social processes that bring a therapy from laboratory bench to medicine cabinet? Who decides what treatment strategies to pursue or how to develop and test medications? Exactly what does it mean to say that a treatment "works"? Like debates about the causes of AIDS, claims and counterclaims about treatments involve fervent struggles for credibility—struggles waged in the shadow of towering uncertainty and driven by urgent need. Progress, and power, derive from the ability to submit credible answers—to push back the bounds of uncertainty, to offer something that "helps," to voice what is "known."

The actors in this drama are as varied as the interests that motivate them and the values that animate them—the researchers hoping to hit on breakthroughs in the basic or applied sciences of AIDS research; the pharmaceutical and biotechnology companies whose stock values might fluctuate by millions of dollars, depending on the latest reports about the successes or failures of their products; the medical professionals who must translate inconclusive and contradictory research findings into workable, day-to-day clinical judgments; the regulatory agencies and advisory bodies that serve as "gatekeepers," ruling on the safety and efficacy of new therapies; the patients who consume the drugs and populate the clinical trials; the reporters and journalists who interpret scientific research findings to various segments of the public; and, of course, the activists who police the whole process and offer their own interpretations of the methods and the outcomes. In the late 1980s, "treatment activism" emerged as the forward wedge of the multifocal AIDS activist movement in the United States, widely hailed—and sometimes damned—for its ingenuity, brashness, aptitude, and muscle.

"There's no doubt that they've had an enormous effect," commented Dr. Stephen Joseph in 1990, soon after leaving the post of New York City health commissioner. "We've basically changed the way we make drugs available in the last year." [143] While the activist impact on the regulatory procedures of the Food and Drug Administration (FDA) has been widely publicized, this remains just one of many items on treatment activists' agenda for the reformation of biomedical science. As the National Research Council of the National Academy of Sciences put it (in a 1993 report otherwise noteworthy for its *skepticism* about the transformative effects of the AIDS epidemic on U.S. society): "Every aspect of the process by which new pharmacologic agents [are] identified, evaluated, regulated, and allocated [has been] tested by the exigencies of [this] epidemic disease. Questions basic to the epistemologic foundations of biomedicine— questions of verifiability, reproducibility, proof, variability, safety, and efficacy—[have all been] subject to debate and reevaluation." [144]

Treatment activists have been pivotal in this rethinking of biomedical truth-making. They have challenged the formal procedures by which clinical drug trials are designed, conducted, and interpreted; confronted the vested interests of the pharmaceutical companies and the research establishment; demanded rapid access to scientific data; insisted on their right to assign priorities in AIDS research; and even organized research on their own, with the cooperation of allied professionals. Starting out on the margins of the system, treatment activists have pushed their way inside, taking their seats at the table of power. Activists now sit as full voting members of the NIH committees that oversee AIDS drug development, as invited participants at the FDA advisory committee meetings where drugs are considered for approval, as members of federal review panels that consider proposals for research grants, and, at local levels, as representatives on the review boards that approve clinical research at hospitals and academic centers.

In addition to moving inward, they have pursued an evolution "backward," as treatment activists themselves have noted. Beginning with a focus on the end stage of the drug development process, they have worked their way back toward earlier and earlier moments— "from drug approval at the regulatory level of [the FDA], to expanded access for drugs still under study . . . , to the design and conduct of the controlled clinical trials themselves. . . ." [145] Most recently, several prominent treatment groups have pushed back even further, to promote, monitor, and criticize the directions of basic AIDS research—the "pure science" investigations in immunology, virology, and molecular biology that are considered the necessary prelude to the applied work of developing and testing specific therapies.[146]

The vigorous participation of self-educated activists—and more broadly, the rise of knowledge-empowered communities that monitor the course of biomedical research—has had momentous effects on the development of AIDS treatments. These developments have transformed the procedures by which drugs are tested, the ways in which test results are interpreted, and the processes by which those interpretations are then used in the licensing of drugs for sale.

The Conduct of Clinical Research. In the postwar era, the assessment of therapies has been linked to the techniques of the randomized clinical trial. Such trials provide crucial "hard data" about treatment effects, but also obscure political decisions about how to measure the risks and benefits of a drug, cloaking them in the aura and mystery of objective science. Widely considered the pathway to objectivity in modern biomedical research, clinical trial results in practice can be subject to enormous amounts of interpretative flexibility. Precisely because the stakes are often high—both in human lives and in stock market values—deciphering clinical trial findings can prove not only a contentious process, but also a highly public one.[147]

Clinical trials are also a form of experimentation that requires the consistent and persistent cooperation of tens, hundreds, or thousands of human beings—"subjects," in both senses of the word, who must ingest substances on schedule, present their bodies on a regular basis for invasive laboratory procedures, and otherwise play by the rules, known more formally as the study protocols. From the standpoint of the researcher, ensuring the cooperation of research subjects is a complicated endeavor because these "bodies" talk back: subjects participate or don't participate and comply with the study protocols or not, depending on their own perceptions of what works and what doesn't, how desperate their own health situation is, and what options are open to them.[148]

It has recently been argued that the history of clinical trials needs to be rewritten to, in effect, "bring the patient back in"—to demonstrate how the capacity to construct knowledge through this particular technique is both enabled and constrained by the research subjects and the resistance they present to the epistemic goals of the clinical investigators.[149] In fact, the AIDS epidemic should be considered a decisive turning point in this revisionist history. AIDS trials are distinctive not only because of the militancy of many of the patients, but because their representatives have mobilized to develop effective social movement organizations that evaluate knowledge claims, disseminate information, and insert laypeople into the process of knowledge construction. The activist representatives of AIDS patients not only facilitate the flow of information to and among them, but also press demands about what should be studied in the first place and how the research protocols should be worded. Highly technical details such as the entry requirements for trials, the types of controls employed, and the endpoints to be used in studies have all been the subject of vociferous debate. Such developments pose substantial complications for the "politics of therapeutic evaluation."[150]

The Interpretation of Studies. "You can't reproduce the real world in a . . . clinical study," acknowledges Dr. Douglas Richman, a prominent AIDS researcher at the University of California at San Diego. "The hope is that you can define things in such a way that you can get some interpretable data in which the bias is sufficiently limited [so] that it's meaningful and it's applicable to other situations. . . ."[151] As Steven Shapin expresses it, any laboratory experiment has credibility only insofar as it is taken to "stand for" some actual conditions in the "real world": for example, "when Robert Boyle put a barometer in the air-pump and then exhausted the air, its behavior was meant to stand for what would happen were one to walk a barometer up to the top of the atmosphere." But the *extent* to which the experiment adequately represents reality is always subject to negotiation—and open to deconstruction.[152] The effect of activist interventions into questions of research design and interpretation has been precisely to "denaturalize" clinical trials—to call the objectivity of the methods into question, to reveal their "artifactual and conventional" status, and to make the results of given trials more open to question.[153]

Few people, including practicing physicians and many academic researchers who conduct clinical trials, can entirely follow all the statistical arguments that constitute the formal evidence invoked in favor of, or in opposition to, a given treatment.[154] Most players therefore become adept at reading the signposts: Where was the study published? Who conducted it? Was it peer reviewed? Is anyone criticizing it? Are there any methodological flaws or "gray areas" that have been pointed out? Has the FDA acted on it? Has the NIH issued treatment guidelines? Do I know of doctors who are prescribing this drug? How are their patients doing? The social power of a study depends considerably on these markers of credibility, and their absence can cause problems for the acceptance of the study's findings.

Into this complex field of claims and counterclaims, markers and precedents, signals and responses, enter the AIDS activists. Activist participation has done nothing less than change the ground rules for the *social construction of belief*—the varied processes by which different groups and institutions in society come to believe that a given treatment is "promising" or "disappointing," "effective" or "junk," "state of the art" or "passé." Activists have become proficient at interpreting the credibility of AIDS trials, and they have educated their base communities about how to scrutinize newspaper reports of "miracle cures" and journal articles about the "definitive" clinical trial. Activists in turn have promoted their own assessments: *that* study makes sense; *this* drug seems to be working. They have argued for rethinking the risk-benefit calculus for life-threatening illnesses, and they have pushed for the rights of patients to accept greater risk in deciding whether to try experimental treatments.

The Politics of Risk and Regulation. In a world that depends heavily on specialized expertise, decisions about risks increasingly are adjudicated by impersonal organizations and institutions. But particularly in cases of controversy and politicization, it becomes harder to "contain" such decisions within normal organizational routines. Thus the regulatory hearings that consider evidence from clinical trials in order to license pharmaceutical products for sale are often heated sites for the negotiation of credibility, risk, and trust.[155] "Regulatory science," as Sheila Jasanoff calls it in her study of agencies such as the FDA and the Environmental Protection Agency, is indeed a legitimate variety of scientific enterprise, but it is a very particular variety—and at least in the United States, a particularly adversarial one at that. Regulatory science differs from research science in its goals, its institutional locus, its formal products, its time frame, and its account-ability.[156]

A distinctive difficulty of regulatory science is that everyone involved in making assessments speaks a somewhat different language. The statistician wants to know if the "null hypothesis" of "no treatment effect" has been disconfirmed to a sufficient degree of statistical certainty. The clinician wants to know if her patients' symptoms show improvement. The pharmaceutical manufacturer is concerned with liability and profit margins. And the regulatory official assesses "safety and efficacy" by measuring compliance with statutory and administrative requirements. Patients and their activist representatives want to know if a drug "works": at times they may demand certainty from institutions ill-equipped to provide it; at other moments they may insist on their willingness—indeed, their *right*—to freely assume the risks of uncertainty and ingest substances about which researchers and regulators have doubts. Should the social priority be "access" or "answers"—rapid approval of experimental therapies or careful consideration of the accumulation of evidence? Are these goals in conflict or can they be advanced simultaneously? Regulators, researchers, doctors, patients, and activists have all held different opinions on these questions—opinions that in some cases have shifted markedly over the course of the past decade.

A small number of drugs, many of them chemical cousins of AZT, have been licensed in the United States as antiviral agents effective against HIV infection or AIDS. (Other drugs have been licensed to fight opportunistic infections and neoplasms that are characteristic of AIDS—the infections and cancers that afflict people with weakened immune systems.) It is universally agreed that none of these drugs is a cure for AIDS. Beyond that, the drugs are shrouded in controversy, and AZT, the drug most widely prescribed throughout the late 1980s and early to mid-1990s, has seen its star rise and then fall. What is "known" and "believed" about these drugs, by whom, and where?

The answers to these questions demonstrate how certainty and uncertainty about treatments—much like beliefs about causation—emerge out of multilateral struggles for credibility. I analyze these struggles by tracing the first decade of AIDS antiviral drug development, from 1984 to 1995, and emphasizing the following issues:

What were the approaches to treatment that emerged upon the "black-boxing" of the HIV hypothesis? How have treatment strate gies changed in relation to advances in virology and immunology?

How did AZT become credible as the treatment of choice for AIDS and for lesser HIV infection? How did a bandwagon form behind the promotion of this drug? Why was the drug recommended for many asymptomatic (outwardly healthy) HIV-infected people in 1989, and why did its value for those same patients come into doubt by 1993? Who has supported AZT, who has questioned it, who has labeled it a "poison," and why?

How did AZT's "cousins" ddI, ddC, d4T, and 3TC become the beneficiaries of novel accelerated mechanisms of drug testing and licensing? What is known about the long-term efficacy of these drugs and about newer, perhaps more promising drugs such as the "protease inhibitors"?

What impact has the "democratization of research" had on the assessment of credibility and the construction of belief about drugs? Specifically, what have been the consequences of lay participation on NIH committees and on community advisory boards for clinical trials? How has the development of a sophisticated activist press that evaluates treatments and regulatory policies affected the research and regulatory processes?

How have activists constructed their credibility as scientific actors in this domain? How have they pressed their critiques of the methods employed in the design and interpretation of clinical trials? How has the engagement with clinical and basic science affected the organization and identity of the movement?

In the debates surrounding treatments, just as in those concerning causation, we see participants engaged in disputes about the *meaning* of evidence that simultaneously are disputes about the *standards* of evidence—about what counts as proof and, crucially, who decides. In this respect, there is an underlying commonality between part one and part two of this book. (Indeed, many of the same players surface in both). At the same time, the causation and treatment controversies are in certain respects quite different, and they reveal distinct mechanisms for the establishment of credibility in science. In both cases, the AIDS movement, broadly construed, has played an important and visible role. But in the causation controversies, the most publicized challenges to mainstream views have come from highly credentialed researchers, and representatives of the AIDS movement have enjoyed more success in *assessing* the claims of others than in *asserting* their own. By contrast, the crucial voices of heterodoxy in the treatment controversies have been those of lay activists.

Given the nature of scientific research, there is a certain logic to this difference. The investigation of the etiology and pathogenesis of illness is closer to the realm of "pure science"—the heavily-defended "core" of scientific practice to which few outsiders can successfully gain entry. By contrast, the investigation of treatments—and in particular the establishment of treatment efficacy through the mechanism of the clinical trial—is in part an "applied" science, located more on the "periphery" of scientific practice. It is more easily accessible to members of the patient community, whose participation in the process is indeed essential and who therefore have an immediate claim to a stake in the process and a basis for the development and assertion of their own expertise. A comparison of AIDS causation controversies and treatment controversies is therefore instructive, for it demonstrates how different kinds of scientific debates generate different possibilities for the manufacture of scientific expertise and credibility.

Conceptualizing AIDS: Some Intellectual Debts

Although books and articles analyzing the AIDS epidemic are legion, few have studied the way that scientific knowledge about AIDS is constructed through controversy and claims-making. Indeed, some of the most well-known discussions of the social dimensions of the epidemic, such as Randy Shilts's *And the Band Played On,* obscure as much as they clarify about the construction of knowledge regarding AIDS.[157] Though moving, Shilts's book offers a teleological account of science: the "certainties" of 1987 are projected backward onto past moments in the epidemic, and those who, at the time, endorsed arguments that would later become authoritative are labeled heroes, while those with views that were destined to fall out of favor are characterized as wrongheaded and even dangerous. Though often damning of the conduct of science in the United States, Shilts never moves beyond the classic liberal position that the institutions of science would function just fine if only "politics" (for example, the anti-gay attitudes of a Republican administration) and personal motivations (such as scientific ambition) could be kept from interfering. Such views are in sharp contrast to theoretical perspectives that portray science as normally and inevitably infused with politics of various kinds—perspectives that suggest we analyze knowledge in relation to interests, strategies, and mechanisms of claims-making.

Other mainstream accounts from a traditional science journalism perspective seem to miss much of what is most distinctive about the case of AIDS. Steve Connor and Sharon Kingman's *The Search for the Virus,* for example, is full of useful information about the scientific arguments and hypotheses advanced over time but has nothing to say about anything happening outside of the scientific field narrowly construed.[158] Bibliometric analyses of AIDS publications are likewise helpful in understanding shifts in emphases over time,[159] while Henry Small and Edwin Greenlee's "co-citation" study of AIDS research shows the linkages among different scientific journal articles and biomedical subspecialties.[160] These accounts, however, begin with the a priori assumption that the "field" that generates AIDS knowledge encompasses only mainstream researchers and mainstream scientific journals. Analyses that, for example, take seriously the role of grassroots treatment publications in the dissemination of scientific knowledge about AIDS are few and far between.[161]

Some of the earliest writers on social aspects of AIDS, including Dennis Altman and Cindy Patton, have perspectives closer to my own, insofar as they devote close attention to questions of scientific controversy, expertise, and the politics of gay communities.[162] Patton's subsequent work in her book *Inventing AIDS* and Altman's in *Power and Community* are crucially concerned with the democratization of knowledge and the politics of expertise in ways that I have found insightful and stimulating.[163] Also related to my own work is that of Paula Treichler, who, in a series of articles, has analyzed the scientific discourse of AIDS to reveal the social construction of medical knowledge. Although she has not comprehensively or systematically analyzed the causation and treatment controversies, her insightful writing on both of these topics has informed my own work.[164] Various analysts, such as Susan Sontag, Simon Watney, and Emily Martin, have studied the discursive construction of AIDS,[165] while Watney and a number of others have provided excellent descriptions of the framing of AIDS in the mass media.[166]

There have been surprisingly few detailed analyses of the AIDS activist movement, though there are notable examples from which I have benefited significantly.[167] While the responses of gay and lesbian communities to the epidemic have been documented fairly thoroughly, other constituencies, such as women, African-Americans, Haitians, prostitutes, and injection drug users, have only recently become subjects of extensive investigation (and others, such as people with hemophilia, remain to be investigated).[168] The innovative role of health professionals in the epidemic has also been given less attention than one might expect, although analysts such as Charles Bosk and Joel Frader, Mary-Rose Mueller, Robert Wachter, and Charles Rosenberg have made important contributions.[169] Finally, a number of authors have studied institutional and organizational dimensions of the social response to AIDS,[170] while others have focused usefully on questions of meaning and social identity.[171]

Several writers, including Stephen Murray and Kenneth Payne, have sought to describe and interpret the initial medical speculation about AIDS in the early 1980s (the subject of my chapters 1 and 2).[172] By contrast, there has been surprisingly little scholarly attention paid to Duesberg and the other HIV dissenters (my chapters 3 and 4), the primary exception being the work of Joan Fujimura and Danny Chou.[173] The early impact of AIDS activism on the conduct of clinical trials (see my chapters 5 through 7) has been discussed in a number of works, most of which appeared in the early 1990s—in greatest analytical detail by Peter Arno and Karyn Feiden.[174] This latter group of analyses, each of which has contributed significantly to my understanding of treatment issues, has its strengths and weaknesses but tends overall to bracket consideration of knowledge claims as such. The authors pay little attention to the constitution of scientific knowledge and the relation between frameworks of knowledge and particular technological products (drugs). By contrast, my analysis of treatment controversies tries to bring together, in a systematic way, concerns with drug testing and approval, scientific strategies, and processes of constructing facts and beliefs.

The extensive literature on the social aspects of AIDS not only informs my analysis at every turn but its existence also provides me with a justification, of sorts, for the gaps and omissions in my own account. Let me briefly enumerate some of the most glaring. First, although the United States occupies a dominant position and English-language sources tend to establish the terms of the debate, the scope of AIDS research is indisputably international. However, the resources of any one investigator are finite, and given an overwhelmingly large subject I have been forced to make choices. Therefore I have generally restricted my focus to the United States, even where such restriction necessarily does some violence to the true empirical boundaries of the "field" constitutive of AIDS knowledge. In considering activism, moreover, I have focused primarily on gay activists, who have been most visible and forceful. Even there I have tended to emphasize (or perhaps overemphasize) the actions and perspectives of New Yorkers and San Franciscans, who have indeed set the tone for national debates. (For more information on sources consulted, refer to the Methodological Appendix.)

Second, in my discussion of treatments in part two of the book, I restrict my attention largely to the development of anti-HIV therapeutic agents (antiretroviral drugs) because this provides me with a relatively well-bounded case study in an area that has received heavy scientific and media attention and a great deal of activist involvement. As a result, I say little about the development of drugs to treat opportunistic infections or boost immune functioning or about the development of vaccines (either preventive or therapeutic) or about non-Western therapies. It should be clear that activists have participated in debates about all of these dimensions of research and treatment, and the debates surrounding them cannot wholly be dissociated from those concerning the antivirals. I leave it to others to explore these topics in detail.[175]

PART 1

THE POLITICS
OF CAUSATION

CHAPTER 1

THE NATURE
OF A NEW THREAT

The Discovery of a
"Gay Disease" (1981–1982)

FIRST REPORTS

When a puzzling new medical syndrome was first reported to be afflicting—and killing—young gay men in certain cities in the United States, there was no particular reason to expect that the cause might be a previously unknown virus. Nor did the deaths immediately take on any great medical significance. Michael Gottlieb, a young immunologist at the teaching hospital of the University of California at Los Angeles, began seeing such cases in late 1980 but found that he couldn't spark the interest of the *New England Journal of Medicine,* the most prestigious medical journal in the country, later to publish hundreds of articles on AIDS. In early 1981 the *New England Journal*'s editor instead referred Gottlieb to the U.S. Centers for Disease Control (CDC), the federal agency in Atlanta, Georgia, responsible for tracking diseases and controlling their spread.[1]

The CDC's first report, published in its *Morbidity and Mortality Weekly Report* in June 1981, noted only that five young men in Los Angeles, "all active homosexuals," had been treated over the course of the past year for *Pneumocystis carinii* pneumonia (PCP).[2] Two of the men had died. The microorganism that causes PCP is ubiquitous but is normally kept easily at bay by the body's immune system; therefore cases of PCP were exceedingly rare, restricted to people who were immunosuppressed because of medical treatment (such as chemotherapy) or who for other reasons had severely malfunctioning immune systems. The CDC report zeroed in on the question of sexuality—"the fact that these patients were all homosexual"—to put forward two tentative hypotheses: that the PCP outbreak was associated with "some aspect of a homosexual lifestyle" or with "disease acquired through sexual contact." However, "the patients did not know each other and had no known common contacts or knowledge of sexual partners who had had similar illnesses."

A few weeks later, the CDC reported twenty-six cases (twenty in New York City and six in California) of young homosexual men suffering from Kaposi's sarcoma, a rare form of cancer normally found in elderly men. At least four of the men also had cases of PCP; eight of them had died.[3] On the basis of this report, Dr. Lawrence Altman, medical reporter for the *New York Times,* wrote a short article about the cases of cancer in homosexuals.[4] Appearing deep inside the newspaper on page A-20, the article sounded what would become one of the most common themes in mainstream media coverage of the epidemic: "The reporting doctors said that most cases had involved homosexual men who have had multiple and frequent sexual encounters with different partners, as many as ten sexual encounters each night up to four times a week." Soon after, Dr. Lawrence Mass, health writer for the *New York Native*—the most widely read gay newspaper in New York City and one of only a few to have a national readership—also addressed the question of promiscuity. In an article about "Cancer in the Gay Community," Mass wrote: "At this time, many feel that sexual frequency with a multiplicity of partners—what some would call promiscuity—is the single overriding risk factor. . . ."[5]

Mass's article also explored a range of possible explanations for what he called (in quotes) "the gay cancer," including "an infectious or otherwise cancerous agent," but he noted that the "current consensus of informed opinion is that multiple factors are involved in the present outbreak of Kaposi's sarcoma among gay males." He quoted Dr. Donna Mildvan, chief of infectious diseases at Beth Israel Medical Center, who reported a colleague's belief that the outbreak of illnesses "has to do with the bombardment, the clustering of a whole range of infectious diseases among these patients which may be exhausting their immunodefensive capacities." And he cited Dr. Alvin Friedman-Kien, a professor of dermatology and microbiology at New York University Medical Center, who had examined some of the Kaposi's sarcoma patients and who had speculated about the possible role of amyl nitrite or butyl nitrite inhalants. These inhalants, street drugs that were sold legally and were popular in gay male communities at the time, were often called "poppers" because consumers would pop open the packaging to release the fumes, which were then inhaled to produce a "rush" or to intensify orgasm. Nitrites were believed to have immunosuppressive effects. On the other hand, they had been prescribed to cardiac patients for years, and no unusual cases of PCP or Kaposi's sarcoma had ever been reported in that population.

By the beginning of 1982, a series of more detailed reports in medical journals such as the *New England Journal*[6] was available as a source of additional information and speculation for researchers and medical practitioners, and for translation into the media, particularly the gay press. Researchers agreed that the telltale marker of these cases of immunosuppression was a deficiency in the numbers of "helper T cells"—or in other accounts, an abnormal ratio of helper T cells to suppressor T cells—types of white blood cells involved in the body's immune response.[7] But questions of etiology and epidemiology were considerably more confusing. For one thing, it was already apparent that the "nationwide epidemic of immunodeficiency among male homosexuals"[8] was in fact not restricted to gay men. According to the CDC's task force on the syndrome, 8 percent of the 159 cases were among heterosexuals, one of whom was a woman. In the pages of the *New England Journal,* Michael Gottlieb and his coauthors, the Los Angeles clinicians who had first reported the syndrome to the CDC, described finding the same syndrome in two exclusively heterosexual men, while Henry Masur and coauthors reported eleven cases of PCP in the New York area—five injection drug users, four gay men, and two men who were both.

Nonetheless, the focus of attention in all the medical literature remained squarely on the male homosexual sufferers, as evidenced by descriptors such as Brennan and Durack's "Gay Compromise Syndrome"[9] and Masur et al.'s more euphemistic "Community-Acquired *Pneumocystis Carinii* Pneumonia."[10] All speculation about causes proceeded from the premise of the centrality of male homosexuality. In Durack's words: "What clue does the link with homosexuality provide? Homosexual men, especially those who have many partners, are more likely than the general population to contract sexually transmitted diseases. Lesbians are not, and this apparent freedom, whatever its explanation, seems to extend to Kaposi's sarcoma and opportunistic infections." Yet the assumption that the syndrome was somehow linked with homosexuality actually did little to immediately clarify the etiology, as Durack and others realized. Noting that "male homosexuals are at increased risk for the acquisition of common viral infections" such as cytomegalovirus (CMV), hepatitis B, and Epstein-Barr virus, Durack described the "obvious problem" with the hypothesis that CMV, or any of these viruses, might be the cause: "It does not explain why this syndrome is apparently new. Homosexuality is at least as old as history, and cytomegalovirus is presumably not a new pathogen. Were the homosexual contemporaries of Plato, Michelangelo, and Oscar Wilde subject to the risk of dying from opportunistic infections?" [11] Durack's supposition was that "some new factor," such as poppers, "may have distorted the host-parasite relationship." Concluding with some "frank speculation," Durack put forward a model essentially identical to the one Mildvan had proposed to the *Native:* that "the combined effects of persistent viral infection plus an adjuvant drug cause immunosuppression in some genetically predisposed men."

This model, which was sometimes called the "immune overload" or "antigen overload" hypothesis, represented the initial medical frame for understanding the epidemic: the syndrome was essentially linked to gay men, specifically to the "excesses" of the "homosexual lifestyle." The epidemic coincided historically, *Newsweek* suggested in the article "Diseases That Plague Gays," "with the burgeoning of bathhouses, gay bars and bookstores in major cities where homosexual men meet." [12] Urban gay men, enjoying "life in the fast lane," had subjected themselves to so many sexually transmitted diseases, taken so many strong treatments to fight those diseases, and done so many recreational drugs that their immune systems had ultimately given up altogether, leaving their bodies open to the onslaught of a range of opportunistic infections. As one Harvard doctor is reported to have put it informally, "overindulgence in sex and drugs" and "the New York City lifestyle" were the culprits. [13] What distinguished gay men from CMV-infected, sexually adventurous heterosexuals, and from cardiac patients inhaling amyl nitrite, and from the many patients who took strong antibiotic or antiparasitic drugs was, these experts suggested, that only gay men (or those gay men living in the "fast lane") confronted all these risks at once.

THE POLITICS OF LIFESTYLE

The speculative focus on "the gay lifestyle" casts light on the very nature of epidemiological science. When a mysterious illness appears in a specific social group, it makes eminent sense to ask what distinguishes that group from others not affected, or less affected, by the illness. The difficulty is that the isolation of "difference" presupposes a common understanding of what constitutes the "background" against which this difference stands out. In this sense, epidemiology is inevitably a "normalizing" science, employing—and reinforcing—unexamined notions of normality to measure and classify deviations from the norm.[14] Faced with a "gay disease," epidemiologists immediately fastened upon the most sensational markers of homosexual difference, trumpeting the cases of men with histories of thousands of sexual partners, while ignoring the cases, also reported by clinicians from the very beginning, of gay men who were monogamous or who engaged in relatively modest amounts of sexual experimentation.[15]

With the advantage of hindsight, it is easy to recognize that the initial link between gay men and the new syndrome—while certainly the single most consequential aspect of the social construction of the epidemic—in fact reflected the confounding influences of what Irving Zola has called the "pathways" from doctor to patient. As Zola concluded from a more general study, it is often the case that apparent epidemiological differences in the incidence of some medical conditions actually derive from "factors of selectivity and attention which get people and their episodes into medical statistics. . . ."[16] There are important reasons why people do or do not seek medical help, yet, as Eliot Freidson has noted, the doctor tends to "assume that the cases he sees are no different from those he does not. And so he develops conceptions of illness that may have an inaccurate and artificial relationship to the world."[17]

To put it simply, some people get better medical attention, which means that medical professionals "attend" to their "unique" conditions. In New York City, if not elsewhere, it appears likely that there were at least as many cases of pneumocystis pneumonia among injection drug users as among gay men at the time of the discovery of the syndrome.[18] But gay men, some of them affluent and relatively privileged, found their way into private doctors' offices and prominent teaching hospitals—and from there into the pages of medical journals—while drug users often sickened and died with little fanfare. Even as cases among injection drug users began to be reported, the "gay disease" frame for understanding the epidemic was already falling into place. Colloquially, the epidemic became known among some medical professionals and researchers in early 1982 as "GRID": Gay-Related Immune Deficiency.[19]

The power of frames as organizers of experience is precisely that they work to exclude alternative ways of interpreting an experience.[20] Because "GRID" was a "gay disease," medical practitioners and researchers sometimes resisted the idea that it might appear elsewhere, and those who proposed that the epidemic could affect other people risked being discredited within the scientific community.[21] Randy Shilts described how, throughout 1981, "there was a reluctance [at the CDC] to believe that intravenous drug users might be wrapped into this epidemic, and the New York physicians also seemed obsessed with the gay angle. . . ." "He says he's not homosexual, but he must be," doctors would confide to one another. One New York pediatrician was ridiculed for his contention as early as 1981 that he was seeing children suffering from the same immune dysfunction as homosexual patients.[22]

But the differences in access to health care and the accident of the initial discovery of the syndrome among gay men are not adequate to account for the potency of this frame or the ease with which it fell into place. If gay men were perceived as *plausible* victims of a medical syndrome, it was in part because in the medical literature their sexualized lifestyle was already depicted as medically problematic. On one hand, epidemiologists and clinicians were genuinely surprised by the appearance of such devastating illness among "previously healthy" homosexual men. On the other hand, they were quick to make use of the existing stock of medical knowledge linking gay men with disease—specifically, the literature on sexually transmitted diseases among gay men that was published in the years just prior to, or coincident with, the onset of the epidemic.[23] This literature, which was often cited by early medical claims-makers discussing the new epidemic of immune dysfunction,[24] described an explosion of venereal diseases among gay men, the apparent aftermath of the "sexual revolution" and gay liberation. Concluding that homosexuality must be considered a risk factor in infectious disease, these articles stressed the need for clinicians to confront what one referred to as "homosexual hazards."[25]

Of course, modern conceptions of gay identity have always been partially medicalized. The very term "homosexual" dates from the nineteenth-century literature of doctors and sexologists. Gay identities have been formed, over the past one hundred years, through the dialectical interplay between an affirmative process of self-definition by homosexuals and the imposition of models by various groups of expert claims-makers.[26] In this sense, what is ironic about the medicalization of gay male sexuality in the years just prior to the beginning of the epidemic is that it presupposed the successes of the gay movement, which were in part directed against an earlier medicalization (or "psychiatrization"). In opposition to a conception of homosexuality as a "mental illness," gay activists had put forward a positive conception of gay identity and the gay community. And in fact, the new medical discourse on gay men took as its starting point a particularly recent conception of the "lifestyle" of the urban gay male; this discourse marked the entry of the modern "gay community" into medical history.

While it cannot be doubted that doctors were genuinely concerned with treating the venereal diseases of gay men, the issue was framed in particular ways that influenced medical perceptions of homosexuality. First, the key phrases that were used—"homosexual hazards," "gay bowel syndrome," "homosexuality as a risk factor"—posed the problem essentially as one of identity and "lifestyle," rather than contraction of specific infections.[27] (It seems far less likely that any medical journal would refer to "heterosexual hazards.") Second, the use of abstract, universalizing terms such as "the gay way of life" masked the considerable diversity of the life experiences and sexual practices of gay men;[28] such stereotypes obscured the fact that researchers had made no attempt even to define, let alone systematically sample, the communities they characterized with rather sweeping generalizations.[29]

Yet this was the understanding of gay male sexuality that informed medical speculation in the early days of AIDS. To be sure, the reasoning behind the immune overload hypothesis was not irrational, and the hypothesis was not absurd: after all, the epidemic *was* being observed mainly among gay men; many of these men *did* have many sexual partners; many sexually active gay men *were* known to contract sexually transmitted diseases, as well as use poppers and other drugs. But the strength of the resulting hypothesis depended on a long chain of implicit assumptions—that the syndrome was in essence linked to homosexuals (and the cases among heterosexuals could be explained

away); that the link to gay men meant that the epidemic was related
to gay men's *sexuality;* that if gay men (by this view) were "promiscuous," then the illness must be a consequence of their promiscuity; and
crucially, that repeated exposure to sexually transmitted pathogens
(and to drugs) was actually capable of causing the immune system
damage being observed. Furthermore, there was the assumption that
the recent reported increases in rates of sexually transmitted disease
and of drug use among gay men were indeed of sufficient magnitude
to explain why the syndrome was emerging when it was.

As an initial hypothesis, immune overload was probably no more
or less reasonable than many in the history of epidemiology or medical
science. Nor was it ever hegemonic. For example, the first editorial on
the syndrome in *Lancet,* the influential British medical journal, speculated on everything from "new or unrecognised environmental pollut-
ants" to "even another infective agent";[30] and such conjecture continued in the medical and scientific literature throughout 1982 and 1983.
Where "immune overload" (or, more generally, what Murray and
Payne call the "promiscuity paradigm")[31] exerted its greatest influence was *outside* the world of mainstream scientific practice. Reinforced by the mainstream media and filtering out into diverse arenas,
the idea of a linkage between homosexuality, promiscuity, and illness
informed an emergent sensibility about the syndrome—a vision, sometimes an unarticulated perception, of the epidemic as somehow the
product of "the homosexual lifestyle." At times it has been voiced as
a direct accusation: as late as October 1987, North Carolina's Jesse
Helms could stand on the U.S. Senate floor and proclaim that "every
case of AIDS can be traced back to a homosexual act."[32] The notion
that gays brought on the AIDS epidemic—and should be held responsible for having done so—has persisted long after the decline of mainstream biomedical support for etiological arguments focusing on "the
gay lifestyle."

The idea that homosexuality "causes" AIDS also indicates the tan-
gle of meanings packed into one short word—"cause"—and the difficulties involved in carrying out a conversation about causation that
cuts across a range of lay and specialist communities. As Jana Armstrong has observed, "the word 'cause' is embedded in the language
of public policy, the language of cell biology, the language of epidemiology. But the word does not mean the same thing in every instance of
its use."[33] Even a glance at a medical dictionary generates confusion:
one such dictionary distinguishes between constitutional causes, exciting causes, immediate or precipitating causes, local causes, predispos-

ing causes, primary causes, proximate causes, remote causes, second-ary causes, specific causes, and ultimate causes.[34] ("Etiology" fares little better, since the definition of that term points back to the word "cause.")

Generally speaking, medical doctors were interested in finding a "primary cause"; that is, "the principal factor contributing to the pro-duction of a specific result"—in this case, the destruction of cell-mediated immune responses. But epidemiologists, in their focus on identifying risk groups, were in effect concerned significantly with "predisposing causes": "anything that renders a person more liable to a specific condition without actually producing it." Outside of the medical and scientific professions, the various usages of the word "cause" not only blurred these meanings but embedded notions of causation within a more general vocabulary of moral blame. Like cholera epidemics, which in the nineteenth-century United States were blamed on the squalid lifestyle of the poor;[35] like gonorrhea, once regarded even by doctors as arising "from the continual irritation and excitement of the generative organs" of prostitutes;[36] like smallpox and leprosy, which were blamed on the "unclean" practices of the U.S. Chinese population in the late nineteenth century;[37] the genesis of the new epidemic of immune dysfunction was considered all too often with a view to assigning culpability. Partly through the power of the medical definitional process, partly through the ideological work of the opponents of gay liberation, gay men increasingly came to be equated with the emergent epidemic—it came to constitute part of their social identity.

CLAIMING THE EPIDEMIC

How did members of the affected communities respond to these formulations? Gay communities in the United States were both contributors to the "gay disease" frame and important critics of it. Initially, rumors of various lifestyle risks—a microbe in the water supply or the ventilation system at the most popular bathhouses, for example—spread rapidly through gay communities.[38] Writers in the gay press showed little tendency, early on, to dispute the homosexual connection, as evidenced by the frequent use of the locution "gay can-cer" (though often in quotation marks) to characterize the epidemic in 1981. This phrasing, however imprecise, effectively served as a ral-lying cry to alert gay men to the presence of a new danger.

Since many of the early reports in medical journals were written by clinicians well connected to gay communities, who were treating the patients in question, many gay people—and particularly health writers such as Lawrence Mass, himself a physician—were inclined toward sympathetic views of the medical and public health authorities. Increasingly, however, many gay writers, especially in the more left-leaning publications, were openly critical of medical researchers' tendency to blame the epidemic on gay promiscuity.[39] Much as an earlier generation of feminists had conceived of medicine as a sexist institution, these writers and activists argued that medical science was a heterosexist and sex-phobic institution that reinforced norms of sexual conformity.

Gay physicians, such as those who were members of Physicians for Human Rights, an organization of gay doctors, found themselves at the fulcrum.[40] On one hand, they were called on to introduce their professional colleagues and epidemiological investigators to many specific aspects of the "gay lifestyle," often running up against a judgmental reception within the biomedical establishment. On the other hand, they felt a sense of responsibility to warn their communities about suspected risk behaviors—but knew they would lose credibility if they were perceived to be "sex-negative" or puritanical, given that gay liberation as a political movement was so closely tied to sexual liberation as a personal ethic.[41]

By early 1982, gay and lesbian activists had created two grassroots organizations that would prove to be pivotal in confronting the epidemic: the Gay Men's Health Crisis in New York City and, across the country, the Kaposi's Sarcoma Research and Education Foundation, later renamed the San Francisco AIDS Foundation. A testament to the high degree of political mobilization and access to resources in gay communities at the time, the appearance of these organizations marked simultaneous attempts to provide services to people suffering from the syndrome, relay relevant information rapidly to gay men at risk, and serve as an organized voice regarding questions of public policy.[42]

In the early period, these organizations took no position on the question of etiology. As the Gay Men's Health Crisis advised gay New Yorkers in an open letter in mid-1982: "Unsettling though it is, *no evidence exists* to incriminate any activity, drug, place of residence or any other factor, conclusively, in the outbreak facing us."[43] At the same time, simply by organizing gay communities to confront—and, in effect, claim—the epidemic, these organizations helped to solidify the popular connection between the syndrome and homosexuality (as even the name "Gay Men's Health Crisis" implied). AIDS became a "gay disease" primarily because clinicians, epidemiologists, and reporters perceived it through that filter, but secondarily because gay communities were obliged to make it their own.

Lifestyle vs. Virus (1982–1983)

THE EXPANSION OF RISK

Sensitive to the fact that gay doctors and activists criticized the informal "GRID" designation, the CDC came up with an official name for the epidemic in May 1982 and first used the term in print in September of that year.[44] This name was chosen specifically for its neutrality—Acquired Immunodeficiency Syndrome, or AIDS: "acquired" to distinguish it from congenital defects of the immune system; "immunodeficiency" to describe the underlying problem, the deterioration of immune system functioning (and specifically, a decline in the numbers of helper T cells, causing the body to lose most of its capacity to ward off infection); and "syndrome" to indicate that the condition was not a disease in itself, but rather was marked by the presence of some other, relatively uncommon disease or infection (like PCP or Kaposi's sarcoma), "occurring in a person with no known cause for diminished resistance to that disease." This was strictly a "surveillance" definition, for epidemiological reporting purposes: it did not imply any knowledge about what AIDS "really was." But in the absence of a lab test for a known cause, this definition at least allowed the CDC a crude measure of the scope of the problem.

The newly defined syndrome would, over the course of 1983, achieve the status of a "Worldwide Health Problem," as the headline of one of Lawrence Altman's articles in the *New York Times* labeled it in November. By that time, AIDS cases would be reported "in 33 countries and all inhabited continents."[45] Though most cases were in the United States or Europe, the most striking aspect of the epidemic's spread was the discovery of AIDS in equatorial Africa. In April the *Washington Post* summarized reports appearing in both *Lancet* and the *New England Journal* that described cases of AIDS in European countries, but among patients who had immigrated from or traveled in countries such as Zaire and Chad. Of twenty-nine such cases in France, six patients had become ill before June 1981—that is, before the epidemic was first reported in the United States.[46] Immediately scientists and reporters in the West picked up on the notion that Africa "could have been the breeding place" for the epidemic.[47]

Despite the globalization of the epidemic and the formal change in terminology, the "gay disease" formulation, in various guises, continued to undergird medical investigation of the syndrome through the first half of 1982. For example, an editorial in the *Annals of Internal Medicine* by Dr. Anthony Fauci, a distinguished scientist who would later become the head of the AIDS program at the National Institutes of Health (NIH), laid out a number of etiological possibilities: "Is there a new virus or other infectious agent that has expressed itself first among the male homosexual community because of the unusual exposure potential within this group? Is this an immunosuppressed state due to chronic exposure to a recognized virus or viruses? Is this illness due to a synergy among various factors such as infectious agents, recreational drugs, therapeutic agents administered for diseases that are peculiar to this population such as the 'gay bowel syndrome' . . . ?" But what Fauci never doubted was that the "critical questions" were: "why homosexual men and why occurrence or recognition only as recently as 1979?"[48]

Suddenly, this whole framework for understanding the epidemic was dramatically challenged. On July 9, the CDC reported thirty-four cases of Kaposi's sarcoma or opportunistic infections among Haitians living in five different states in the United States. None of those interviewed reported homosexual activity, and only one gave a history of injection drug use.[49] The following week the agency reported three cases of PCP in people with hemophilia, all of them recipients of a blood product called Factor VIII, "manufactured from plasma pools collected from as many as a thousand or more donors."[50] The CDC refrained from drawing conclusions, but noted that the occurrence of the hemophilia cases "suggests the possible transmission of an agent through blood products." Since bacteria were screened out of Factor VIII in the production process, while smaller particles such as viruses could potentially escape the screen, the "agent" in question would almost certainly have to be a virus.

Mass, writing in the *Native,* quickly noted the significance of these findings: of all the existing etiological hypotheses, "only that of viruses would seem able to provide a unitary hypothesis that could explain the sudden appearance of AID [the *Native*'s term at that time] in a growing number of distinct populations." But he also acknowledged the alternative possibility: Perhaps, he suggested, "we are dealing with a number of superficially similar epidemics, each with its own primary etiology." [51]

GERMS AND MAGIC BULLETS

One syndrome, one cause; many syndromes, many causes: these options suggested not just different etiological hypotheses, but opposing theoretical approaches to the understanding of human illness. Indeed, one of the most intriguing aspects of the early popularity of the immune overload hypothesis was that so many clinicians would readily forsake the approach to disease causation frequently described as the cornerstone of contemporary biomedicine: the principle of "one disease, one cause, one cure." As Allan Brandt has expressed it: "In this paradigm, individuals become infected with a parasite that causes dysfunction of some sort; disease is defined as a deviation from a biological norm. Social conditions, environmental phenomena, and other variables are generally discounted as causes of disease. The physician dispenses 'magic bullets' that restore the patient to health." [52]

Ever since the bacteriological revolution of the late nineteenth century, when germs replaced "miasmas" as the preferred explanation for illness, medical research typically has focused on the discovery of discrete microbial causes for specific diseases. To be more precise, two separate assumptions have been welded together: that most illnesses have a single, fundamental cause, rather than multiple necessary causes; and that the search for the cause of illness should focus primarily on microbes, very secondarily on lifestyle issues, and only incidentally on environmental causes related to the larger organization of the society. Of course, the monocausal/microbial approach has always had its critics. Writing in 1959, René Dubos characterized the "doctrine of specific etiology" as "unquestionably the most constructive force in medical research for almost a century," but noted that "few are the cases in which it has provided a complete account of the causation of disease." Citing the failures, "despite frantic efforts," to find cures for diseases such as cancer and mental illnesses, Dubos argued that the "search for *the* cause may be a hopeless pursuit because most disease states are the indirect outcome of a constellation of circumstances. . . ." [53]

Modern-day epidemiologists, more open to multicausal approaches to disease, may speak of a "web of causation" or may endorse "ecological" and "synergistic" models of illness that emphasize the complex interrelationships among environmental and host factors.[54] But in laboratories, examining rooms, and medical school classrooms, the doctrine of specific etiology holds sway. Many analysts have seen in the monocausal/microbial model of disease the clue to medicine's ideological function within a capitalist society: it encourages people to attribute their illnesses to invisible particles rather than to occupational hazards or defects of social organization.[55] But to understand why clinicians and researchers themselves reach for such explanations, the suggestions of sociologist Andrew Abbott may be more to the point.

First, the germ theory of disease focuses public attention on medicine's greatest triumphs and away from arthritis, heart disease, cancer, and other chronic problems that have proven less amenable to therapeutic success. Second, one of the chief legitimating values of medicine (like other professions) is its perceived efficiency; and as opposed to environmental explanations, monocausal/microbial ones lend themselves to neat and straightforward solutions ("Take two pills every four hours").[56] The search for microbes enhances the power of laboratory researchers, who alone have the tools to conduct it. The search for environmental causes is, by contrast, frequently beyond their ken. In short, the commonly expressed preference of clinicians and biomedical researchers for simple, monocausal, microbial models may in an immediate sense have less to do with medicine's role in legitimating society than with doctors' and scientists' roles in legitimating scientific medicine.

In light of the prevailing explanatory preference, early clinical fascination with "the homosexual lifestyle" is all the more noteworthy. Of course, perceptions that illness is linked to lifestyle have become more common in recent years, with increasing attention to the relation between such factors as stress or eating habits and the development of various diseases. But to the extent that doctors endorsed a multicausal lifestyle model, they were going against the prevailing medical currents. It is well worth asking whether they would have been as likely to do so had it not been for the perception that "the gay lifestyle" was peculiarly laden with a potential for medical hazard.

DISSENT AT THE FRONT LINES

Once put squarely on the table, the notion of a single, unifying cause of AIDS carried with it immediate practical implications. The virus theory, now described by the *Los Angeles Times* as "a potentially much more serious candidate for the cause," was also a scary one, as it "raised the specter" of a communicable disease that might potentially affect anyone.[57] Or as *Newsweek* warned in August, "the 'homosexual plague' has started spilling over into the general population."[58] With the news, toward the end of 1982, of a case of AIDS having developed in a blood transfusion recipient twenty months old (one of whose donors was found to have AIDS)[59] and of other cases in the female sexual partners of intravenous drug users with AIDS,[60] the viral hypothesis gained increasing credibility. It wasn't that the lifestyle theories were immediately abandoned: for example, a news report in the influential *Journal of the American Medical Association* (*JAMA*) surveying the controversy in late September 1982 claimed straightforwardly that "it seems unlikely that a virus alone is inducing AIDS," and devoted significant attention to the poppers theory and others, as well as to two researchers' discovery of a genetic marker in patients with Kaposi's sarcoma.[61] However, the greater the number of risk groups, the less relevant seemed the details of "lifestyle," and the more attractive the notion of a unifying cause that could account plausibly for all manifestations of the syndrome.

In response to this challenge, advocates of the immune overload hypothesis struggled to fortify their claims. A central player was Dr. Joseph Sonnabend, a South African–born physician and researcher. A specialist in infectious diseases, Sonnabend had also done research in England on the drug interferon, put in a stint at Mt. Sinai School of Medicine as an assistant professor of microbiology, and served as the director of venereal disease control for the New York City Department of Health. At the time the epidemic emerged, Sonnabend was practicing as a community doctor in New York's Greenwich Village, largely treating the sexually transmitted diseases of his many gay male patients.[62] Sonnabend had little inclination toward simple, monocausal models of illness. As he would later put it, his South African medical education had stressed that "if you want to understand sickness, you have to understand the environment in which sickness occurs."[63]

Writing in the *Native* in September 1982, Sonnabend sought support for his views by warning his readers that endorsement of the viral hypothesis could result in antigay discrimination and prejudice: "To publicly propose that any minority group carries a specific infectious agent capable of causing severe immunodeficiency and cancer is an act of tremendous seriousness. Given the potential repercussions, it verges on the irresponsible that the suggestion is made on the basis of evidence that remains conjectural."[64] The "conjecture," in Sonnabend's view, rested on twin assumptions, both of them debatable: that the same disease was present in "at least four disparate groups" (Haitians, intravenous drug users, hemophiliacs, and gay men) and that the disease was actually new in each group. While Sonnabend was careful to make clear that he was not ruling out these possibilities, his central thrust was to question them by suggesting that there might be various syndromes of immunodeficiency, all with similar symptoms. But rather than attempt to explain the cases of AIDS in the "newer" risk groups, Sonnabend focused attention on immunodeficiency in gay men. He proposed a variant of the original immune overload hypothesis, involving repeated infection with CMV and the reactivation of infection with Epstein-Barr virus. The bottom line, for Sonnabend, was summarized by the title of the *Native* article "Promiscuity Is Bad for Your Health." "This is not a moralistic judgment," Sonnabend insisted, "but a clear statement of the devastating effects of repeated infections."

As a neighborhood doctor, Sonnabend had limited resources with which to establish credibility, so his first step was to recruit allies.[65] His advantage, as he later saw it, was his location on the front lines: "I was in the situation, as a physician to many of the men who actually developed the disease, to observe the guys in their setting. . . ."[66] But his problem was that, within the research establishment, he was isolated:[67] "I had this very unique access to information. But it was just myself, a lonely business. There were no takers, because I didn't have an important position in some medical center. . . . However, I did contact David Purtilo, the chairman of pathology at the University of Nebraska. Purtilo was known to me as an expert on Epstein-Barr virus."[68]

With Purtilo and another researcher, Steven Witkin, Sonnabend published an article in *JAMA* in May 1983, presenting his claims to a wide medical audience. (This article was later reprinted in the New York Academy of Science's 1984 volume on AIDS, as well as in *JAMA*'s "official" 1986 anthology of the epidemic, *AIDS: From the Beginning.*)[69] Challenging the "prevailing view" that a novel infectious agent caused AIDS, the authors reminded their readers of "another acquired immunodeficiency syndrome," called Neapolitan disease, which "resulted from malnutrition and various viral infections." Similarly, the authors contended, multiple factors that included "recurrent cytomegalovirus (CMV) infections and immune responses to sperm are likely major causative factors" among promiscuous homosexual men. But on the crucial question of other "risk groups," the authors had little to say: "We cannot, at this time, explain why AIDS is thought to be occurring in Haitians, hemophiliacs, and others. Acquired immunodeficiency has many causes, including malnutrition, hormonal alterations, use of opiates and other intravenous drugs, and acute viral infections." [70]

Also in early 1983, Sonnabend became the editor of a new medical journal, *AIDS Research,* and declared its first issue "an appropriate occasion to review an alternative hypothesis regarding the genesis of AIDS." Here Sonnabend devoted more attention to the other "risk groups," noting that "transfusions are themselves immunosuppressive," since they expose the recipient to a variety of antigens in the donated blood, and that many Haitians are subject to tropical infections, as well as to poverty and malnutrition, both of which are highly correlated with illness. Sonnabend argued that "the risk groups are too broadly defined," and that focused epidemiological research was needed to tease out the specific risk factors (such as exposure to sexually transmitted pathogens in the case of gay men) actually linked to AIDS. Epidemiologists could also assess his model, he suggested, by comparing the prevalence of CMV in populations with and without AIDS.[71]

But Sonnabend had no epidemiologists at the ready, and in the absence of data, his hypothesis was, at best, informed speculation. Much the same could be said about all the "immune overload" theorists. Two years into the epidemic, there was little specific evidence in support of the claim that immune overload caused AIDS in gay men, let alone in other risk groups. Some research had reported on the health effects of poppers, including one study showing that of eight outwardly healthy gay men with signs of T-cell abnormalities, most were consumers of amyl nitrite.[72] But the numbers were too small to warrant strong conclusions. More generally, epidemiologists and statisticians found it "exceedingly difficult to disentangle nitrite use from such other risk factors as the frequency of sexual encounters and the multiplicity of sexual partners." [73] While the interwoven nature of these epidemiologically correlated behaviors could be taken as evidence of an overload model, it could just as easily reflect spurious associations. As Mass pointed out in a discussion of the limits of epidemiological thinking, "On the superficial basis of numbers alone . . .

wearing handkerchiefed Levi's and having Judy Garland records in one's collection might also seem risky."[74]

MEDICAL UNCERTAINTY
AND GAY SKEPTICISM

As the number of AIDS cases continued to rise, increasingly fearful gay men struggled to make sense of the shifting and indeterminate medical claims and to sort out the implications for their everyday lives. Toward the end of 1982, *Gay Community News* (*GCN*), a left-leaning weekly based in Boston, cited the "growing consensus among experts that AIDS is transmissible . . . and most likely through sexual contact."[75] Expressing the paper's sex-positive philosophy, writers in *GCN* were suspicious of views that blamed gay men for becoming sick, whether voiced by medical authorities or by gay men themselves. One prominent political analyst, Michael Bronski, wrote disapprovingly of the president of Gay Men's Health Crisis, quoting him as saying: "Something we have done to our bodies—and we still don't know what it is—has brought us closer to death."[76] Another writer in the same issue of *GCN* applauded the views of Jim Geary, head of the Shanti Project, a San Francisco organization: "The reason [we] get sexually transmitted diseases is not because we have multiple sexual partners. . . . It's because we don't take the necessary precautions in having sex."[77]

The question of how to translate etiological uncertainty into guidelines for personal safety was deeply troubling to gay communities across the United States. Nowhere did the debate rage more fiercely than in the pages of the *Native* in late 1982. The *Native*'s editor and publisher, Chuck Ortleb, introduced side-by-side commentaries by stressing the paper's democratic impulse and the need for the general public to assess scientific and public health debates: "The articles printed on these pages provide good examples of the level of debate prevailing in medical circles. . . . Confusing? Contradictory? Of course. But then, so is much of the discussion surrounding the present health crisis. It's a discussion that we feel virtually everyone should be involved in—gay people as well as non-gay, laymen as well as physicians, policy-makers as well as the citizenry. . . ."[78]

One view in the debate was offered by Peter Seitzman, president of New York Physicians for Human Rights, the gay doctors' association.[79] His argument was straightforward, if not altogether reassuring:

"The available evidence overwhelmingly suggests that AIDS is caused by some as yet undiscovered transmissable [sic] agent," probably a virus. Since the transmission pattern appeared to be similar to that of the hepatitis B virus, prevention guidelines would be "precisely the same as those for avoiding hepatitis B," namely, never use a syringe used by someone else and reduce promiscuity. Eager to avoid any implication of antisex attitudes, Seitzman reassured his readers that he himself had been "no more of an angel than Mae West." But he concluded by affirming the virtues of "monogamy as a survival technique," declaring that promiscuity is not immoral "but simply dangerous."

The "opposing" commentary by Michael Callen and Richard Berkowitz in fact arrived at roughly similar, if far more forceful, conclusions, but began with radically different etiological premises. It was also quite different in tone. Callen and Berkowitz identified themselves as twenty-seven-year-old men, both "victims of AIDS," each with a history of having been "excessively promiscuous." Although the article didn't say it, they were also both patients of Dr. Sonnabend and they endorsed his immune overload hypothesis. (Callen would go on to become the most prominent "long-term survivor" of AIDS in the United States, a familiar figure at rallies and demonstrations; until his death in 1993, he remained an activist and an ally of Sonnabend's.) Entitled "We Know Who We Are: Two Gay Men Declare War on Promiscuity," the article was nothing short of a manifesto: "Those of us who have lived a life of excessive promiscuity on the urban gay circuit of bathhouses, backrooms, balconies, sex clubs, meat racks, and tearooms know who we are. . . . Those of us who have been promiscuous have sat on the sidelines throughout this epidemic and by our silence have tacitly encouraged wild speculation about a new, mutant, Andromeda-strain virus. We have remained silent because we have been unwilling to accept responsibility for the role that our own excessiveness has played in our present health crisis. But, deep down, we know who we are and we know why we're sick." [80]

Turning to the medical evidence in favor of the different causal hypotheses—which they had evaluated on the basis of "personal experiences," their talks with researchers and doctors, and their "own readings in both the medical and the lay press"—Callen and Berkowitz argued that "AIDS is not 'spreading' the way one would expect a single-viral epidemic to spread." The confinement of AIDS to specific risk groups, they maintained, should lead us to look for the specific explanation for each group's immunosuppression. In practical terms, whatever theory one chose to believe, "the obvious and immediate solution to the present crisis is the end of urban male promiscuity as we know it today," the authors concluded. "The party that was the '70s is over," and anyone who defended promiscuity on political or ideological grounds was simply in denial.

Sharp responses to Callen and Berkowitz were quickly forthcoming, both in the *Native* and in other lesbian and gay publications. Charles Jurrist, writing "In Defense of Promiscuity," argued in his reply that the uncertainty of scientific knowledge about causation had to be factored into any evaluation of personal risk. While granting that the immune overload hypothesis "is the most plausible of the several theories concerning the origins of AIDS," Jurrist reminded readers that the hypothesis was far from proven: "It therefore seems a little premature to be calling for an end to sexual freedom in the name of physical health." [81]

Others, such as Michael Lynch, writing in the pages of the Canadian lesbian and gay newspaper *The Body Politic,* were even more assertive in defending sexual freedom against medical moralism. These writers put the issue in historical and political context: The medical critique of gay promiscuity was simply the latest of many attempts to portray gay sexuality as diseased. At stake in the debate was "gay identity" itself. Gay men had fought to construct an affirmative identity, an essential part of which involved strong defense of sexual freedom and a critique of puritanical attitudes. And many of those they had fought against were doctors and medical researchers. Given this history, it followed that the debate about gay men and their sexual practices was thoroughly intertwined with an older power struggle: who was to say what it meant to be gay—the doctors, or gay men themselves? [82] As Lynch poignantly expressed it: "Like helpless mice we have peremptorily, almost inexplicably, relinquished the one power we so long fought for in constructing our modern gay community: the power to determine our own gay identity. And to whom have we relinquished it? The very authority we wrested it from in a struggle that occupied us for more than a hundred years: the medical profession." [83]

In the absence of a cure for AIDS, or even an agreed upon cause—and in the aftermath of an initial scientific framing of AIDS as a "gay disease" linked to promiscuity, a formulation that aroused the wrath of many in gay and lesbian communities—the credibility of doctors, biomedical researchers, and public health authorities suffered greatly in those communities. Increasingly gays were prompted to respond by insisting on their own right to intervene—to weigh the evidence, pass judgment, and remind the medical establishment at every pass whose lives were really on the line. Gay doctors like Mass sought a moderate position; writing in the *Native* in response to Lynch's commentary in *The Body Politic*, he acknowledged: "To an enormous extent, what Lynch is saying is true. Mainstream medicine and psychiatry have in fact been largely responsible for contemporary stereotypes of homo-sexuals as 'abnormal,' 'perverse,' and 'sick.' At the same time, how-ever, mainstream medicine and psychiatry continue to serve vital health needs." Maintaining that the problem was not with medical science but with "the political abuse of that science," Mass advised his readers to "be critical but remain open to well-qualified medical advice." [84] But for those on either extreme of the promiscuity debate, from Lynch to Callen and Berkowitz, the watchword was self-reliance. Become your own expert: ultimately, that was the only reasonable hope gay people might have of surviving. "Rely on no single source for your information," exhorted Callen and Berkowitz: "not your doctor, not this newspaper, not the Gay Men's Health Crisis, not the Centers for Disease Control." [85]

Of course, it goes without saying that this strategy of collective em-powerment presumed the existence of gay doctors, gay newspapers, and a Gay Men's Health Crisis. To be sure, the spreading disease would decimate the ranks of existing gay leadership. But ironically, the gay response to AIDS both presupposed and furthered the social development of lesbian and gay communities and their political clout—a process that Dennis Altman has called "legitimation through disaster." [86] Gay men and lesbians had long confronted homophobic attitudes, antigay discrimination, and heterosexist presumption on a daily basis in the workplace, in religious settings, in encounters with family members, on television, and in the movies. But in organizing to meet these challenges, lesbians and gay men had developed political and social institutions that were poised to respond to the new threat when it erupted. Moreover, gay communities were dominated by white, middle-class men—people with influence in society and access to an array of social, cultural, and political resources. It's no surprise that gays were hotly debating the details of causation theories while intravenous drug users—often the poorest of the poor—sat on the sidelines: these were the realities of power in the United States in the 1980s. Even people with hemophilia, a diverse group that had the benefit of a preexisting national lobby, did not mobilize forcefully in response to the emergence of the epidemic. In this early period, Haitians were the only other group to challenge medical claims; they objected to the portrayal of Haiti as a possible origin of the epidemic and combated wild epidemiological speculation about the role of voodoo rituals in the transmission of AIDS. And most of the opposition came not from the grassroots but from politicians in Haiti and Haitian doctors living in the United States.[87]

The distinctiveness of gay communities' approaches to the emergence of the epidemic is brought out in Cathy Cohen's comparative analysis of gay and African-American responses. Although gay communities were hit harder, both gays and African-Americans came to be disproportionately represented in the statistics of illness and death as the epidemic proceeded. Both of these social groups were marginalized, and historical memory inclined both of them to distrust federal biomedical institutions. Yet "the indigenous norms and structures of these communities" promoted different political outcomes: "In the Gay community AIDS has become associated with the community's struggle for rights and entitlements. In the Black community much of the response to AIDS is based on a framing of the disease that still emphasizes behavior and the individual actions of those who have AIDS, making it much more difficult to transform AIDS into a political issue for the community."[88] As Cohen has described, established African-American organizations eschewed "ownership" of the problem of AIDS. It was often up to black gays and lesbians—those who stood at the intersection of these two social groups—to try to mobilize African-American communities and start up new organizations, while simultaneously confronting racism within gay communities.[89]

The Triumph of Retrovirology (1982–1984)

GALLO'S FAMILY OF VIRUSES

Writing in 1988, Robert Gallo, the NIH scientist who would share credit for discovery of what was to become known as the "human immunodeficiency virus," reflected back on the scientific effort to understand AIDS. Gallo concluded that progress had been made possible by "two general earlier developments": "*first,* by major advances that took place in basic sciences, particularly in immunology

... and molecular biology . . . ; and *second,* by the opening of the whole field of human retrovirology that, oddly enough, occurred only a few years before the AIDS epidemic. . . ." To this Gallo added, "There is no doubt in my mind that if AIDS came upon us full force in the 1960s or even in the early 1970s, we would still be wandering in the dark regarding most of what we know today."[90]

Gallo's "odd" fact can be put in different terms: At the moment when people began to suspect that AIDS might be caused by an infectious agent, there existed a small group of prominent scientists working in a very specialized area who were inclined to imagine that a "retrovirus" might be the cause, who were motivated to pursue that speculation, and who were well equipped to do so. Only in the 1960s had researchers discovered that the genetic material of certain viruses consists of RNA (ribonucleic acid) rather than DNA (deoxyribonucleic acid, often called the "blueprint of life"). Normally, viruses infect cells and turn them into virus factories, causing the cells to produce new viruses according to the specifications of the viral DNA. The virus's DNA is copied into RNA, which is then used to manufacture viral proteins; once the new viruses are assembled, they are ejected and go off to infect other cells. When viruses were found that consisted of RNA rather than DNA, they presented a puzzle to scientists, because it was unclear how the viruses could replicate. In 1970, however, in work that would win them the Nobel Prize, researchers David Baltimore at the Massachusetts Institute of Technology and Howard Temin at the University of Wisconsin independently discovered that these RNA viruses contained an enzyme, which they termed "reverse transcriptase," that copied the viral RNA into DNA. This DNA then served as the blueprint for the manufacture of new viruses. So while in normal viruses the sequence was "DNA to RNA to new viruses," in these unusual viruses there was an extra step: "RNA to DNA to RNA to new viruses." To describe the transcription from RNA to DNA and back again, virologists coined the term "retrovirus."[91]

During the "War on Cancer" in the 1970s, researchers such as Gallo at the NIH's National Cancer Institute (NCI) investigated links between animal retroviruses and various forms of cancer. However, until the late 1970s, no retroviruses were known to cause disease in humans. At that time, both Gallo and a group of Japanese researchers claimed credit for the discovery of one believed to cause adult T-cell leukemia, a rare form of cancer found mostly in Japanese fishing villages.[92] Gallo named the retrovirus the human T-cell leukemia virus, or HTLV. This work earned him the Lasker Prize, the highest award in biomedicine short of the Nobel Prize. He found another virus in the same family in 1982, which he claimed caused a different type of leukemia; in consequence, the two viruses became known as HTLV-I and HTLV-II.

As Gallo described it in retrospect, when he first heard about the new syndrome in gay men in 1981, he had no reason to think it might be linked to a retrovirus and indeed had little interest in the issue.[93] Or as Joan Fujimura has suggested more generally, scientists construct and pursue "do-able problems": they do not venture off in any direction at random, but rather structure their work by finding effective ways of integrating and coordinating the relationship between the experimental procedures at hand, the organization of their laboratories, and the social worlds through which they move.[94] Given that the initial hypotheses focused on homosexual lifestyle risks, many virologists simply saw no particular reason to be interested.

By Gallo's account, his curiosity was piqued only in 1982, when James Curran of the CDC briefed NIH researchers about the epidemic, expressing to them his own belief that the syndrome was caused by an infectious agent, and stressing that one hallmark of the syndrome was the helper T-cell deficiency.[95] This was enough for Gallo to hypothesize that the epidemic might be caused by HTLV or by a retrovirus of the HTLV family—by a close relative, that is, of the two viruses whose discovery had already brought him considerable acclaim within the world of virology. After all, HTLV specifically infected helper T cells; moreover, HTLV was known to be transmitted in blood and semen, which seemed also to be plausible transmission routes of the putative agent in AIDS. Finally, there was some precedent for a retroviral role in a condition like AIDS, since a feline retrovirus was linked to immune deficiency in cats. Gallo became convinced that AIDS was an HTLV-linked disease. Only some years later would he do an about-face and make an intriguing confession: "That hypothesis, as it turned out, was wrong. Nonetheless, it was fruitful, because it stimulated the search that led to the correct solution."[96]

Gallo had little patience for alternative hypotheses that were common at the time. The medical tendency to, as he put it, "round up the usual suspects"—CMV, Epstein-Barr virus, and the like—seemed to him unlikely to provide an explanation for what was, after all, a *new* epidemic. Nor was he impressed by the popular hypothesis of immune overload. Interestingly, he objected not just on empirical grounds—

that immune overload seemed unlikely to account for manifestations in all the risk groups—but also on the basis of his understanding of causality in disease processes: "Whereas some complex diseases . . . are believed to involve different steps and sometimes different factors, most human disease (even some cancers) can be thought of as involving a primary causal factor. Certainly this has been the case for most past epidemic disease for which we in time did learn the cause."[97]

Committed in general to what Dubos called the "doctrine of specific etiology," Gallo dedicated his laboratory to an investigation of his hypothesis: that AIDS was caused by the virus he was already working with and had invested in, HTLV. Within weeks of embarking on this search, Gallo's assistants found the leukemia virus in the T cells of two U.S. gay men, a Haitian woman who died of AIDS in France, and a Frenchman who had received a blood transfusion.[98] Gallo sent two papers describing the findings to *Science* magazine, the preeminent general science publication in the United States. His colleague, Myron ("Max") Essex at the Harvard School of Public Health, sent along a third paper also reporting signs of HTLV infection in AIDS patients.

THE FRENCH VIRUS

Meanwhile, across the Atlantic, a similar search for a retroviral cause of AIDS was proceeding according to different premises. In Paris, a group of physicians had been meeting informally to discuss the epidemic, and one of them, an immunologist named Jacques Leibowitch, who was familiar with Gallo's work on HTLV, had become convinced that a retrovirus was the cause. Skeptical of arguments about poppers and promiscuity,[99] Leibowitch specifically hoped to demonstrate "that the cause of AIDS was not homosexually related."[100] But neither Leibowitch nor any of his colleagues knew how to look for a retrovirus, so they set out to enlist the support of Luc Montagnier, chief of viral oncology at the famous Pasteur Institute, a private, nonprofit research institution founded by Louis Pasteur in 1887.

The physicians' group had a hunch that if a virus was causing the depletion of T cells, then there might be higher levels of virus present in people who were at an earlier stage of illness, before most of their T cells had been killed off. So they sent Montagnier samples of lymph tissue from a gay male patient with "lymphadenopathy syndrome"—a condition of chronically swollen lymph glands, increasingly prevalent among gay men and believed by many to be a precursor to AIDS. Montagnier's research team extracted T cells from the tissue and put them in an incubator with nutrients, hoping to grow a virus. When tests showed the presence of reverse transcriptase, the enzyme that is the distinctive marker of retroviruses, they knew they had found something. The reverse transcriptase activity rose and then fell—a sign that the virus was killing its host cells—but by adding fresh cells from new sources, the French researchers were able to maintain the culture. With the aid of electron microscopy, the Pasteur group also succeeded in photographing viral particles.

When Montagnier contacted Gallo in early 1982 and informed him of his findings, Gallo encouraged him to submit his paper to *Science,* so that Gallo's, Essex's, and Montagnier's papers could all appear together. Since *Science* allows its authors to suggest appropriate peer reviewers, Gallo told Montagnier he would be happy to review the Pasteur Institute's findings for the magazine. In his comments to *Science,* Gallo urged rapid publication, stressing the importance of Montagnier's work. But in addition, as reporter John Crewdson has described in a highly critical exposé of Gallo's work, Gallo offered to write the abstract, which Montagnier had neglected to include. Gallo's abstract identified the French virus as a "C-type retrovirus," similar to Gallo's HTLV.[101] Gallo had effectively enlisted the Pasteur researchers behind his own HTLV.

The papers appeared in *Science* in May 1983,[102] where, as Crewdson noted, they "made a considerable splash."[103] But few people paid much attention to Montagnier's paper, which followed the other three in the pages of *Science;* it appeared simply to confirm the findings of the American researchers. As Jay Levy, a virologist at the University of California at San Francisco Medical School (UCSF), who had also embarked on a search for a retroviral causative agent, later recalled, "The write-up in the *Science* papers sounded like the French virus and the Gallo virus were the same."[104]

But Montagnier and his collaborators suspected otherwise. Their photographs didn't especially resemble HTLV. And when they exposed their virus to HTLV antibodies, they didn't observe any "cross-reaction"—as they should have, if the virus were really a close cousin of HTLV. Most crucially, their virus killed T cells in the test tube. HTLV caused its host cells to multiply wildly—the hallmark of cancer. Of course, the French had no actual proof at this point that the virus they had found was indeed the cause of AIDS. But they were increasingly convinced that theirs was a previously undiscovered retrovirus, not HTLV or even a member of the same family; and they set out to demonstrate its causal relationship to the epidemic.

By fall 1983, at the virology conference held each September in Cold Springs Harbor, New York, Montagnier could report finding his virus—which he was now calling "LAV," or lymphadenopathy-associated virus—in about 60 percent of patients with lymphadenopathy syndrome and 20 percent of those with AIDS. None of these patients appeared to be infected with HTLV. At the conference, Gallo angrily disputed Montagnier's findings, claiming that the French measurements had to be in error. (Much later, Gallo would write: "I have come increasingly to regret that the tone or spirit of my questioning that day was too aggressive and therefore misunderstood.")[105] What Gallo did not mention to the conference-goers was that, despite his own lab's best efforts, he and his associates had been unsuccessful in finding HTLV in the majority of samples from AIDS patients that they had been studying over the past several months.[106]

AN ADDITION TO THE HONOR ROLL?

The events of the subsequent seven months are obscure, and—despite intensive scrutiny by journalists and a half dozen official investigations by various reputable bodies—the facts may never fully be known. What appears beyond dispute is that, shortly after the Cold Springs Harbor conference, Montagnier forwarded to Gallo a sample of LAV for him to study. Then, the following April, reports of Gallo's discovery of a "third variant" of HTLV began to appear in the pages of U.S. newspapers. Just months after insisting that HTLV was the cause of AIDS—while increasingly having trouble finding it in AIDS patients—Gallo presented the world with a new virus, "HTLV-III," which he claimed was a member of the HTLV family. Later, in January 1985, investigators would determine that Gallo's HTLV-III samples had a 99 percent genetic similarity to Montagnier's LAV—that is, the viruses were much too similar to have come from separate sources. The implications were clear: Whether the consequence of accidental contamination of viral cultures—a common problem in virology labs—or of outright theft and misrepresentation, the Pasteur Institute's LAV had found its way into Gallo's cultures. Almost beyond a doubt, Gallo had in fact "discovered" Montagnier's virus.[107]

Yet none of this was known in 1984. Indeed, there was little said about Montagnier on April 23 that year, when Margaret Heckler, President Ronald Reagan's secretary of health and human services, stood before a roomful of reporters. "The probable cause of AIDS has been found," she announced with some fanfare: "a variant of a known human cancer virus, called HTLV-III." Just a few days earlier, Lawrence Altman, the *New York Times*'s medical reporter, had received a scoop from CDC Director James Mason, who told him that a virus discovered in France, called LAV, was the likely culprit; the *Times* had run the story on the front page.[108] "There was so little excitement in the scientific community when the French came up with their announcement last May," noted Mason, claiming he did not understand why it had taken so long for the importance of the Pasteur Institute's work to be recognized. But at the press conference on Tuesday, Mason's boss had a different tune to play.

"Today we add another miracle to the long honor roll of American medicine and science," said Heckler. "Those who have said we weren't doing enough," she added, in response to widespread complaints of inactivity on AIDS by the Reagan administration, "have not understood how sound, solid, significant medical research proceeds." As Randy Shilts described it, the researchers on the podium with Heckler "blanched visibly when she proclaimed that . . . a vaccine would be ready for testing within two years."[109]

Heckler made only brief reference to the Pasteur Institute scientists, describing them as "working in collaboration with the National Cancer Institute"; she indicated her belief that LAV and HTLV-III "will prove to be the same."[110] Nor was mention made of UCSF virologist Jay Levy, who was also close on the heels of a virus linked to AIDS. (He would submit his paper to *Science* the following month.)[111] Pressed by puzzled reporters, Gallo added: "If it [the virus] turns out to be the same I certainly will say so. . . ."[112] Heckler emphasized the crucial role of the U.S. research, noting that only Gallo had succeeded in reproducing large quantities of the virus, which was necessary for the development of a blood test that could detect viral antibodies.[113] Hours earlier, the U.S. government had filed a patent application for just such a test.[114]

The *New York Times*, in an editorial printed a few days afterward, was not slow to draw implications from the episode. "In the world of science, as among primitive societies, to be the namer of an object is to own it," the *Times* noted wryly, pointing to the dispute between

"LAV" and "HTLV-III." Since the blood screening test was not yet in commercial operation and no vaccine had yet been produced, "what you are hearing is not yet a public benefit but a private competition—for fame, prizes, new research funds." [115]

"STRONG EVIDENCE OF A CAUSATIVE INVOLVEMENT"

Certainly one of many unusual aspects of the whole affair was that Heckler's press conference was held before Gallo's findings had even been published in a peer-reviewed forum—normally a serious breach of professional scientific etiquette in itself. Those who wanted more substantial information about Gallo's claims had to wait until May 4, when four articles by Gallo's group appeared in the pages of *Science*. This too was extraordinary. As Gallo later commented, "Getting one paper in *Science* is a lot. Getting two is fantastic. Getting three was a record. We had four at one time." [116]

Gallo used these articles to put forward a series of interconnected claims: that he had found a new virus; that he had succeeded in mass-producing it; that the virus was related to HTLV; that antibodies to the virus could be detected in blood; and, most crucially, "that HTLV-III may be the primary cause of AIDS." In the second of the four papers, Gallo and his coauthors focused specifically on the etiological argument. After reviewing the evidence in favor of an infectious agent as the cause of the syndrome, Gallo reminded his readers that "we and others have suggested that specific human T-lymphotropic retroviruses (HTLV) cause AIDS." [117] Gallo's wording was also significant: he had redefined HTLV, from "human T-cell *leukemia* virus" in 1983, to "human T-*lymphotropic* retroviruses" in 1984. While the original name denoted the relation between a single retrovirus and a specific form of cancer, the new name described a family of viruses more vaguely characterized as "T-lymphotropic," that is, having an affinity for T cells. Gallo had reinvented "HTLV" so as to more plausibly encompass his new virus as a relative of HTLV-I and HTLV-II.

Moving on to HTLV-III, Gallo described detecting the virus in, and isolating it from, "18 of 21 samples from patients with pre-AIDS [the so-called lymphadenopathy syndrome], three of four clinically normal mothers of juvenile AIDS patients, three of eight juvenile AIDS patients, 13 of 43 . . . adult AIDS patients with Kaposi's sarcoma, and 10 of 21 adult AIDS patients with opportunistic infections." Although

ideally one would expect to find a primary causative agent in every
case of a disease, Gallo noted that "the incidence of virus isolation
reported here probably underestimates its true incidence since many
tissue specimens were not received or handled under what we now
recognize as optimal conditions." In contrast with these findings that
associated the virus with the expression of AIDS was the striking absence of HTLV-III in cases where AIDS was also absent. Out of 115
clinically normal heterosexual blood donors, not a single one showed
signs of the virus. And out of 22 clinically normal gay male donors,
only one tested positive for the virus, and that person developed AIDS
within six months. These studies, Gallo and his coauthors concluded,
"provide strong evidence of a causative involvement of the virus in
AIDS." [118]

What in fact had Gallo established? Four years later, in response to
challenges about whether the virus had been proven to cause AIDS,
Gallo would maintain: "In my opinion all of the sufficient data was
available at the time the cause was first announced in the spring of
1984." [119] But this was a difficult position to sustain, at least on the
basis of Gallo's published findings. Gallo had shown that, in specific
small samples, laboratory signs indicating the presence of his virus
were often correlated with the expression of AIDS at what were believed to be two different stages of disease progression ("pre-AIDS"
and AIDS). Moreover, there were no such signs of virus in clinically
normal people, suggesting that the virus or viruses had some special
relationship to AIDS. But just because HTLV-III and LAV were often
correlated with the syndrome, did that mean they were causing it?
AIDS, after all, was a syndrome whose hallmark was the presence of
a range of opportunistic infections; perhaps HTLV-III and LAV were
viruses that were contracted by people who *already* had weakened
immune systems. Gallo would have been in a better position to respond to this challenge if he had had more cases like that of the clinically healthy but infected gay man who later developed AIDS. But the
other 21 of his 22 "clinically normal homosexual donors" all tested
negative for the virus, so there was really no evidence that HTLV-III
infection was a precursor to immune system damage. (Three out of 4
of the "clinically normal mothers of juvenile AIDS patients" tested
positive for the virus, but these numbers were small, and Gallo did
not report that any of the women had subsequently developed AIDS
symptoms.) [120]

When asked ten years afterward whether he had been able, at

the time of publication, to rule out the possibility that HTLV-III was an opportunistic infection, Gallo acknowledged that he could not. But "the evidence was overwhelming in my mind," Gallo recalled. "Science is never 100 percent. It's not mathematics. You play not on hunches, but on data that becomes overwhelming in your mind. . . ." [121] To make a credible claim for "strong evidence of a causative involvement," Gallo was in fact relying heavily on the *plausibility* of HTLV-III as a pathogenic agent, given what was known about the virus and about AIDS. At least in vitro, HTLV-III killed helper T cells. And the central manifestation of immune system damage in people with AIDS was precisely the low numbers of those same helper T cells. Still, at this point, little was known about the effects of HTLV-III in vivo.

KOCH'S POSTULATES
AND THE PROOF OF CAUSATION

Epidemiologists and biomedical researchers rely on a range of principles to establish causation in disease. However, since the acceptance of different versions and interpretations of these principles of causation has itself become one of the stakes in the controversy over the causation of AIDS, these principles cannot be independently invoked as neutral measures. The most well known causation criteria are called "Koch's postulates," named after Robert Koch, the nineteenth-century German microbiologist. The postulates consist of four steps that are easily stated. First, the causal agent must be found in all cases of the disease. Second, the agent must be isolated from a carrier and grown in pure culture. Third, when the culture is injected into a susceptible laboratory animal, the animal must contract the disease. Finally, the causal agent must then be recovered from the diseased animal.

The precise relevance of Koch's postulates to contemporary biomedical research (particularly with regard to viruses, which were unknown at the time of Koch's own work) is in dispute, and this dispute has been magnified as a result of recent debates about the causation of AIDS. Many have proposed that researchers nowadays must work with "modern" or revised versions of the postulates, and have argued that Koch himself did not intend them to be followed rigidly.[122] Nevertheless, Koch's postulates remain a well-known reference point for considering questions of etiology in scientific medicine.

For instance, Richard Krause, the director of the National Institute of Allergy and Infectious Diseases of the NIH, gave a conference talk in the summer of 1983 on "Koch's Postulates and the Search for the AIDS Agent," noting that "technical difficulties" often "impede the fulfillment" of all of Koch's postulates, but concluding: "If we abide by the scientific guidance of Koch's postulates, we are sure to discover the cause of AIDS." [123] Similarly, Lawrence Altman focused squarely on Koch's postulates in an article, published later in 1984, on "How AIDS Researchers Strive for Virus Proof." [124] Altman presented Koch's postulates as an important medical tradition that researchers have looked to for a century, but he noted that doctors are sometimes forced to rely on immunological or other experimental evidence when Koch's postulates cannot fully be satisfied. With less equivocation, James D'Eramo wrote in the *New York Native* soon after the Heckler press conference: "The definitive classical proof that a virus or bacterium causes disease rests on causing the disease in animals by injecting them with the putative agent. AIDS has yet to occur in a laboratory animal." [125] Dr. Nathan Fain, the medical writer for the national, West Coast–based gay newsmagazine the *Advocate,* made roughly the same claim in May when he explained why "work must continue to prove beyond all doubt that the candidate virus does cause AIDS." [126]

Clearly, if Koch's postulates are the benchmark, then Gallo's May 1984 articles in *Science* by no means established HTLV-III as the cause of AIDS. But since the criteria for proving causation have been contested, it may be useful to assess the credibility of Gallo's claims-making by looking at a relatively weak version of the causation criteria presented in a recent epidemiology textbook. According to Mausner and Kramer, the likelihood that an association is causal can be evaluated by examining several criteria.[127] First, there is the strength of the association, which they describe as the "ratio of disease rates for those with and without the hypothesized causal factor": here Gallo's evidence is compelling but far from perfect, since he was able to isolate the virus only in fewer than half of the samples from people actually diagnosed with AIDS. Second, the "dose-response relationship": does a higher dose of the causal factor result in higher rates of disease expression? Gallo had no data on this point. Third, the consistency of the association across different studies: clearly this was yet to be determined. Finally, is the association a "temporally correct" one, meaning that the cause precedes the expression with a sufficient "induction period" or "latency period"? With the exception of the one virus-positive, clinically healthy gay man who developed AIDS within six months, Gallo had no relevant data to report.

Given the state of the evidence in early 1984, perhaps a more plausible claim was that of Jay Levy, whose results in isolating what he called "ARV," or AIDS-associated retrovirus, were published in August.[128] Levy found signs of ARV in about half his AIDS patients and in about 20 percent of clinically healthy homosexual men, but in only 4 percent of clinically healthy heterosexuals. Levy recalled agonizing over how to phrase his conclusion: "I called a good friend of mine . . . who's an editor, and I said, 'How do I do this? I don't want to say it *isn't*, but I don't want to say it *is*.'"[129] In the end, Levy's wording was cautious: "Although no conclusion can yet be made concerning their etiologic role in AIDS, their biologic properties and prevalence in AIDS patients certainly suggest that these retroviruses could cause this disease."[130]

But for Gallo, the notion that he had proven the virus to be the cause became something crucial to defend, particularly as his credibility on other claims was challenged. In 1985, the Pasteur Institute sued the U.S. government in a patent dispute over the discovery of the virus, and in 1987 the heads of the two governments, Jacques Chirac and Ronald Reagan, signed an agreement splitting the royalties for the commercial antibody test. Especially after it became apparent that Montagnier's LAV had found its way into Gallo's viral cultures—a point that Gallo would formally concede in 1991—Gallo gradually backed off from claiming any primacy. And although Gallo continued to present the discovery of HTLV-III as a natural outgrowth of HTLV research,[131] he was eventually forced to accept the prevailing view that, from a genetic standpoint, the new virus was not reasonably classifiable as an HTLV virus. In response to the confusing array of acronyms then in use—HTLV-III, LAV, ARV, HTLV-III/LAV, and others—the Human Retrovirus Subcommittee of the International Committee on the Taxonomy of Viruses rebuffed Gallo and agreed on a new, compromise, name in 1986: HIV, human immunodeficiency virus. (Levy and Montagnier signed the agreement; Gallo and his close associate, Max Essex, dissented.)[132]

THE FRAMING OF AIDS

The naming of the virus by the Human Retrovirus Subcommittee marked the initial stabilization of "HIV" as a unitary object of medical knowledge.[133] But even before this point, the illness AIDS had become a relatively stable cultural entity whose social meanings, however fluid and multiple, had at least begun to congeal. Over the course of a few years, AIDS had come to be "framed," or constructed, within the context of strong beliefs and attitudes about sexuality, promiscuity, and homosexuality and through recourse to a wide range of analogies: Was AIDS like cancer? Was it like herpes? Was it like hepatitis B? Was it an HTLV-like illness? AIDS itself had also come to serve as a frame for understanding other events and social behaviors. Perhaps most notably, as sociologist Steven Seidman has argued, "AIDS . . . provided a pretext to reinsert homosexuality within a symbolic drama of pollution and purity."[134]

These framings, and the associated stigma, had also provided possibilities for gay men to assert claims for "ownership" of the epidemic (however ambivalently), or at least some of the public responses to it.[135] Indeed, the same social networks and institutional linkages that had permitted rapid amplification of a virus also gave rise to the organization of a concerted grassroots response. Lesbians, subject to what Erving Goffman has called a "courtesy stigma," or stigma by association, acted as collaborators with gay men in these efforts, often playing leadership roles.[136] This extraordinary success of gay and lesbian communities in establishing their right to speak about the epidemic would fuel a willingness and capacity to challenge the knowledge-making practices of biomedicine in the coming years.

Biomedical researchers, and in particular virologists, had also staked out claims to "ownership" of AIDS, and had done so through powerful findings concerning a probable causal agent. The credibility of AIDS research would rapidly become linked to the credibility of this particular causal claim: between 1984 and 1986, the retroviral hypothesis would achieve near-hegemonic status among scientists. It would also, by and large, be taken for granted in the communities affected by the epidemic, in the mass media, and among the lay public. The pathways, mechanisms, and consequences of the "black-boxing" of HIV are the topics of the next chapter.

CHAPTER 2

HIV AND THE CONSOLIDATION OF CERTAINTY

The Construction of Scientific Proof (1984–1986)

THE BLOSSOMING OF AIDS RESEARCH

Scientific research on AIDS expanded at a rapid clip during the mid-1980s. From only a couple dozen publications in 1982, the literature grew by more than six hundred new publications in 1983, eleven hundred in 1984, sixteen hundred in 1985, and twenty-seven hundred in 1986. The annual growth rate ranged between 47 and 75 percent, at a time when the level of biomedical publication in general increased at a rate of only 3 or 4 percent a year.[1] In 1982, AIDS articles appeared in three different languages and were published in the journals of five different countries; the 1985 contributions, by contrast, included forty-three countries and twenty-one languages (however, articles were published predominantly in the English language, in U.S. and British journals).[2]

That AIDS research became a scientific growth industry in these years is not surprising in itself. After all, the exponential curve of the cumulative scientific literature roughly matched the exponential curve of the cumulative number of AIDS cases reported to the World Health Organization.[3] That is, the development of scientific interest in AIDS simply paralleled the epidemic's toll. But these general statistics on overall growth of the literature do not tell the full story. The official announcement of the discovery of the probable cause of AIDS, marked by the Heckler press conference and the publication of Gallo's articles in *Science,* dramatically transformed the nature of published research on AIDS.

Some specific numbers suggest this transformation.[4] Fully a quarter of all 1983 publications on AIDS were concerned, at least in part, with the topic of etiology. By 1985 the number had declined to about 10 percent and by the following year to about 5 percent. The percentages can be deceptive: in absolute numbers there continued to be a constant production of about 150 papers a year that discussed etiology. But in relative terms these papers came to constitute a smaller and smaller fraction of the whole. Meanwhile, during the same period, the percentage of papers concerned with the virus soared, rising from 2 percent in 1983, to 5 percent in 1984, to 20 percent in 1985, to 37 percent (almost 2,000 publications) in 1986. (Research focusing on "the virus" included articles on HIV under its various apparent guises, such as HTLV-III, LAV, and ARV, as well as articles on "HIV-2" ["HTLV-IV," "LAV-2," and so on], a second retrovirus linked to AIDS, discovered by Montagnier in West Africa in October 1986.[5] With the discovery of HIV-2, the original virus was dubbed "HIV-1," although many continued to refer to it simply as HIV.)

Interest in etiology trailed off, while interest in the virus itself exploded: these facts, taken as a whole, are consistent with what is intuitively apparent—that the hypothesis "HIV causes AIDS" enjoyed a rapid and successful transition to the status of scientific fact. But this leaves many questions unanswered. Why did other scientific writers come to accept Gallo's claim? What evidence was considered? What evidence was disputed? What additional evidence, if any, proved decisive in the minds of researchers? Did anyone challenge the reigning hypothesis?

CITATION AND THE
CONSTRUCTION OF FACTS

Paula Treichler, a discourse analyst and cultural critic, has questioned the realist presumption that the HIV hypothesis became fact simply "because it's true." With reference to Gallo and his close associates, Treichler has argued: "By repeatedly citing each other's work, a small group of scientists quickly established a dense citation network, thus gaining early (if ultimately only partial) control over no-menclature, publication, invitation to conferences, and history."[6]

Yet Treichler provided neither evidence nor elaboration to support this claim. To consider the acceptance of Gallo's hypothesis more care-fully, I performed a content analysis of those scientific articles pub-lished in seven major journals in 1984, 1985, and 1986 that cited Gallo's crucial 1984 article published in *Science* (the one specifically advancing the causal argument).[7] Within the pages of these journals during the period 1984–1986, there were 244 articles that cited Gallo, ranging from 19 in *Nature* to 66 in *Science*. These were the pivotal years, as evidenced by the citation trend in all scientific publications: Gallo's article was cited 116 times in 1984 and 410 times in 1985; this dropped off slightly to 384 citations in 1986 and then more sharply to 341 citations in 1987 and 284 citations in 1988. Like most influential scientific articles, Gallo's enjoyed a brief period of heavy use during which more and more people found reason to invoke it—after which point the claims enunciated within it presumably became too much a part of common knowledge for citation to be necessary.[8]

In my content analysis I investigated four factors: first, whether sci-entists and clinicians referenced Gallo's article in order to support *qualified* claims about the causal role of the virus ("HIV is the virus widely believed to cause AIDS") or *unqualified* claims ("HTLV-III, the etiological agent in AIDS, . . ."); second, whether qualified and un-qualified claims were made more (or less) frequently over time; third, whether articles authored or coauthored by Gallo or any of his 1984 coauthors were more (or less) likely to make unqualified claims than those written by other authors; and fourth, whether the articles that made unqualified claims were more likely to cite later articles in con-junction with Gallo's in order to back up those claims. (For details on how this analysis was carried out, see the Methodological Appendix.)

Table 1 shows a striking shift over the three-year period. Only 3 percent of the 1984 articles that cited Gallo (2 out of 59) did so in conjunction with unqualified claims about the virus being the cause. Fifty-eight percent of them cited Gallo to support qualified claims, while 34 percent cited Gallo for other reasons and without making etiological claims. By the following year, the percent citing Gallo to make unqualified claims had jumped to 25 percent (26 out of 106). And by 1986, 62 percent (49 out of 79) of the articles cited Gallo to make unqualified claims, and only 22 percent did so in conjunction with qualified claims.[9]

Table 1 *Patterns of Causal Claims in References to Gallo et al. (1984) in Seven Major Journals*

Year	Type of reference	N	%
1984	Explicit unqualified reference to the virus as the cause	2	3.4
	Implicit unqualified reference to the virus as the cause	2	3.4
	Qualified reference to the virus as the cause	34	57.6
	Explicit reference to possibility that the virus may not be the cause	1	1.7
	Article not cited in conjunction with a causal claim	20	33.9
	Total	59	100.0
1985	Explicit unqualified reference to the virus as the cause	26	24.5
	Implicit unqualified reference to the virus as the cause	2	1.9
	Qualified reference to the virus as the cause	62	58.5
	Explicit reference to possibility that the virus may not be the cause	0	0.0
	Article not cited in conjunction with a causal claim	16	15.0
	Total	106	99.9
1986	Explicit unqualified reference to the virus as the cause	49	62.0
	Implicit unqualified reference to the virus as the cause	3	3.8
	Qualified reference to the virus as the cause	17	21.5
	Explicit reference to possibility that the virus may not be the cause	0	0.0
	Article not cited in conjunction with a causal claim	10	12.7
	Total	79	100.0
	Grand Total	244	

A glance at some of the more authoritative sources within the sample reveals the trend over time. A review article by the Council on Scientific Affairs of the AMA, published in October 1984, spent nearly two pages reviewing various etiological hypotheses and then concluded: "At the present time, the retrovirus etiology of AIDS is the hypothesis for which there is the most convincing evidence." However, "even though the time may be close at hand when the definitive cause of AIDS is established, there is yet much to be explained." The authors noted several questions: "Why has AIDS been largely confined to certain groups while the majority of the population does not appear to be at much risk of acquiring the disease? Why does frank AIDS develop in only a small percentage of patients with the lymphadenopathy syndrome?" [10] A year later, several prominent epidemiologists from the CDC wrote an article for *Science* reviewing the literature on the epidemiology of AIDS, noting in the opening paragraph that, in 1984, "a retrovirus variously termed lymphadenopathy-associated virus (LAV), human T-lymphotropic virus type III (HTLV-III), or AIDS-associated retrovirus (ARV) was isolated and *shown to be the cause of AIDS* [emphasis added]." [11] Similarly, a group of investigators with the Division of Virology of the Food and Drug Administration (FDA) wrote in the *Annals of Internal Medicine* in late 1985: "The role of the human T-lymphotropic virus type III (HTLV-III) in the development of the acquired immunodeficiency syndrome (AIDS) is firmly established"—citing only the three "discovery" papers published, respectively, by Montagnier in 1983, Gallo in 1984, and Levy in 1984. [12]

Expressions of doubt or skepticism—let alone support for other hypotheses—were extraordinarily rare throughout this period from 1984 to 1986. The *Lancet*'s initial editorials reporting on the Heckler press conference and on Gallo's articles in *Science* criticized the public fanfare and argued for a sober assessment of the facts. The journal noted that the finding of a virus "is no proof of causality," given the possibility "that these viruses are simply passengers—yet another opportunistic infection to which these patients are susceptible." [13] "Nevertheless," the editorial went on to say, the fact that two laboratories had isolated the viruses from AIDS patients and that the viruses had been identified in many of the risk groups and rarely in controls "[lends] credence to our prejudice that viruses such as these are likely to be the guilty party."

One article in the *New England Journal*, published in August 1984, noted in passing that "further evidence is necessary to substantiate [the] possibility" of a retroviral cause. [14] More serious doubts tended to be voiced only in short letters to journals. Arthur Ammann of UCSF Medical School called for a "cautious appraisal" in a September 1984 letter to *JAMA*. Arguing that "there is no historical precedent for believing that a single infectious agent is capable of abolishing a normal immune system," Ammann suggested that AIDS might conceivably be

the consequence of "multiple infections" involving HTLV-III acting
synergistically with other viruses, such as CMV. Before concluding
that HTLV-III is the sole cause, he cautioned, "a great deal more evidence must be obtained." [15] But interventions such as these failed to
gather any allies, and they largely vanished from the pages of the
prominent medical and scientific journals after 1984.

What role did Gallo play in pushing the argument that his virus
was the cause of AIDS? Articles authored or coauthored by Gallo or
his coauthors certainly accounted for a substantial part of this literature—about a third of all publications in the sample for 1984 and
1985 and a quarter of them for 1986. (Of course, in many of these
cases where the names of Gallo and/or his coauthors appear somewhere in the middle of a lengthy list, Gallo's lab most likely played a
marginal role, perhaps no more than supplying viral samples.) But an
interesting finding, revealed in table 2, is that, in terms of the pattern
of making qualified or unqualified claims, there are no statistically
significant differences [16] between the papers influenced by Gallo's
group and those with other authorship. As Treichler has asserted,
Gallo's group may have strengthened the credibility of their claim simply by publishing so many papers about AIDS and referencing their
1984 paper at every turn. But in referencing it, they were no more or
less likely to make either qualified or unqualified etiological claims
than other scientific researchers who cited it during the same years.
They promoted their product—but they did not, in any crude or bla-
tant sense, oversell it in terms of its causal implications.

On the other hand, Gallo and his collaborators were less circum-
spect than Montagnier's group, who, as late as March 1985, wrote
cautiously in *JAMA:* "Although the precise role of LAV in the pathogenesis of AIDS remains to be confirmed, the present report, together
with the recent description of HTLV-III and AIDS-related virus, provides growing evidence in favor of a T-lymphotropic retrovirus as the
causative agent in AIDS." [17] And in November 1985, Montagnier reminded his readers that "cofactors"—factors in addition to the primary cause, such as antigens or foreign proteins—might often work
together with LAV to cause AIDS.[18] Montagnier, in other words,
sought to incorporate some of the claims contained in earlier hypotheses, such as the immune overload hypothesis, within a new explanation that gave star billing to LAV.

A remarkable aspect of the change that took place over the three-
year period is that the trend is observable even among those papers that

Table 2 *Patterns of Causal Claims in References to Gallo et al. (1984) in Seven Major Journals ("Gallo authors" versus "No Gallo authors")*

Year	Type of reference	Gallo authors		No Gallo authors	
		N	%	N	%
1984	Explicit unqualified reference	2	10.0	0	0.0
	Implicit unqualified reference	0	0.0	2	5.1
	Qualified reference	11	55.0	23	59.0
	Explicit reference—may not be cause	0	0.0	1	2.6
	No causal claim	7	35.0	13	33.3
	Total	20	100.0	39	100.0
1985	Explicit unqualified reference	9	24.3	17	24.6
	Implicit unqualified reference	0	0.0	2	2.9
	Qualified reference	21	56.8	41	59.4
	Explicit reference—may not be cause	0	0.0	0	0.0
	No causal claim	7	18.9	9	13.0
	Total	37	100.0	69	99.9
1986	Explicit unqualified reference	13	65.0	36	61.0
	Implicit unqualified reference	0	0.0	3	5.1
	Qualified reference	4	20.0	13	22.0
	Explicit reference—may not be cause	0	0.0	0	0.0
	No causal claim	3	15.0	7	11.9
	Total	20	100.0	59	100.0
	Grand Total	77		167	

do not cite any subsequent research. Table 3 shows all papers in the sample from 1985 and 1986 that made a causal claim when citing Gallo's paper (as opposed to citing him for some other reason). These papers (ninety in 1985 and sixty-nine in 1986) are divided into two groups: those that cited Gallo alone or Gallo in conjunction with other previous or roughly contemporaneous "discovery" papers, such as work by Montagnier and Levy; and those that cited Gallo in conjunction with at least some later research. One might expect that papers also citing later research would be more likely to make unqualified claims. While that apparently is not the case in 1985, it seems to be in 1986. (The numbers are too small for the results to be statistically significant, but twelve of fourteen such articles made unqualified claims.)[19] However, two points deserve note. First, only a minority of

Table 3 *Patterns of Causal Claims in References to Gallo et al. (1984) in Seven Major Journals (Articles from 1985 to 1986 That Cite Early Papers versus Those That Cite Later Research)*

Year	Type of reference	Citations of early papers only		Citations of later research	
		N	%	N	%
1985	Explicit unqualified reference	21	28.8	5	29.4
	Implicit unqualified reference	2	2.7	0	0.0
	Qualified reference	50	68.5	12	70.6
	Explicit reference—may not be cause	0	0.0	0	0.0
	Total	73	100.0	17	100.0
1986	Explicit unqualified reference	37	67.3	12	85.7
	Implicit unqualified reference	3	5.5	0	0.0
	Qualified reference	15	27.3	2	14.3
	Explicit reference—may not be cause	0	0.0	0	0.0
	Total	55	100.1	14	100.0
	Grand Total	128		31	

the articles that made unqualified claims about the virus being the cause (five out of twenty-six in 1985 and twelve out of forty-nine in 1986) pointed to *any* later research when making such claims. In both years, most articles that made unqualified claims referenced the early set of papers only. Second, even among those articles that failed to cite any subsequent research, the original trend is apparent: between 1985 and 1986 the ratio of qualified to unqualified claims shifts markedly.[20] These articles would seem to follow Gallo's own lead, gradually reinterpreting the significance of the early papers by imputing to them a stronger causal claim than even their authors made at the time of their publication.

To be sure, one might argue that people who failed to cite the subsequent research have been influenced by it nonetheless. Perhaps when researchers cited the early papers as having "proven" that HIV causes AIDS, they intended these citations to serve as a kind of shorthand or synecdoche that symbolically represented the larger body of published scientific literature. For this reason alone, it makes sense to attend to the other research findings published in this time period that supported the HIV hypothesis. However, many of the subsequent articles that were co-cited with Gallo's provide little additional evidence. The two most commonly cited articles (each cited three times by articles in the sample making unqualified claims)—Samuel Broder and Gallo, published in the *New England Journal* in November 1984, and Flossie Wong-Staal and Gallo, published in *Nature* in October 1985[21]—are review articles summarizing the literature on the "HTLV family" of viruses. The only additional etiological evidence that Broder and Gallo provided appeared in a brief mention of unpublished data from Gallo's lab showing (1) that HTLV-III had been found in semen and saliva in addition to blood, and (2) that HTLV-III had, by this point, been isolated from over 95 persons and could be recovered over 90 percent of the time from patients with "pre-AIDS." These latter data from Gallo's lab were eventually published by S. Zaki Salahuddin et al. in the *Proceedings of the National Academy of Sciences*,[22] though in this paper the Gallo group also reported that they still were unable to isolate the virus from half of the patients with full-blown AIDS. The Wong-Staal and Gallo paper is essentially the same in terms of its contribution to the question of causality. The authors simply reviewed the original *Science* articles and the additional findings published by Salahuddin et al. in the *Proceedings*.

Both review articles pointed to the Salahuddin article for the new evidence, and that paper was also cited on its own by other authors in the sample. But turn to that study and the citation pathway neatly reverses direction. The authors declared that "it is clear that HTLV-III is causatively involved in the immune disorder AIDS," and they explicitly advised the reader to refer back to Broder and Gallo for a summary of the evidence.[23] Findings such as these certainly support Treichler's claim—that Gallo and his close associates established a network of citations that served to create the impression of greater certainty than Gallo's own data warranted. In circular fashion, each article points to a different one as having provided the definitive proof; the buck stops nowhere. Still, one can find places where Gallo did a better job of summarizing the existing evidence. For example, in a less frequently cited article in the journal *Blood*, Wong-Staal and Gallo reviewed two types of evidence in addition to the serology studies.[24] First, in an unpublished study from Gallo's lab, out of ten blood donors whose recipients later developed AIDS, ten tested positive for HTLV-III antibodies. Second, an "animal model" was provided when chimpanzees were deliberately infected with HTLV-III.[25] The chimps "mounted an immune response to the virus, and some developed enlarged lymph nodes analogous to the lymphadenopathy syndrome that often precedes AIDS." According to Wong-Staal and Gallo, these various results, accompanied by the knowledge that HTLV-III kills T cells in the test tube, "unambiguously establish HTLV-III as the etiologic agent of AIDS."[26]

BLOOD AND CHIMPS

Whether they made qualified or unqualified claims, other authors, including the Montagnier group, pointed to similar types of evidence: serology studies, transfusion studies, and chimpanzee studies.[27] Why these types of studies? Implicitly or explicitly, researchers had Koch's postulates—or similar criteria—in the backs of their minds.[28] Two points, if established, would greatly enhance the credibility of the HIV hypothesis: that the virus could be found in all (or some reasonable percentage of) cases of the syndrome and that the virus, when transmitted accidentally to another human or when injected deliberately into an animal, caused the same condition. Even Gallo himself, who would in subsequent years dismiss the applicability of Koch's postulates when critics complained that they were not satisfied in the case of HIV, invoked them in his paper with Wong-Staal. Describing the "unpublished observations" of ten seropositive blood donors whose recipients later developed AIDS, Wong-Staal and Gallo commented that "nature has indirectly fulfilled one of Koch's postulates by documenting transmission of the agent prior to development of the disease."[29]

What kind of case is presented by these various studies on serology, transfusion cases, and animals? Most crucially, how do they address the alternative explanation—that HTLV-III/LAV/ARV is simply an opportunistic infection common among people with severe immunodeficiency? The serology studies were perhaps the weakest in this regard: researchers were unable to find the virus in many cases of full-blown AIDS, and they were unable to show, on the basis of blood testing, that infection preceded immunosuppression. One study by the Montagnier group presented some important data. The researchers detected LAV antibodies in seventeen of twenty-five AIDS patients, thirteen of thirteen homosexual men with "pre-AIDS," and only one of one hundred random healthy blood donors. But their innovation was to also look for antibodies in patients with immunodeficiencies that were genetically caused. Out of twenty-three such patients, none tested positive for antibodies to LAV, "supporting the contention that LAV is unlikely to represent simply another opportunistic infection" in people who are already immunodeficient.[30]

The chimpanzee study was subject to various interpretations. Out of three chimps injected with plasma from an AIDS patient, two developed antibodies to HTLV-III. One of them developed lymphadenopathy and a "transient decline" in the ratio of helper T cells to suppressor T cells. As of a year later, none of them had developed any opportunistic infections. Shinji Harada and coauthors, summarizing the etiologic evidence in *Science*, wrote with reference to this study that HTLV-III "causes a similar disease in chimpanzees";[31] but technically no chimp had developed AIDS (and for a decade, no chimp would).[32] Donald Francis and his coauthors were more cautious, claiming only that the chimp study "offers the possibility of proof that LAV/HTLV-III is the cause of AIDS." "Time will show," they added, if the chimps actually develop the full syndrome.[33]

Studies of donors and recipients of blood transfusions (or blood products used by hemophiliacs) went the furthest in confronting the question of whether the virus was the primary cause.[34] For example, Paul Feorino and his coauthors wrote in the *New England Journal* in May 1985 that they had isolated HTLV-III from six transfusion recipients who had developed AIDS and from twenty two of twenty five donors who were identified as being "high-risk."[35] In one of the six cases, both the presumed donor and the recipient had AIDS at the time the study was performed, "raising the question whether HTLV-III/LAV might represent an opportunistic infection in both." But in the other five cases, while the recipients all had AIDS, the donors were asymptomatic "carriers" of the virus. Since the donors were healthy, the virus was apparently not an opportunistic infection in their cases. And the recipients had no other known risk factors besides receipt of a tainted transfusion.

Before calling the case closed, however, one might examine an analogous study performed by prominent researchers (Harold Jaffe, Donald Francis, and others), reported in *Science* a month *before* the Heckler press conference.[36] This group found antibodies in nine of 117 donors to twelve patients with transfusion-associated AIDS. Grouping the donors into twelve sets corresponding to the twelve patients who received their blood products, the researchers discovered that nine of the sets each included a donor who could have been the source of infection. In six of the nine sets, the antibody-positive donor fit other epidemiological and immunological criteria as a person at risk for AIDS, and four of those six had lymphadenopathy when interviewed for the study. The irony, however, is that these scientists were *not* testing for antibodies to HTLV-III. They were studying *HTLV-I*, the virus that, in 1983, Gallo was promoting as the cause of AIDS. A month later, everyone would simply forget about HTLV-I—but the transfusion data presented in support of that virus was nearly as good[37] as what the Feorino group would present a year later as "further evidence of the etiologic role of HTLV-III/LAV"—and Jaffe would be the second author listed on Feorino's paper.

HIV as "Obligatory Passage Point"

THE POWER OF A HYPOTHESIS

Why, over the course of 1984, 1985, and 1986, did AIDS researchers so overwhelmingly come to accept as given a hypothesis that—while highly plausible and consistent with many facts known about the epidemic—was not "conclusively" proven, according to the standards of evidence they claimed to support? Nothing suggests any vast conspiracy to stifle debate, though critics would later claim as much. One reasonable explanation would eventually be proposed by Gallo himself, in response to a challenge by the HIV dissenters: "As anybody in the business knows who works [with AIDS], there is more evidence that this virus causes AIDS than you have with the vast majority of diseases [that we] long ago have accepted"[38] as caused by viruses.

Of course, it wasn't that the HIV hypothesis was problem-free. Savita Pahwa and his coauthors (who included Gallo) noted one crucial "paradox" in the *Proceedings of the National Academy of Sciences* in late 1985:[39] the virus, presumed to do its dirty work by infecting and killing T cells, could be found, using "the most sensitive methods available," only in a tiny fraction of any AIDS patient's T cells—sometimes as few as one in one hundred thousand cells. An important part of the prima facie case against the virus had been its propensity to kill T cells in the test tube. But in living human beings, the virus simply could not be found in enough T cells to account straightforwardly for their disappearance in AIDS patients.

Still, the virus hypothesis had considerable evidence behind it and only a few findings seemed anomalous; no other hypothesis about AIDS had a track record anywhere nearly as impressive. What's more, the virus gave researchers a mission. Within months of the publication of Gallo's articles in *Science,* other scientists began to report their findings—on the prevalence of HTLV-III/LAV antibodies in various populations, on the detection of the virus in various body fluids, on the patterns of transmission of the virus, on possible antiviral treatments, on the development of vaccines against the virus. Especially in 1984, such researchers typically were careful to make qualified claims, noting that the virus was "believed" to be the cause or was the "probable" cause. But in practice, the qualifications meant next to nothing, because the virus—and the virus alone—is what all of them were busy spending their time studying. The phrasing of one article in the *New England Journal* was typical: "Now that HTLV-III has been identified as the probable cause of AIDS, it is possible to confirm the modes of transmission and document the spectrum of clinical disorders caused by this agent."[40] At last, the authors seemed to be suggesting, we all have something to do. A plausible candidate had been proposed by eminent virologists, and most researchers were content to endorse their judgment.[41]

Clinicians, and researchers in other fields, who read the professional literature simply to keep up with the latest findings, not to critically evaluate the analyses and methodologies, were even less likely to raise questions. As Harry Collins has suggested on the basis of recent social studies of science, there is typically "a relationship between the extent to which science is seen as a producer of certainty and distance from the research front."[42] Any fuzziness in the data that might have been observable by a trained epidemiologist or virologist was likely to be missed by the doctor treating AIDS patients, who turned to the *New England Journal of Medicine* just to get the bottom line.

If a scientist as eminent as Gallo had been pushing an alternative explanation, then most likely there would have been more debate and closer scrutiny of the etiological evidence. But no challenge of that sort existed. The more time passed and the more that scientists became invested in research on HIV, the clearer became the virus's social role as what Bruno Latour has called an "obligatory passage point"—a necessary way station between social actors and the satisfaction of their interests. A meeting of the Conference of State and Territorial Epidemiologists in June 1985 might be singled out as the defining moment that the HIV hypothesis became a social fact. Conference members approved a series of resolutions, adopted soon afterward by the CDC, that redefined "AIDS" to make diagnosis dependent on a positive antibody test result along with the presence of any one of an expanded list of opportunistic infections and cancers.[43] People whose antibody test came back negative would in most cases be diagnosed as AIDS-free, even if they, too, suffered from one of the conditions on the list.[44]

Those who did challenge the hegemonic position risked strong resistance and career repercussions. The story of Shyh-Ching Lo, a young virologist at the Armed Forces Institute of Pathology, is instructive in this regard. When in 1986 he reported finding a "novel virus" in tumor cells taken from AIDS patients with Kaposi's sarcoma, Lo "brought a heap of abuse down on his head," in the words of a reporter for *Science*.[45] Lawrence Altman treated the story as important, and the *Times* gave it front-page treatment.[46] But skeptical AIDS researchers, including Gallo, lashed out at Lo, claiming he had failed to justify his claims. Lo pressed on, discovering the agent in various body tissues of AIDS patients; when he injected it into four silverleaf monkeys, they all died within nine months. Furthermore, Lo was able to isolate the agent from six HIV-negative patients who had symptoms similar to those of AIDS. Yet his articles were rejected by more than half a dozen journals before finally seeing the light of day in the *American Journal of Tropical Medicine and Hygiene* in 1989.[47]

Eventually, it became apparent that the agent Lo had isolated was not a virus but a primitive organism called a mycoplasma.[48] Since mycoplasmas are common contaminants of tissue cultures, it remained debatable whether the mycoplasma had really come from the AIDS patients. But only in 1990, when Montagnier independently began talking about a possible role for mycoplasmas as a cofactor in AIDS, did researchers belatedly begin to take Lo seriously. Until that time, Lo—despite his credentials as a virologist—could not make his voice heard over the chorus supporting the reigning theory.

SCIENCE, THE MEDIA, AND THE CONSTRUCTION OF SOCIAL REALITY

What cannot be overstated is that the HIV hypothesis was not simply a scientific powerhouse. It was also—crucially—a *social* phenomenon. Immediately after the discovery of the probable cause of AIDS was announced, the hypothesis began its work of transforming the world and reshaping people's lives. Within two years, the first patients began taking azidothymidine (AZT), an antiretroviral drug that—at least temporarily—prevented the virus from replicating;

prescribed for many thousands of patients, AZT has earned millions of dollars for its manufacturer, Burroughs Wellcome. Even before that, thousands of people were touched irrevocably by the machinery of antibody testing, which sorted them into polar categories of "positive" and "negative." Gay communities were quite simply split into two groups; and despite frequent and sincere criticism of the tendency, antibody status became a decisive marker of identity—the sort of attribute gay men mentioned in personal ads, along with skin color and sexual predilections, to describe who they were and who they sought. In response to a belief in the HIV hypothesis, thousands of people changed the way they had sex—supposedly one of the most intractable aspects of human behavior. Even a practice as thoroughly unthinkable, in the contemporary U.S. political context, as providing intravenous drug users with clean needles suddenly became a reasonable, if controversial, health strategy that sane politicians might propose or endorse. Within a few years, the HIV hypothesis quite simply restructured the world, altering what millions of people did and said.

The mass media both mirrored and facilitated the process by which HIV became a social fact.[49] A content analysis of selected articles from the *New York Times* suggests the trend over the period from 1984 to 1986. (I examined all twenty-one articles published in the latter half of 1984 that discussed both AIDS and the virus; in 1985 and 1986 news coverage skyrocketed, and I examined every fifth such article, in chronological order: forty-three articles in 1985 and fifty-one in 1986.[50])

In the second half of 1984, articles that discussed both AIDS and the virus were cautious in their conclusions (see table 4). Out of twenty-one such articles, eighteen made only qualified claims about the virus as the cause. By 1985, a striking shift had occurred: Out of forty-three articles in the sample for the year, twelve made only qualified causal claims and eight made only unqualified claims. Seventeen articles (41 percent) made *no* explicit claims yet clearly conveyed their implicit endorsement—in sixteen of seventeen cases by the unqualified use of the phrase "the AIDS virus" in reference to HIV.[51] By 1986, the number of articles making only qualified claims had dropped to five out of fifty-one; ten articles made only unqualified claims; and the number of implicit claims rose to thirty-three (65 percent of the total). The decline in the use of qualifiers and the growing reliance on phrases such as "the AIDS virus" (or, more problematically, "the AIDS test") tell a clear story: reporters took for granted that the cause of AIDS was known. They had their doubts, to be sure, about whether Gallo

Table 4 *Patterns of Causal Claims in Sample of* New York Times *Articles Referring to Both AIDS and the Virus*

Dates	Type of reference	N	%
7/84–12/84	Only unqualified references to virus as cause	1	4.8
	Only qualified references to virus as cause	18	85.7
	Mixed qualified and unqualified references	1	4.8
	Implicit claim that virus is cause	0	0.0
	References to possibility virus may not be cause	1	4.8
	No causal claim	0	0.0
	Total	21	100.1
1/85–6/85	Only unqualified references to virus as cause	1	11.1
	Only qualified references to virus as cause	5	55.6
	Mixed qualified and unqualified references	2	22.2
	Implicit claim that virus is cause	1	11.1
	References to possibility virus may not be cause	0	0.0
	No causal claim	0	0.0
	Total	9	100.0
7/85–12/85	Only unqualified references to virus as cause	7	15.6
	Only qualified references to virus as cause	7	21.9
	Mixed qualified and unqualified references	1	3.1
	Implicit claim that virus is cause	16	50.0
	References to possibility virus may not be cause	1	3.1
	No causal claim	2	6.3
	Total	34	100.0
1/86–6/86	Only unqualified references to virus as cause	6	27.3
	Only qualified references to virus as cause	3	13.6
	Mixed qualified and unqualified references	0	0.0
	Implicit claim that virus is cause	12	54.5
	References to possibility virus may not be cause	0	0
	No causal claim	1	4.5
	Total	22	99.9
7/86–12/86	Only unqualified references to virus as cause	4	13.8
	Only qualified references to virus as cause	2	6.9
	Mixed qualified and unqualified references	0	0.0
	Implicit claim that virus is cause	21	72.4
	References to possibility virus may not be cause	2	6.9
	No causal claim	0	0.0
	Total	29	100.0
	Grand Total	115	

NOTE: 1984 results derive from full population data, while 1985 and 1986 results derive from samples drawn from the full populations.

was the one who should receive credit for discovering it, but that the virus was indeed the cause was only very rarely questioned.[52]

Articles in the *Times* in mid-1984, such as one by Judy Glass on June 3, discussed the reports of a viral cause in tentative terms. Glass quoted a medical professor who asked whether the virus was "the chicken or the egg"—the real cause or just another opportunistic infection.[53] In October, Lawrence Altman sounded a more definitive note: researchers had "taken a major step toward fulfilling Koch's postulates" by transmitting the virus to chimpanzees.[54] From about that time onward, articles by Altman—the *Times*'s main authority on AIDS—stopped expressing any doubts. In the second half of 1984, Altman wrote six articles about AIDS and the virus which made only qualified claims about its causal role and one that made both unqualified and qualified claims. In 1986, out of the seven articles in the sample that were by Altman, none made any qualifications. Two made unqualified claims only, while five simply implied that the virus was the cause (in four cases by referring to HIV as "the AIDS virus"). Altman did, however, write articles that discussed some of the anomalies in the HIV hypothesis, such as the mystery of why so few T cells appeared to be infected with the virus.[55]

THE APPEAL OF A VIRUS

Elsewhere in society, the viral hypothesis found a ready audience. Gay communities in general and AIDS organizations in particular were little inclined to dispute the causal role of HIV. As early as December 1984, in an information packet distributed to local health care providers, the San Francisco AIDS Foundation made its views plain: "A multiplicity of theories concerning AIDS causation has given way in most quarters to the conclusion that a specific retrovirus is the causative agent."[56] More often, as Dennis Altman has pointed out, politically liberal groups have tended to endorse environmental, multicausal models of illness and to criticize the "single bullet" approach.[57] In this case, however, AIDS organizers had good reason to find the HIV hypothesis attractive. Increasingly, gay men had been under attack, accused by various right-wing spokespersons of pursuing a "promiscuous" lifestyle that was in reality a "deathstyle."[58] Fears that they would be quarantined en masse had become widespread among gays. Indeed, Dr. Edward Brandt, Reagan's assistant secretary of health in 1983, has since indicated that the Reagan administration gave serious consideration to the idea of a mass quarantine at that time.[59] But while the talk about lifestyle had seemed to lay the groundwork for victim blaming in the larger society, the viral hypothesis had more neutral moral implications. Pursuing a lifestyle was seen as a choice; contracting a virus seemed more like plain bad luck.

Not that the acceptance of the viral hypothesis served to sever altogether the popular connections between etiology and culpability. On the contrary, AIDS still was all too frequently perceived as a phenomenon whose very existence demanded a guilty party. But attention now tended to focus on the virus itself and the question of its origins. Had HIV originated in Africa, as many Western scientists maintained (to the displeasure of many Africans)? Did Cubans fighting in Angola bring the disease to Haiti? Was HIV the product of genetic engineering by the CIA or the U.S. Army, as fringe groups in the United States, along with official Soviet media sources, proposed? Had HIV or a simian form of it been unwittingly introduced into Africans via vaccines (against smallpox, malaria, or polio, depending on the theory) prepared from monkey tissue and administered in WHO vaccination programs in Africa? But while debates over these and other theories about origins of the virus raged and sometimes held various parties, nations, or continents culpable for the origins of the virus, to a significant degree they left gay men unscathed.[60]

Furthermore, the viral hypothesis provided gay communities with an important repertoire of responses to the widespread panic over casual transmission of AIDS. Opinion polls in 1983 and 1984 suggested that large numbers of people in the United States believed that AIDS could be transmitted by coughs and handshakes, drinking glasses and shared toilet seats.[61] Many people acknowledged that they were shunning contact with gay people against the possibility that those people might have AIDS, and gay rights groups were reporting a rise in cases of antigay discrimination in the workplace, in housing, and elsewhere in the society. Increasing knowledge about the highly specific routes of HIV infection offered a ready answer. The solution was not to avoid the risk *groups,* AIDS educators asserted, but to avoid the risk *practices*—principally, sex without a condom and the sharing of syringes. Given the near-total protection of the blood supply with the advent of the antibody tests, AIDS advocacy groups could plausibly claim that it was *easy* to protect oneself from getting AIDS. More radical public health measures such as quarantine were therefore unnecessary.[62]

Finally, the viral hypothesis resonated with the "safe sex" (or "safer sex") strategies that were already being promoted in gay male communities by 1983. Although many commentators had continued to stress the importance of limiting the number of sexual partners, others had focused on a different solution: taking standard steps to prevent the spread of sexually transmitted diseases, such as using condoms or avoiding ejaculation inside the body. Michael Callen and Richard Berkowitz had emphasized these points in a forty-page booklet, "How to Have Sex in an Epidemic," that enjoyed considerable circulation in gay communities on both coasts.[63]

Given evidence that HIV could indeed be blocked by condom use, the viral hypothesis solidified a "sex-positive" AIDS education strategy. While mainstream public health officials continued to counsel monogamy, the fledgling grassroots AIDS organizations put forward a different message that was both pragmatic and scientifically based: have as much sex as you like, as often as you like, with as many different people as you like, and as long as you follow a set of rules to prevent the transmission of HIV, you will be (almost entirely) safe. (Monogamy, by contrast, was a far less credible prevention measure, the grassroots AIDS educators pointed out: especially in communities where HIV was prevalent, monogamous unsafe sex might be quite dangerous, while monogamy in the context of safe sex was essentially redundant.)

Despite frequent opposition from government funders concerned about sexually explicit language and images, the grassroots AIDS educators set out to "eroticize" safe sex—to make it seem not only normative behavior, but attractive and sexy. Techniques of safe-sex education and even the precise definitions of safe sex became, in effect, a "zone of control" that emerging community-based organizations carved out of the larger terrain of the viral hypothesis. That they were experts on safe sex was acknowledged early on: in the midst of the 1984 controversy over whether to close down the gay bathhouses in San Francisco, a state superior court judge who heard arguments on the case mandated that the San Francisco AIDS Foundation would define which activities practiced in bathhouses were safe and which were not.[64] Yet to a significant extent, assumptions of their expertise came to depend on the widespread acceptance of claims about HIV transmission and its causal role in AIDS. Without the belief in HIV as the cause, AIDS organizers could have continued to promote their safe sex guidelines, but only as plausible measures that seemed likely to work. With HIV, the idea of safe sex rested on the shoulders of scientific authority.[65]

ALTERNATIVE VIEWPOINTS

Certainly dissenting voices spoke out, and more so in the gay and lesbian press than anywhere else. The *Advocate*, the most mainstream of the major news sources on AIDS, was the least critical of researchers. Nathan Fain, the magazine's health writer, considered the question of causality closed after the reports of the chimpanzee studies. "What all this means to the man and woman on the street," wrote Fain, "is that . . . convincing proof now exists that there is one virus that is the sole triggering mechanism of AIDS." Cofactors might also be necessary to cause the full syndrome, but—as the headline put it—"The Proof Is In on a Virus." [66]

GCN, more inclined toward suspicion of experts and no friend of Robert Gallo's, took a more cautious position. Christine Guilfoy, one of the chief writers on the topic, referred to the causal claim in qualified terms throughout 1984 and 1985. A year after the Heckler press conference, in April 1985, Guilfoy wrote: "Although many believe HTLV-III plays a primary role in the development of AIDS, it is still unresolved how the virus works and what cofactors, if any, play a role." [67] Particularly by the second half of 1985, however, writers in GCN tended to refer to HTLV-III without further explanation of its relationship to AIDS. It was simply assumed that the reader understood what this virus was and why it was being written about. Of course, referring to HTLV-III carried different implications than speaking of "the AIDS virus," as mainstream reporters were apt to do. Like the gay press generally, GCN avoided (and often criticized) the phrase "AIDS virus" for its implied conflation of two states: seropositivity and illness from AIDS.

GCN was also a place where alternative views could gain expression. In late 1986, John Lauritsen, a survey researcher and writer who had coauthored a pamphlet warning gay men about the dangers of poppers,[68] raised the question of whether HIV had definitively been proven to cause AIDS: "Notwithstanding the thousands of assertions that have appeared in the popular media and in government press releases, the fact remains that medical science has a series of tests that any microbe must pass before it can be considered the cause of a particular disease. These tests are known as 'Koch's Postulates,' and the 'AIDS virus' has soundly flunked them." [69] Concluding that HIV cannot be the cause of AIDS, Lauritsen reopened an old can of worms: "There must be something in the gay lifestyle that is causing gay men to develop AIDS." Consistent with his earlier focus on poppers, Lauritsen targeted "the 'recreational drugs' . . . that became a prominent feature of the urban gay male lifestyle beginning in the early 1970s."

The true voice of dissent, however, was the *New York Native,* for which Lauritsen most regularly wrote. Indeed, the *Native* and its publisher Chuck Ortleb increasingly located themselves on the fringes of the emerging AIDS movement, precisely through their incessant skepticism (some would claim, paranoid doubt) about the HIV hypothesis.[70] Writing in the *Native* in fall 1994, Joseph Sonnabend, proponent of the immune overload hypothesis, advised gay men not to read too much into the HTLV-III antibody test: "It should be emphasized at this point that the question of whether HTLV-III plays any role in the pathogenesis of AIDS must remain open."[71] The following year, Sonnabend expanded on his views in an interview in the *Native,* speculating about the motivations and interests behind the emphasis on HTLV-III as the sole cause of AIDS and questioning the certainty of expert pronouncements: "Unlike what Dr. Anthony Fauci and Dr. Robert Gallo tell us, we are very far from understanding this disease. Very little is known. The sort of smugness that emanates from the government scientists is offensive, considering what is at stake. . . ."[72]

The *Native* treated Sonnabend respectfully as its resident authority, but when it was Gallo's turn to be interviewed, he had no such luck. In August 1984, James D'Eramo tried to corner Gallo on the question of whether HTLV-III had been proven to be the sole cause of AIDS:

[D'Eramo:] What about fulfilling Koch's postulates . . . ?
  [Gallo:] . . . Koch did not fulfill those postulates in much of the work he did. They're hardly ever fulfilled in viral and fungal diseases, and hardly ever in parasitic diseases. . . . What's the remaining part of Koch's postulate that is not fulfilled anyway?
[D'Eramo:] It's the animal model.
  [Gallo:] . . . you don't need an animal model in immunological diseases. Those of us who know a little bit about retroviruses realize that in some retroviruses you can't go outside the species to reproduce the disease.

In frustration at D'Eramo's questioning of the causal claim, Gallo finally challenged him directly, asking, "Why does anyone resist this data?" Gallo continued: "All I can say is that they don't know the data, they don't understand it, or they may not know some of the data that aren't published yet. Nobody at high levels in science is arguing about this data."[73] Often outspoken, Gallo probably never considered the impact of his tone on readers of the *Native* or on its staff. Nothing could have been better calculated to offend the sensibilities of the *Native* and inflame its constituency than Gallo's implication that the scientific debates were over the heads of laypeople, who should rest content to leave it up to the experts.

Meanwhile, the *Native* committed itself to a range of rival theories about the causes of AIDS. The process had its origins back in 1983, when the newspaper began promoting the view that AIDS was linked to an epidemic disease in pigs, called swine fever. This hypothesis was first floated by a postdoctoral fellow at the Harvard School of Public Health, named Jane Teas. In a 1983 letter to *Lancet,* Teas proposed that AIDS might be caused by a variant of the African Swine Fever Virus (ASFV), which had never been known to infect humans. Teas had done no research on AIDS or swine fever, but she was struck by the apparent similarity in symptoms as well as by the Haitian connection: AIDS seemed to have appeared in Haiti in 1978 and swine fever in 1979. She speculated: "Perhaps an infected pig was killed and eaten either as uncooked or undercooked meat. One of the people eating the meat who was both immunocompromised and homosexual would be the pivotal point, allowing for the disease to spread to the vacationing 'gay' tourists in Haiti."[74]

In 1983, at a time when the question of etiology was still open, Teas's letter prompted some response. Two groups of researchers, one Haitian, the other Belgian and Dutch, wrote letters to *Lancet* saying they had looked for antibodies to ASFV in small samples of AIDS patients but with negative results in all cases.[75] Later the 1984 AMA review article on AIDS would acknowledge the swine fever hypothesis as one of many legitimate ideas that simply failed to pan out.[76] Teas, however, felt that the responses to her hypothesis were inadequate, and she became convinced that the scientific establishment was shutting her out. She had written to both the CDC and the U.S. Department of Agriculture, but received no "satisfactory" response from either organization. When Chuck Ortleb, the *Native*'s publisher, approached her, she was happy to promote her ideas and to voice concern about the "hostility" and closed-mindedness of government science.[77]

Teas was the sort of person who would have minimal credibility in mainstream scientific circles—after all, she casually admitted that she began "knowing nothing about AIDS" and that she taught herself about swine fever in an afternoon's reading.[78] But to Ortleb, this kind of self-education by nonexperts epitomized the critical attitude toward scientific authority that he had been promoting in the pages of his newspaper. Through a series of articles, Ortleb pushed the swine fever angle, asking why government researchers were so slow to follow it up and insinuating that the government was acting at the behest of the pork industry.[79]

In a striking demonstration of the perceived importance of the gay press in the eyes of the public health officialdom, James Mason, the conservative Mormon director of the CDC, flew to New York in early 1984 to try to reason with the *Native*'s publisher. Mason even gave Ortleb a scoop—two weeks before he spoke with the *New York Times*—about LAV being the probable cause of AIDS. But Ortleb became convinced that Mason was trying to divert his attention and "coopt" him, and though the *Native* began reporting on LAV and HTLV-III, the newspaper also continued to promote Ortleb's pet theory.[80]

Ortleb's single-handed campaign eventually succeeded in inducing New York State health authorities to search for ASFV in AIDS patients and in generating some coverage of the hypothesis in more mainstream newspapers such as the *New York Times*.[81] But when further supportive evidence of a causal role for ASFV was not forthcoming, Ortleb was on to the next rival theory, and then the next—Lo's mycoplasma, Duesberg's heretical views, and in recent years the claim that AIDS and chronic fatigue syndrome are different forms of the same disease. Over time, the *Native*'s star began to fall, and Ortleb became an increasingly controversial figure within the AIDS movement. Cultural critic and AIDS activist Douglas Crimp complained in 1987: "Rather than performing a political analysis of the ideology of science, Ortleb merely touts the crackpot theory of the week, championing whoever is the latest outcast from the world of academic and government research."[82]

MARKERS OF CREDIBILITY

Despite speculation about swine fever and mycoplasma, despite challenges from people like Lauritsen and Ortleb, and despite some scientific interest in cofactors, the basic fact remained: The proposition "HIV causes AIDS" was hegemonic in U.S. science and society as 1986 came to a close. That year, the American Medical Association had published in book form an authoritative collection of articles on AIDS that had appeared in recent years in its journal, *JAMA*.[83] Although the collection included the Sonnabend, Witkin, and Purtilo article from 1983 (buried near the end in a "Special Reports" section), it contained no articles published later than 1983 that questioned the relationship between HIV and AIDS. For the back of the book, the AMA's Task Force on AIDS had reviewed "the complete list of published articles" on AIDS in the medical and scientific literature, with the goal of preparing "a brief bibliography that could serve as a source document to guide the interested reader through the massive body of literature on AIDS." The section on etiology contained fifty-six references, of which fifty-four alluded to a retroviral cause of AIDS in the title. Only one of the fifty-six articles proposed an alternative etiology—an article by J. J. Goedert on the role of recreational drugs in causing AIDS. Even the Sonnabend, Witkin, and Purtilo article—included in the collection itself—failed to make it into this definitive bibliography.

Another important benchmark of the credibility of the HIV hypothesis was the influential *Confronting AIDS,* a survey of knowledge and a blueprint for action published by the National Academy of Sciences' Institute of Medicine. Prepared by a blue-ribbon panel consisting of prominent virologists, clinicians, public health experts, and social scientists, the 352-page report encapsulated the official, credible body of knowledge about AIDS *circa* 1986. Though ostensibly a study of "the AIDS epidemic," the report might more accurately be called "Confronting *HIV*"; early in the introduction, it explained that "AIDS" is only a surveillance definition used for epidemiological purposes and that the term "does not include the full spectrum of conditions now known to be associated with HIV infection."[84]

Nonetheless, in a section entitled "The Causative Agent of AIDS," the report did briefly review the growing evidence that HIV caused the syndrome. First, antibodies reactive to viral proteins were found in "nearly all instances" of people with AIDS, while tests of people not in "high-risk" populations were "uniformly negative." Moreover, the prevalence of antibodies in different groups corresponded with what was known about the geography and timing of the epidemic. Second, the virus itself could be isolated from the white blood cells of most people who were antibody positive; the authors added parenthetically that "the failure to isolate the virus from all infected persons is most likely due to technical limitations in the lymphocyte culture methods and to the depletion of target cells in the advanced stages of the disease." Finally, the blood transfusion data were compelling: they "clearly showed that the virus could be transmitted to a previously uninfected person who could then develop AIDS. . . ."[85]

Elsewhere in the report, however, the authors acknowledged a good deal of uncertainty. They noted that it remained mysterious precisely *how* HIV caused the characteristic depletion of T cells, given the small percentage of cells that appeared to be infected.[86] This was a problem but not an insoluble one, the report implied, noting that many researchers had begun speculating about the "indirect" means by which HIV could be causing T-cell loss. Montagnier, for example, had proposed that HIV initiated an autoimmune mechanism, whereby the immune system of the infected person was "fooled" into killing its own T cells; and other hypotheses were equally complex.

Another question was whether HIV worked alone to cause AIDS or whether some "cofactor" or "cofactors" might also be involved. But despite raising these various questions about how HIV caused disease and whether HIV worked alone, the main thrust of the report was to focus squarely on the problem of HIV infection. Thus chapter 6 of the report, "Future Research Needs," divided research priorities into the following categories: structure and replication of HIV, natural history of HIV infection, epidemiology of HIV infection, animal models for HIV infection, antiviral agents, vaccines against HIV, and social science research.[87]

John Lauritsen, who titled his review of *Confronting AIDS* in the *Native* "Caveat Emptor," noted: "For those who are true believers in the 'AIDS virus' ideology, a number of disconcerting bombshells are detonated in this book. To begin with, the report acknowledges that it is impossible to isolate HIV from many AIDS patients and that some AIDS patients show no evidence of ever having been infected with the virus."[88] Yet as Lauritsen was no doubt painfully aware, the "bombshells" simply failed to echo in the larger society or even in the sectors of it that concerned themselves principally with the epidemic. In a few short years, an industry had grown up around AIDS, encompassing doctors and researchers, service providers and grassroots educators, lawyers and writers, politicians and policymakers—a complex of individuals, groups, and formal organizations. And within this industry, HIV was the common link between actors and interests. The virus was the "obligatory passage point" that stood between people and the grants they sought to obtain, the programs they endeavored to establish, and the propositions they wanted to advance. In its transformation into scientific fact and social reality, "HIV causes AIDS" had become a "black box"; and when people like Sonnabend or Lauritsen tried to reopen the box and review the evidence and arguments, theirs were isolated voices with minimal credibility. It would take someone with considerably more scientific capital to focus significant scientific and extrascientific attention on the question of whether HIV had in fact been proven to cause AIDS.

CHAPTER 3

REOPENING
THE CAUSATION
CONTROVERSY

From Deafening Silence
to the Pages of *Science* (1987–1988)

How does a controversy that seemed to have been closed come to be reopened? What sort of tactics enable someone to disrupt the smooth transfer of knowledge from hypothesis to fact to common sense? The story of Peter Duesberg, who became the premier "HIV dissenter," is an enlightening one. Like other prominent researchers, Peter Duesberg proceeded to AIDS from prior work on retroviruses and their relation to cancer. Born in Germany in 1936, Duesberg received a Ph.D. in biochemistry from the University of Frankfurt; in 1970, he joined the faculty of the University of California at Berkeley in the Department of Molecular and Cell Biology.

In the 1970s, as millions of dollars were poured into the "War on Cancer," cancer research increasingly came to be dominated by what Joan Fujimura has called the "bandwagon" of oncogene theory.[1] This theory held that certain genes within each cell had the potential to cause cancer. Closely tied to oncogenes were the cancer-causing retroviruses, which, it was argued, contained genes that could turn normal cells into cancer cells. Duesberg not only mapped the genetic structure of retroviruses but was the codiscoverer of the first known oncogene, called *src* (pronounced "sark"). These accomplishments established him as a figure of note in his field.

To date, Duesberg has authored or coauthored more than 200 professional publications. A survey of the "Medline" database, which lists scientific publications that are medically relevant, shows more than 150 articles, literature reviews, monographs, and letters authored or coauthored by Duesberg.[2] A study of the *Science Citation Index,* a crude but not uninformative indicator of a scientist's perceived importance in the eyes of peers,[3] reveals that publications with Duesberg as first author have been frequently cited over the years, though particularly in the late 1970s. Between 1975 and 1979, for example, 76 of his publications were cited more than one thousand times. By comparison, during the same period, publications by his contemporary[4] and colleague, Robert Gallo (that is, those with Gallo as first author), received over eight hundred citations. These figures put both scientists in the exceptional category, since articles listed in the *Science Citation Index* are cited on average only a handful of times a year—indeed, many are not cited at all.

Over the course of his career, Duesberg has received a number of awards and prizes, including being named the 1971 California Scientist of the Year. In 1986, the NIH awarded him an Outstanding Investigator Award, a special research grant for high achievers. In April of that same year Duesberg was elected into the National Academy of Sciences (NAS)—the cream of the crop, numbering about fifteen hundred of the top scientists in the United States. But Duesberg's career has not been without controversy. Indeed, in recent years, he had increasingly positioned himself as somewhat of a maverick, challenging the same conventional wisdom that he had earlier helped to construct. By the mid-1980s, Duesberg had become known as a dissenter from oncogene theory. "We have this nice idea of the oncogene model as some kind of switch" that turns on cancer, Duesberg told *Forbes* magazine, "but it has yet to be proved."[5] In 1985 Duesberg published a formal challenge to oncogene theory in *Science.*[6] Not everyone accepted Duesberg's argument, but neither did Duesberg suffer professional consequences as a result of his heterodox position. Indeed, both his Outstanding Investigator Grant and his induction into the NAS followed on the heels of his dissent.

POSING THE CHALLENGE

In many respects, the concerns Duesberg expressed in his article in *Cancer Research,* published in March 1987, were an extension of those he had voiced earlier. Entitled "Retroviruses as Carcinogens and Pathogens: Expectations and Reality," this sixteen-page review article with 278 references presented no original research but continued the argument that Duesberg had been trying to put forward: that retroviruses are simply not "the vessels of evil they have been labeled to be." In recent years, the general hypothesis that viruses were linked to cancer had been gaining ground, in part because many viruses (both retroviruses and ordinary DNA viruses) had been isolated from tumors and leukemias, particularly in animals. Duesberg pointed out, however, that many of these same viruses "were subsequently found to be widespread in healthy animals and humans." In his view, only a specific subset of these viruses were actually oncogenic (cancer-causing): those containing a class of genes called *onc* genes. Retroviruses lacking these *onc* genes, according to Duesberg, were harmless and ubiquitous; they could "coexist with their hosts without causing any pathogenic symptoms." [7]

Without question, had Duesberg stopped there his article would have been ignored by everyone outside of a narrow specialist community. But Duesberg had another point to make, one that would occupy the final third of the article. The scientist later recalled: "As I was writing . . . AIDS just sort of literally exploded into the news media, and an article on retroviruses not at least taking a position [on] AIDS would have been rather incomplete. . . ." [8] From Duesberg's perspective, the identification of the HIV retrovirus as the causal agent in AIDS was highly problematic. First, he pointed to the considerable disparity between the number of people estimated to be infected with HIV and the number of people who actually had AIDS. In the United States, where one to two million people were believed to be HIV positive, the annual incidence of AIDS among the virus-infected groups was only 0.3 percent. In Haiti and Africa, where estimates of infection ran even higher, the annual incidence was estimated at less than 0.01 percent. Since the introduction of the hypothesized agent so rarely appeared to cause disease, Duesberg claimed that Koch's third postulate had not been satisfied.

Second, Duesberg argued that it was implausible that a retrovirus would cause illness years after infection. He noted that many people infected with HIV report having a brief, mononucleosis-like illness a few weeks after infection, and that this is what might reasonably be expected from a retrovirus. By contrast, the claim that HIV also caused AIDS some years later was hard to reconcile with the claim that HIV directly killed T cells: "We are faced with two bizarre options: Either 5 year old T cells die 5 years after infection or the off-spring of originally infected T cells die in their 50th generation, assuming a generation time of one month for an average T cell." Furthermore, Duesberg noted that, in a study published in 1986 and conducted by Gallo and his associates, viral RNA was detected in only one of every ten thousand to one hundred thousand T cells in infected persons. In Duesberg's view, it was absurd to claim that a virus expressing itself in so few cells could be causing so much damage, since the body is constantly manufacturing new T cells. Even if the virus were to kill every ten-thousandth T cell every twenty-four hours, "it would hardly ever match or beat the natural rate of T-cell regeneration." [9] Finally, Duesberg argued that there was no "simian model" for AIDS as required by a strict interpretation of Koch's postulates. Studies of chimpanzees and monkeys deliberately infected with HIV showed that these primates failed to develop a condition like AIDS (although such primates did develop viral antibodies, along with a mononucleosis syndrome similar to that in humans, shortly after infection).

What, then, did it mean to test HIV antibody positive? For Duesberg, it meant that one was *protected* against the effects of HIV: The purpose of antibodies is precisely to protect the body against the spread and expression of a pathogen. Having antibodies to HIV was therefore like being vaccinated against the virus. Until the immune system had created these antibodies, the person infected with HIV might suffer from the mononucleosis syndrome; but once the person tested positive for antibodies (normally within weeks after infection), he or she was safe—at least from HIV. HIV didn't harm its hosts; it was simply one of the many viral infections sustained by people with AIDS or at risk for AIDS, as was Epstein-Barr virus and CMV (found in 80 to 90 percent of them) and herpes (found in at least 75 percent). Perhaps AIDS was caused by one of these other infectious agents, perhaps it was caused by something other than a virus; Duesberg had no way of knowing. But HIV alone "is not sufficient to cause AIDS and . . . there is no evidence, besides its presence in a latent form, that it is necessary for AIDS." [10]

A CONTROVERSY TAKES PUBLIC SHAPE

Most scientific publications, sociologists of science have pointed out, are destined to die a lonely death. Given the tremendous number of publications that appear each year, it is inevitable that the average paper is ignored by the vast majority of scientists. Only a minority of papers are cited by many others; fewer still become the object of direct debate. As a general rule, one need not invoke a complicated explanatory apparatus to account for the fact that a scientific paper may sink beneath the surface of professional attention without causing much of a splash.[11]

Duesberg's paper might have been particularly inclined in that direction because many of the points he was making were not especially new. Such questions as how the virus could cause the near-elimination of T cells when only a few seemed to be infected had been raised before; this particular anomaly had made it into the National Academy of Sciences' *Confronting AIDS* and had even been discussed in the gay press. But arguably Duesberg's essay was different, and it might have been expected to generate a livelier response. It was written by an eminent scientist whose articles typically had been cited by dozens of other scientists each year. It was published in a respected journal. It had enormous implications if correct in its arguments. And it constituted nothing short of a declaration of war on some of the most prominent virologists in the world. Yet had it not been for the pressure exerted by outsiders who wrote about Duesberg in the alternative and mainstream press, the scientific community might never have addressed Duesberg's claims. Indeed, throughout the latter part of 1987 and early 1988, it was precisely the "AIDS establishment's" apparent avoidance that most incensed the HIV dissenters—and that provided them with their best ammunition.

The first apparent published mention of Duesberg's article came in a cover story by John Lauritsen in the June 1, 1987, issue of the *New York Native*. As the issue's cover advertised, the focus of the article was to encourage people with AIDS not to take the medication AZT.[12] Recently approved for AIDS patients, AZT was believed to inhibit replication of the virus in infected cells by interfering with the process of reverse transcription. AZT, in other words, made sense as a treatment for AIDS only if AIDS was caused by HIV. This is precisely what Lauritsen disputed, and much of the article was devoted to the proposition that "HIV Is Not the Cause of AIDS."[13]

With the discovery of the virus, "dogma rapidly came to prevail"; "all other research efforts were shunted aside, ostracized, under-funded," Lauritsen complained. Against this dogmatism, it was—until now—impossible for dissenters to make their voices heard: "Since 1984, there have been a few of us who stated in print that epidemio-logical evidence, together with the failure of HIV to fulfill any of Koch's postulates, made it most unlikely that HIV could be the sole cause of AIDS. . . . We were isolated. Some AIDS researchers did not believe in the 'AIDS virus' ideology, but, in the interests of self-preservation, they remained silent." But now that a prominent scien-tist had entered the fray, "all this has changed"; and the HIV dissenters could emerge from their isolation. As Latour has noted, "the power of [scientific] rhetoric is to make the dissenter feel lonely"; this is pre-cisely what happens to the "average person" who tries to challenge highly technical scientific texts.[14] The most obvious solution is to re-cruit credible allies who can provide rescue from isolation. Lauritsen had found just such an ally.

"Unless HIV's champions can do some very fancy explaining," Lauritsen concluded, "Duesberg's article has unambiguously relegated the 'AIDS virus' etiology to medical history's trash heap of falsified hypotheses." Insisting that "Gallo and the other 'AIDS virus' ideo-logues" must respond to Duesberg's article "fully and in detail," Lau-ritsen did his best to up the ante in the controversy: "If the Public Health Service and the media remain silent about Duesberg's article, and persist in expounding the discredited HIV mythology, then gay men will have cause to be gravely concerned. This would mean that the government and their confederates in the medical establishment are not acting in good faith, that nothing they say can be trusted, that their interests are hostile to ours. Their silence would raise the possibility of a horrible hidden agenda."[15]

Soon after this article appeared, Lauritsen went to interview Dues-berg at the NCI, where Duesberg was working while on sabbatical from the University of California. The interview was published both in the Native and, sometime later, in its more literary offshoot, Chris-topher Street; the Native ran photos of Gallo and Duesberg on its cover, with the headline "Which Man Is Right?" The interview re-corded a fascinating duet between Duesberg and Lauritsen, with Duesberg voicing his support for Lauritsen's claim that AZT is poison-ous ("It is a poison. It is cytotoxic.")[16] and Lauritsen feeding Dues-berg suggestions about what might cause AIDS. When Duesberg shrugged off a direct question on causation ("Well, that's a difficult one. . . . I really wonder what it could be"), Lauritsen put forward the idea advanced earlier by various proponents of a multifactorial etiology that AIDS might have different causes in different groups. Duesberg chimed in: "Absolutely. And in Africa I don't think anybody knows what kind of AIDS exists, or *whether* AIDS exists. In the case of the drug users, I could well see that an infection of toxins—and the drugs are impure; no one knows where they come from—is hell for the immune system. And also medical injections—streptomycin or penicillin—are also not good on a regular basis. They are immunosuppressive themselves. Perhaps it is a simple question of lifestyle." [17]

While assuring Duesberg that it was not incumbent on him to come up with an alternative hypothesis—"It's quite enough to have falsified theirs"—Lauritsen nonetheless pushed Duesberg's speculations further. He described for Duesberg what he called the "profile" of the average AIDS patient—a profile whose characteristics supposedly included long-term drug abuse, promiscuity, and repeated cases of sexually transmitted disease:

[*Lauritsen:*] Looking at that profile . . . I think it would be surprising if
              such people did not become seriously sick from their lifestyle.
[*Duesberg:*] I would be surprised, too. The number of contacts, the num-
              ber of things they inject. You wonder how they could do it. [18]

By the end of the interview, Duesberg appeared to be sliding out of his formal position of agnosticism and toward an endorsement of a lifestyle model similar to the immune overload hypothesis that had been so popular in the first years of the epidemic—indeed, a particularly judgmental version of that hypothesis.

According to James Kinsella's study of AIDS and the media, the *Native*'s publisher, Chuck Ortleb, quickly took it upon himself to conduct a "phone-calling campaign" to promote Duesberg's arguments. [19] But the *Native*—a paper whose fascination for unorthodox and speculative theories had left it with tarnished credibility even among its intended readership of gay men, let alone elsewhere—had only minimal power to spread the word about Duesberg or to evoke much alarm about a "horrible hidden agenda." Duesberg's claims did begin to circulate in gay communities; they were picked up, for example, by Charles Shively, writing about various alternative AIDS theories in *Gay Community News.* [20] But only with Katie Leishman's September

1987 article in the popular magazine *Atlantic Monthly* did Peter Duesberg begin to hit the mainstream. Dubious of official pronouncements about the epidemic, Leishman's article ranged widely, exploring the possibilities of insect transmission and presenting a sympathetic portrait of Jane Teas's unappreciated efforts to push the African swine fever hypothesis. Near the end of the article, however, she also turned to Duesberg and Koch's postulates, noting that Duesberg "is so certain of his claim that he has offered to be inoculated with HIV." [21]

Soon afterward, Duesberg made his first of what would prove to be several appearances in a British television documentary series called *Dispatches*. In an episode entitled "AIDS—The Unheard Voices," produced by a group called Meditel and broadcast on November 13, the narrators cited Duesberg to suggest that discrimination against antibody positive people, however deplorable on its own terms, was particularly irrational if HIV were not even the true cause of AIDS. [22] Though controversial in Britain, the show attracted little notice in the United States. Meanwhile, Harvey Bialy, the editor of a journal called *Bio/Technology*, had become interested in Duesberg's arguments, and Bialy invited Duesberg to write a summary of his *Cancer Research* article. Adopting a journalistic style, Duesberg complained that "the 'deadly AIDS virus' has been sold to the public as the cause of AIDS with the confidence and authority that is usually derived from absolute scientific proof." [23]

In the immediate aftermath of the Leishman piece and Duesberg's own article in *Bio/Technology*, Duesberg began to be recognized in U.S. media circles as a credible and "quoteworthy" dissenter on the subject of AIDS. [24] By the end of 1987, gay newspapers such as *Gay Community News* and San Francisco's *Bay Area Reporter* were publishing articles specifically about Duesberg—and about the failure of his colleagues to respond to him. "How come researchers continue to study HIV but have not refuted Duesberg's theory?" asked the subhead to the *GCN* article. "I've asked questions they apparently can't answer," Duesberg was quoted as saying. [25]

Before long the story had acquired its own momentum. In January, Celia Farber, a journalist with the pop music magazine *Spin*, featured Duesberg in a long interview in her column called "AIDS: Words from the Front." [26] In the interview, Duesberg suggested that researchers such as Gallo found themselves simply unable to retreat from their original claims because the "stakes are too high now": "Every progress report from their laboratories is discussed by Dan Rather and

Barbara Walters, *Newsweek,* and *Time* magazine. . . . To say that now, maybe, the antibody wasn't worth committing suicide for or burning houses for, would be very embarrassing."[27] Even more provocatively, Duesberg delivered a stinging critique of the political economy of contemporary biomedical research, questioning the motives of AIDS researchers: "Scientists researching AIDS are much less inclined to ask scrutinizing questions about the etiology . . . of AIDS when they have invested huge sums of money on companies that make money on the hypothesis that HIV is the AIDS virus. . . . Gallo stands to make a lot of money from patent rights on this virus. His entire reputation depends on this virus. If HIV is not the cause of AIDS, there's nothing left for Gallo. If it's not a retrovirus, Gallo would become irrelevant."[28]

As a reporter for the journal *Science* would later put it: "In the world of biomedical research, where ties to industry are pervasive but mentioning the fact is not, these are fighting words."[29]

INTERESTS, INVESTMENTS, AND "FALLEN ANGELS"

Such charges made for good copy, but Duesberg's point was actually more subtle: virologists had "invested" in the HIV hypothesis—not just financially, though this was true in some cases, but personally, professionally, and psychologically. The following year, in a speech at a scientific gathering, Duesberg put forth this analysis as a full-fledged, revisionist history of retrovirology's desperate search for "clinical relevance." "On the basis of promises and expectations, the retrovirologists . . . have become the darlings of molecular and clinical biology in the last twenty years," Duesberg explained. Retroviruses were expected "to hold keys to cancer and other diseases," yet despite massive funding, the promise had not been fulfilled. Earlier in the century, virologists enjoyed spectacular successes against polio and smallpox. But "in the 1970's and 80's, virology suffered from the same fate that inorganic chemistry suffered in the early part of the century, when no new elements were left to be discovered!" Virology became "a thoroughly academic discipline, without significant clinical factors."[30]

With more and more virologists at work using ever more sophisticated tools, it was inevitable that they would "succeed" in finding viruses that appeared to be linked to diseases that in fact have other causes, Duesberg argued. In this sense, virologists had become "the victims of their own weapons." Having found one such virus in AIDS patients, virologists were now fanatically invested in the claim that the virus caused the syndrome: "An 'AIDS virus' is perhaps the last hope for the clinical relevance of the highly visible, highly decorated and powerful retrovirus establishment." [31]

Duesberg was the first to note that it would have been simpler for him to pursue a sure thing, a "succession strategy" (to use Bourdieu's terminology), [32] as opposed to a high-risk "subversion strategy" of scientific advancement. "Clearly the value of my very considerable investment in retroviruses would be much compounded by a clinically relevant retrovirus, which should thus motivate me to believe in HIV!" Duesberg told the gathering. "But since all work on retroviruses in the last 25 years has shown that latent retroviruses are harmless, and that virtually all retroviruses in wild animals and in humans are latent, I have lost faith in the central dogma of the program . . . ," said Duesberg, characterizing himself as a "fallen angel, like Lucifer." [33]

THE DUESBERG STORY GOES MAINSTREAM

With charges that AIDS experts were reaping millions of dollars from a discredited hypothesis, it didn't take long for the story to hit the newspapers. On January 7, the *New York Post* became the first daily newspaper to print an article specifically on the Duesberg controversy, called "AIDS Experts on Wrong Track: Top Doc." [34] Writer Joe Nicholson, the *Post*'s medicine and science editor, cited Duesberg's offer to have himself injected with HIV, and he also quoted Gallo's protestation that "no serious scientist is interested in this." Nicholson paid considerable attention to Duesberg's credentials, noting that this "top scientist" had been studying viruses for twenty years, was a member of "the elite National Academy of Sciences," and had spent the preceding year on a scholarship at the NIH, "the world center of AIDS research." But Nicholson failed to mention that Duesberg's work at NIH was on cancer, not AIDS; nor did he justify his initial identification of his protagonist as "AIDS expert Dr. Peter Duesberg," given that Duesberg had neither conducted any laboratory research on AIDS nor had any professional contact with AIDS patients.

Perhaps predictably, the *Post*'s more upscale competitor was quick to follow up and to do so in a more skeptical vein. "A Solitary Dissenter Disputes Cause of AIDS," wrote the *New York Times*'s Philip Boffey, in a short (728-word) article published not in the front section but on the medical science page in section C. [35] The article pitted

Duesberg's "provocative argument" against "virtually all of the lead-ing scientists engaged in AIDS work [who] believe that Dr. Duesberg is wrong," and it quoted Anthony Fauci of NIH as saying: "The evi-dence that HIV causes AIDS is so overwhelming that it almost doesn't deserve discussion any more." Boffey also suggested that Duesberg's claims might be old hat: "AIDS experts insist that the issues raised by Dr. Duesberg have been considered at length within the scientific community. They cite plausible mechanisms whereby a tiny fraction of infected cells could disable vast numbers of additional cells."

A two thousand–word article by Joel Shurkin appearing soon after-ward in the *Los Angeles Times* lent considerably more credibility to Duesberg's views.[36] In an implicitly equalizing move, Shurkin referred to a debate between "two camps," the "dissidents" and the "AIDS Establishment," which "disagree not so much on the basic facts as on their interpretations." Shurkin's discussion of disagreement between scientists tended to convey a certain legitimacy upon Duesberg's argu-ments. For example, one AIDS researcher "who refused to be quoted by name" said that Duesberg was factually incorrect and that the virus had indeed been found in all patients. But another researcher "said the truth is somewhere in between." Such disagreement had the effect of suggesting that there was a legitimate spectrum of opinion on these questions and that Duesberg's views, however unpopular, were not beyond the reaches of plausible scientific theorizing.

Just as Duesberg's name was inching further into the mainstream media, *Spin* published a follow-up piece, an interview with Gallo in which the virologist responded—heatedly—to Duesberg's views.[37] (William Booth, the news writer for *Science,* later characterized Gallo's "ranting and raving" as "bizarre," but added that the inter-view was tape-recorded without Gallo's knowledge.[38]) Should one keep an open mind on the question of the causation of AIDS? inter-viewer Anthony Liversidge, a New York City science writer, asked Gallo.

> [*Gallo:*] No. I don't think anybody needs to keep an open mind on that. It is silly, OK?
> [*Liversidge:*] Is there any flaw in [Duesberg's] logic that is easy for you to point out?
> [*Gallo:*] No. He's a good fellow. It's a useless interchange. Really totally useless. He's an organic chemist. I would never argue with him about electronic spin resonance in a molecule of organic compound.

Gallo went on to say, "This is just so trite that it is a waste of my goddamn time. I'm busy." Everyone knew that HIV was the cause of AIDS: "Call 5,000 scientists and ask." [39]

Gallo's central complaint about his colleague was that Duesberg was simply not qualified to comment on the question. Or as Gallo bluntly told his interviewer: "Arguing with Peter is like you arguing with me." Furthermore, said Gallo, Duesberg had misinterpreted published evidence and ignored crucial arguments about the role of HIV in causing AIDS: "Hasn't Duesberg ever understood indirect mechanisms in cell killing? There are immune responses to the virus that destroy the proliferation of the T cell. That's crystal clear now. It is not just a matter of the virus going in and killing the cell directly. Does that take a genius?" Finally, Gallo was furious at Duesberg for failing to recognize the human consequences of his arguments: "Peter can do a lot of disservice. He has now indicated to people that they can go out and fuck around and get infected by this virus and not worry. That's the part where I am mad at Peter. Peter is joking about very serious matters that are going to alter some people's behavior." [40]

Celia Farber capped off Liversidge's interview by appending an ironic comment, noting that a few years earlier, when Gallo introduced Duesberg at a university talk, he characterized Duesberg as having "a rare critical sense which often makes us look twice, then a third time, at a conclusion many of us believed to be foregone." And Farber quoted Duesberg's response to the Gallo interview: "I must say, of all the scientists I've known, Gallo's reactions are the most unscientific." [41] In fact, Gallo was a convenient foil for Duesberg. Though this would change in the years to follow, at the moment Gallo was the AIDS establishment figure that everyone loved to hate. As rumors had spread that Gallo might have stolen Montagnier's virus, Gallo had come to be a symbol of expertise gone bad: untrustworthy, patronizing, and resentful of challenges. Just the past month, *Gay Community News* had spotlighted his attitude toward the AIDS activist group ACT UP in its "Quote of the Week" feature: "I don't care if you call it ACT UP, ACT OUT or ACT DOWN, you definitely don't have a scientific understanding of things," Gallo had reportedly told activists. [42]

GAY DESPAIR, GAY SUSPICION

If gay men in early 1988 were apt to distrust Gallo, they were also inclined to be open to heretical views. This was a particular moment in the history of the AIDS epidemic in gay communities, one marked both by profound desperation and the emergence of a new wave of militant activism. Gay men were wracked with frustration by the slow rate of progress in the development of treatments for AIDS, and those testing positive for HIV antibodies were increasingly pessimistic about their likelihood of avoiding illness and eventual death. Earlier on, the claim that AIDS was caused by a virus had resonated with gay concerns about avoiding discrimination and stigmatization. But this changed with reports by public health officials that the percentage of those infected with the virus who would go on to develop AIDS was not, as first believed, a small minority of 5 or 10 percent but in fact appeared to be at least 70 percent and might, in the absence of new treatments, rise as high as 100 percent. These tidings led to a deepening gloom between 1985 and 1988.[43] For the largest and most established gay communities, where local newspapers routinely reported that one out of every two gay men probably was infected,[44] such news can only be described as devastating. AZT at this point was prescribed only for people who already had AIDS (at a cost of about ten thousand dollars a year per person—and it was failing to keep them alive for very long). Some vocal spokespersons in gay communities, particularly in New York, argued that AZT did more harm than good. And there were no approved medications that antibody-positive people could take to keep them from progressing to an—apparently inevitable—AIDS diagnosis.

One response to these difficult times was a rebirth of activism, epitomized by the actions of groups like ACT UP and the San Francisco–based advocacy group Project Inform, that focused on eliminating the bottlenecks in the federal drug approval process, challenging the pharmaceutical houses over price-gouging for medications, and—as a popular slogan had it—getting "drugs into bodies."[45] But a second response to the mood of desperation was a surge of interest in heretical views about AIDS. The AIDS establishment had failed to deliver; perhaps it was time to listen to some new voices. Understandably enough, cofactor theories were particularly attractive since they offered hope that not all those who were HIV antibody positive would actually develop AIDS. But more radical theories that disputed the HIV-AIDS link altogether had a certain appeal as well. Indeed, when Duesberg, along with Joan McKenna (director of an independent organization called the Institute for Thermobaric Studies, in Berkeley, and an advocate of the view that AIDS is actually a disguised form of syphilis), was invited to speak at a public forum in San Francisco's heavily gay Castro district in January 1988, they were met by a standing-room-only crowd of six hundred. Many more were turned away at the door, according to *San Francisco Chronicle* reporter Randy Shilts, "reflecting the growing currency that a number of unconventional theories about the cause of AIDS are gaining in the gay community."[46] Duesberg himself "received a hero's welcome" at the forum, in the words of an article published in the *San Francisco Sentinel*, a gay news-weekly.[47]

That Duesberg should inspire the admiration of the gay masses was not without irony, given that the researcher at this point appeared to endorse the same immune overload hypothesis that, earlier in the epidemic, had often been characterized as homophobic and had been criticized for "blaming the victim." But initially people knew little about Duesberg. When interviewed by the *Sentinel,* Duesberg refused to give an alternative explanation for what causes AIDS, saying only, "I can't answer that." Shortly afterward, however, the *Oakland Tribune* quoted him as explaining: "I suspect we are dealing with an environmental lifestyle disease that has hit drug users, hemophiliacs and some gay communities the hardest. The trauma of anal intercourse could also be a factor. They could have used too many drugs, been too promiscuous, or had their immune systems weakened by venereal diseases, foreign antigens and antibiotics."[48] More damningly, the February 2 *Village Voice* quoted Duesberg as saying that the epidemic was "caused by a lifestyle that was criminal twenty years ago."[49] Days later, this remark became *GCN*'s "Quote of the Week."[50]

As statements such as these became known, Duesberg lost any chance of sustaining large-scale support in gay communities. By February 1988, negative articles about Duesberg began to appear, including the *Voice* article, written by medical reporter Ann Fettner, called "Dealing with Duesberg: Bad Science Makes Strange Bedfellows." Duesberg's views on causation, Fettner wrote, constituted "a stunning regression to 1982, when everything under the sun, and gay practices in particular, were being blamed for the outbreak of the disease."[51]

Yet even as Duesberg's stock was beginning to fall in gay communities, he was gaining considerable attention in the mass media and even in some government circles. On February 9, the refusal of mainstream AIDS researchers to confront Duesberg was blasted by Jack Anderson, the syndicated columnist and well-known muckraker. According to Anderson, Harvey Bialy, the editor of *Bio/Technology,* had been planning a workshop called "How Does HIV Cause AIDS?" and a senior White House domestic policy analyst named Jim Warner had offered to cohost it. Warner was reported to be "frustrated about the inadequate response he had gotten to Duesberg's theory"; sponsorship by the White House "would guarantee the attendance of Gallo and other experts." Yet shortly before the conference was to take place, it was abruptly removed from the White House calendar. According to one editor at *Bio/Technology,* "The impression was that the pressure came from the NIH." When Anderson asked about the conference, Warner replied, "I can't talk about that." Anderson also noted that Gallo refused to return his phone calls.[52]

THE ESTABLISHMENT HITS BACK

For the AIDS experts who thought Duesberg's arguments were pernicious nonsense, there were two choices, both of them fraught with some peril. They could continue to ignore Duesberg, at the risk of appearing closed-minded, imperious, or unscrupulous, and hope that he would eventually go away or that the media would simply lose interest. Or they could engage him directly and seek to show him up, at the risk of granting him further credibility or, at a minimum, publicity. "Many AIDS researchers refuse to comment publicly because they fear it will legitimize Duesberg," said NIH's Anthony Fauci, quoted in a March 1988 news article in *Science.*[53]

Yet to many scientists, the political costs of ignoring Duesberg increasingly seemed to overshadow the risks inherent in engaging with him. Apparently in a move to undercut Duesberg's complaint of being marginalized, Dr. Frank Lilly of the Albert Einstein College of Medicine, the chairman (and the only openly gay member)[54] of the President's Commission on the HIV Epidemic, an advisory body appointed by President Reagan the year before, responded to Duesberg's requests for an opportunity to make his views known by inviting him to testify at the commission's hearings in February. However, in what would prove to be a common theme in responses to Duesberg in the years to follow, commission members blasted Duesberg for the sin of playing to a public audience. One member, Dr. William Walsh, lectured Duesberg: "I would hope that you would press your theory within the scientific circles and not carry this uncertainty to the public. . . . Don't

confuse the public—don't confuse the poor people who are suffering
with this disease."[55] This appeal to Duesberg to avoid publicizing his
dissent enraged Katie Leishman, who had promoted Duesberg earlier
in the pages of *Atlantic Monthly*. She blasted the commission for its
treatment of Duesberg, in an op-ed piece published in the *Wall Street
Journal* entitled "The AIDS Debate That Isn't." Leishman reserved
particular ire for Walsh: "The suggestion that the public and patients
must be protected from confusion is not merely condescending but
faintly sinister."[56]

From the vantage point of the AIDS researchers and public health
officials who were on the receiving end of all this criticism, the situation was rapidly getting out of hand. Into the fray stepped the American Foundation for AIDS Research (AmFAR), a prominent independent foundation that raised money for AIDS and dispensed it to a
range of university-based and community-based research projects.
With strong ties both to gay community representatives and mainstream researchers, AmFAR was well situated to play mediator. Am-
FAR sponsored a forum held at George Washington University in
Washington, D.C., on April 9 and invited a range of panelists.[57] Anthony Fauci, the most prominent government scientist present, had
reservations about agreeing to participate but decided to come because
"the scientific community can't afford to ignore [Duesberg] any
longer."[58]

At the forum, after Duesberg summarized what he termed the "paradoxes" of the HIV hypothesis, panelists and audience members hit
back hard. Panelists insisted that Duesberg was simply wrong to say
that viruses always cause disease within months and never do so in the
presence of antibodies. And they noted that with the advent of a new
technique for manipulating DNA called the polymerase chain reaction
(PCR) it was now possible to find HIV in nearly 100 percent of samples
from people with AIDS—though still not in every case, as Duesberg
was quick to observe. As to the presence of HIV in so few T cells, Fauci
stated that HIV also infected other immune system cells called macrophages and might hide in bone marrow cells.[59] Fauci was particularly
vehement in response to suggestions that AIDS really was linked to lifestyle: "What kind of risk behavior does the infant born of an infected
mother have?" he asked. "And what about the 50-year-old woman
who received a blood transfusion from an infected donor?"[60]

Perhaps the most interesting data were presented by Warren Winkelstein, an epidemiologist from Berkeley's School of Public Health.
Winkelstein's numbers came from the San Francisco Men's Health

Study, a prospective study of one thousand single men, gay and straight, twenty-five to fifty-four years old, who had been recruited by statistical sampling methods several years earlier, and who were reexamined every six months.[61] One of several prominent "cohort studies" on HIV infection in the United States and around the world, the San Francisco Men's Health Study offered data of a kind that was simply not available at the time that closure had first been reached on the subject of HIV as the cause of AIDS.

In direct response to Duesberg's claims about Koch's postulates, Winkelstein organized his comments around what he described as a modern-day reformulation of those postulates, which consisted of five criteria. First, the "prevalence of disease should be significantly higher in those exposed to the factor than in unexposed controls." Winkelstein didn't have any data specifically on the prevalence of AIDS in the larger population, and his study (originally designed to examine progression to AIDS) had excluded from the outset any men already diagnosed with AIDS. But he did perform clinical and lab tests on his subjects upon entry, looking at a range of indicators considered to be predictors of AIDS, and the antibody-positive men had significantly higher prevalence rates for eighteen of the twenty-one indicators studied.

The second criterion was that incidence of disease (new cases) should be significantly higher in those exposed to the causal factor. This was precisely what Winkelstein had found. Thirty months into the study, of the 399 subjects who were antibody positive upon entry (all of them gay or bisexual), 13 percent had developed AIDS. Thirty-six subjects had seroconverted (become antibody positive) over the course of the thirty months; of these men, 8.3 percent had developed AIDS. And among 374 homosexual or bisexual men who remained seronegative throughout the thirty-month period, not a single person developed AIDS. Winkelstein estimated the probability that this association between antibody status and AIDS could have occurred by chance at less than one in a million.

According to the third criterion, a "spectrum of host responses" should follow exposure to the agent "along a logical biological gradient"; Winkelstein explained that this was demonstrated by the gradually declining T-cell counts in the antibody-positive group. Fourth, the disease must follow exposure to the causal agent: this criterion was confirmed by retrospective analysis of frozen sera that had been collected from gay men in San Francisco in 1978 for a hepatitis B vaccine study; analysis of the sera showed that gay men in San Francisco were already infected before cases of the disease were known. And finally, elimination of the agent should decrease the incidence of cases: Winkelstein acknowledged that this criterion had yet to be satisfied, but he predicted that the decline in HIV transmission among gay men would eventually cause a corresponding decrease in the incidence of new AIDS cases.[62]

During a lively question-and-answer period that followed the formal presentations, Anthony Liversidge, the interviewer who had elicited choice comments from Gallo, asked an important question about Winkelstein's data. Might not the same correlation between HIV infection and AIDS illness hold, asked Liversidge, if HIV were simply another opportunistic infection and not the actual cause of AIDS? Winkelstein acknowledged the point but argued that all the other evidence indicating a causal role for HIV made it highly unlikely that the correlation was "merely coincidental."[63]

Opinion about the forum ranged widely in the gay and alternative press, from Ann Fettner's forthright denunciation of Duesberg as "homophobic" to Lauritsen's dismissal of the panel as a "kangaroo court."[64] Interestingly, the AmFAR forum attracted a fair amount of attention in scientific publications but little in the mass media.[65] (Possibly the mainstream reporters had lost interest once the apparent conspiracy of silence had ended, while by this point the larger scientific community was very much concerned about the potential ramifications of the controversy.) The position of reporters for both *Science* and *Nature*, the two most influential general science publications in the world, was that Duesberg had effectively been shown up. William Booth, writing his second article about Duesberg for *Science*, pointed to "vigorous head-shaking and audible groans" as Duesberg made his case. "If the . . . session accomplished anything," said Booth, "it was to confirm Duesberg as odd man out."[66]

Writing in *Nature*, Rebecca Ward noted that the base of Duesberg's "credibility" all along had been "mainly among patient populations with the greatest interest in learning that HIV infection does not lead inevitably to a fatal disease," rather than among his scientific peers. At the forum, "Duesberg's quest for scientific credibility for his unorthodox theories . . . lost ground." Ward concluded with a prediction about the future course of the controversy, again distinguishing between Duesberg's popular credibility and his credibility in scientific circles: "Duesberg's theories will no doubt continue to receive attention from groups already mistrustful of the scientific establishment's response to AIDS. But scientific acceptance for his ideas about AIDS, never very high, seems to be sinking." [67] Little could Ward or Booth have guessed that, more than five years later, Duesberg would not only remain at the center of debate but would have garnered some backing from reputable *scientists* for his stance.

AMASSING CREDIBILITY

Part of Duesberg's capacity to attract credible support hinged on moving the debate more fully into respectable scientific circles. In April he published a brief restatement of his arguments in the British publication *New Scientist* [68] (this was only weeks after the journal's editors, in an editorial called "And Yet It Kills," described Duesberg as "reveling in some peculiar form of intellectual self-indulgence"). [69] But Duesberg's real coup was to force the AIDS establishment to debate him in the august pages of *Science*.

Here Duesberg was aided by Bialy, editor of *Bio/Technology*, who in March had written a letter to Dr. Daniel Koshland, the editor of *Science* and a colleague of Duesberg's at Berkeley: "I am very tired of hearing AIDS establishment scientists tell me they are 'too busy saving lives' to sit down and refute Peter's agruments [sic] (although each one assures me they could 'do it in a minute if they had to'). . . . I urge you to use your offices to get Fauci or Gallo or Levy or Hazeltine [sic], or Essex to prepare a rebuttal of Peter's arguments that is as carefully argued and referenced as his paper in Cancer Research." To simply dismiss Duesberg and hope he will eventually go away, concluded Bialy, "is a disservice and a disgrace to the very principles of scientific inquiry that you helped to teach me some twenty years ago." [70]

Koshland solicited a short statement from Duesberg ("HIV Is Not the Cause of AIDS") and one coauthored by William Blattner (an NCI scientist), Gallo, and Temin ("HIV Causes AIDS") and ran the two statements, along with each party's response to the other, as a "Policy Forum" in the July 29, 1988, issue of *Science*. In their response to Duesberg, Blattner, Gallo, and Temin made what they saw as a crucial distinction between etiology (the cause of a disease) and pathogenesis (the processes by which the disease develops, including the mechanisms by which the etiologic agent causes the disease to be expressed). When he disputed whether HIV directly killed T cells and whether HIV was present in enough cells to cause immune system damage,

Duesberg was raising questions about pathogenesis. But while "there are many unanswered questions about the pathogenesis of AIDS, ... they are not relevant to the conclusions that HIV causes AIDS."[71] Recalling this turn in the debate some years later, Gallo would be adamant: "Never in the history of medicine have you had to solve pathogenesis before you could talk etiologically."[72]

Why, then, were the authors so certain that HIV caused AIDS? In their contribution ("HIV Causes AIDS"), they made their case succinctly—though drawing less on virology, their area of expertise, than on epidemiological arguments: "The strongest evidence that HIV causes AIDS comes from prospective epidemiological studies that document the absolute requirement for HIV infection for the development of AIDS." Serology studies in the United States and around the world had demonstrated that wherever researchers found HIV, they would later find AIDS cases. The authors gave other examples. Over 95 percent of HIV-infected infants developed AIDS by the age of six, while their uninfected siblings never did. HIV, and not any other known infectious agent, was linked to transfusion-associated AIDS. And once HIV began to be screened out of the blood supply, the incidence of transfusion-associated AIDS began to decline, at least among newborns who received transfusions. The authors provided one telling anecdote involving a baby that received a transfusion of HIV-tainted blood from a donor who later developed AIDS. The baby developed AIDS without any other risk factors, while the baby's mother and the baby's twin remained healthy. Blattner, Gallo, and Temin "conclude that there is overwhelming evidence that HIV causes AIDS."[73]

Duesberg, however, was less than impressed by his colleagues' arguments. Epidemiology establishes correlations, Duesberg argued; it never proves causation. He went on to state than in order to establish a plausible causal model, researchers must make some sort of case that the putative cause is indeed *capable* of causing the disease in question. Pathogenesis, therefore, is never entirely dissociable from questions of etiology. In the past, when researchers have made causal claims in the absence of genetic or molecular evidence of activity, the results included, in Duesberg's words, "some of the most spectacular misdiagnoses in virology."[74]

That said, Duesberg proceeded to address the epidemiological evidence presented by his interlocutors. First, he took exception to the claim that AIDS followed "in a predictable sequence" from HIV infection in all populations, noting once again that the incidence of AIDS, expressed as a percentage of the group believed to be seropositive, seemed to vary widely between groups and between countries. Second, it was "presumptuous" to argue that HIV, rather than any other potential cause, was linked to AIDS in blood transfusion cases and in congenitally infected children. In the case of transfusions, how did we know that the recipients had no other risk factors during the years between infection and the development of AIDS? Besides, most of them were hemophiliacs, "persons with health risks . . . that are not representative of healthy individuals." As to the children, "96% had other health risks": their mothers were prostitutes or drug users, or the children had received blood products. So why assume that *HIV* was the culprit? These cases would be more convincing, Duesberg maintained, if the study authors had included a control group of matched antibody-negative persons and shown that they developed none of the AIDS indicator diseases or symptoms.

THE CONSEQUENCES OF CONTROVERSY

What degree and what forms of credibility had Duesberg garnered in 1987 and 1988? On one hand, Duesberg's name and ideas, along with those of other dissenters, continued to surface in a variety of media and contexts. The gay magazine *Christopher Street* (owned, like the *Native,* by Chuck Ortleb) promoted alternative hypotheses of etiology in several more articles in 1988,[75] and Duesberg entered the left-wing press with a positive treatment in the newsweekly *In These Times.*[76] In a segment on AIDS treatments shown on the *MacNeil/Lehrer News Hour,* a San Francisco correspondent interviewed Duesberg, along with adversaries such as Winkelstein and Don Francis of the CDC.[77] Jack Anderson wrote another column, focusing on Duesberg, Joseph Sonnabend, and Michael Callen, describing a "raging debate" over what caused AIDS, which was being enacted "behind the scenes of the AIDS crisis."[78] Duesberg was also featured in a lengthy article in the popular scientific magazine *Discover,* which noted that he "doesn't look like a troublemaker" and that "even the Presidential Commission on AIDS recently listened to his testimony."[79]

Moreover, there were signs throughout 1988 that Duesberg's views resonated with a small but not insignificant popular audience, particularly some gay men in cities throughout the United States. Volunteers at the San Francisco AIDS Foundation information hotline reported a "small but growing number of calls about alternative theories regarding the cause of AIDS." [80] And a number of activists were speaking out about the need to keep an open mind on the question of etiology. Michael Hirsch, founder of an advocacy group for HIV-positive people called Body Positive, was quoted in *Christopher Street*: "Body Positive feels very strongly that all possible theories and treatments should be explored. . . . Putting all our eggs in one basket is dangerous, as in the situation with HIV. AIDS has taught us that we have to assume responsibility for our own health. . . . We need to know about people like Duesberg and [Stephen] Caiazza [a proponent of the syphilis theory of AIDS causation], but the media is not going to tell us about them." [81]

Finally, "AIDS establishment" scientists were increasingly forced, however reluctantly, to acknowledge the existence of controversy. "What is the evidence that HIV-1 is the cause of AIDS? It is late in the history of HIV-1 to bring this point up for review," complained Gallo in an overview of "HIV—The Cause of AIDS" published in 1988 in the *Journal of Acquired Immune Deficiency Syndromes*. "However, in the past year or so, those of us in the United States have seen the HIV-1 cause of AIDS conclusion repetitiously, though not always thoughtfully, attacked by a few colleagues." The acceptance of their views, warned Gallo, "may lead to an irresponsible, carefree spread of the virus and progressive decline in the credibility of scientists, physicians, and health care workers." [82]

But the most authoritative public representations of knowledge about AIDS showed little impact of the so-called "raging debate" beyond, in certain quarters, a perceptible hardening of positions. The 1988 update to the National Academy of Sciences' *Confronting AIDS* is instructive. In 1986, the report had questioned whether the term "AIDS" was still adequate to capture the full spectrum of conditions associated with HIV infection; by 1988, the authors were unequivocal: the actual disease being fought was the disease of HIV infection. "It is now clear that the 'AIDS epidemic' is really an epidemic of HIV infection, and when referring to the epidemic in general, we use the terms interchangeably." [83] In 1986, the NAS authors had reviewed, without much passion, the evidence in support of the HIV hypothesis; but the 1988 update declared in boldface type: "The committee believes that the evidence that HIV causes AIDS is scientifically conclusive." [84] The establishment line was presented without mention of dissent—yet the adamant tone of the presentation in comparison to that of two years earlier suggested that Duesberg's opposition had mobilized scientific experts.

Another marker of authoritative knowledge was the report of the presidential commission, which appeared in 1988. Like the NAS, the commission tended toward a phenomenological merging of "HIV" and "AIDS," declaring in its "Executive Summary" that "the term 'AIDS' is 'obsolete.'" The commission maintained that "'HIV infection' more correctly defines the problem. The medical, public health, political, and community leadership must focus on the full course of HIV infection rather than concentrating on later stages of the disease." [85] Such formulations, of course, left little room for doubt concerning the etiologic role of HIV. The phrase "HIV disease," the codification into language of a hegemonic belief, made it harder even to think the question of whether causality had been proven.

Consolidation and Refinement (1989–1991)

"RED FLAGS" AT THE ACADEMY

Over the course of the next several years, Duesberg remained the most prominent of the "HIV heretics," and he engaged in a persistent struggle to keep his views before the eyes of a professional readership. By June 1988, before *Science*'s "Policy Forum" had even appeared in print, Duesberg had submitted another article, this time to the *Proceedings of the National Academy of Sciences* (*PNAS*). The house organ of the same academy that had published *Confronting AIDS, PNAS* was unlikely to be receptive to Duesberg's views. Yet by virtue of having been inducted into the academy a few years earlier, Duesberg enjoyed a privilege unique in the world of scientific research: NAS members generally could publish in the *Proceedings* without submitting themselves to the rigors of formal, anonymous peer review. Instead, members were asked simply to show each submission to a knowledgeable colleague who could vouch for its worth and validity.

This special treatment was discretionary, however, and in practice *PNAS* suspended the policy in the case of manuscripts that raised the "red flag"—the managing editor's term for "things that have the possibility of ending up on the front page of the *Washington Post*." [86] The ambiguities of this policy had caused headaches for *PNAS* editors before, most notably in 1972, when the renowned scientist and academy member Linus Pauling was prevented from asserting in the journal's pages that vitamin C could cure cancer. As Evelleen Richards has argued in a study of the Pauling controversy, *PNAS*'s gatekeeping practices reveal in particularly stark outline the "social character of the publication process" in science.[87]

Duesberg's article was eventually published by *PNAS* in February 1989,[88] with a second one to follow two years later[89]—yet the behind-the-scenes politicking attracted more attention than the articles themselves. Writing another news report for *Science,* William Booth described the "60 pages of correspondence" generated by "nearly 8 months of protracted, often testy, occasionally humorous negotiations" between Duesberg and Igor Dawid, the chairman of the editorial board. Dawid's predecessor, Maxine Singer, had rejected Duesberg's 1988 submission outright on the grounds that it repeated the arguments in *Cancer Research* and therefore lacked originality. Maintaining that the article had one hundred new references, Duesberg pressed his case, and Dawid, having taken over from Singer, passed the paper along for peer review by three anonymous reviewers, all of whom raised objections to the manuscript. "For the next 6 weeks," said Booth, "by express mail and by fax machine, Duesberg and Dawid duked it out," with Duesberg agreeing to a number of changes and clarifications. Booth suggested that Dawid eventually surrendered to the inevitable; he quoted from Dawid's correspondence: "At this state of protracted discussion I shall not insist here—if you wish to make these unsupported, vague, and prejudicial statements in print, so be it. But I cannot see how this could be convincing to any scientifically trained reader."[90] In truth, what Dawid may have failed to see was that Duesberg could later use the very fact of having been published in the *Proceedings* as capital to advance his position.

Anthony Liversidge, writing a longer piece for *The Scientist,* raised the more nettlesome questions about "just what constitutes fair play in the science publishing arena." On one hand, it seemed problematic to have a special publication policy for academy members that was applied only selectively. On the other hand, what was the point of insisting that the paper be peer reviewed if in the end the journal was going to publish it anyway, despite the fact that all three reviews were unfavorable? Liversidge quoted Walter Gilbert, a professor of molecular biology at Harvard and winner of the 1980 Nobel Prize for his work on DNA sequencing methods, who criticized the *PNAS* editors for giving Duesberg "too much of a rough going." But opponents of Duesberg, such as Gallo—who said he hadn't read the paper because "I have to work for a living"—simply chalked up the incident to the peculiarities of *PNAS*'s policies: "The *Proceedings* is a great journal, but you can't stop a member from publishing unless it is totally off the wall." [91]

ARENAS OF CONTROVERSY

Besides the articles in the *Proceedings*, there were three other important arenas in which the controversy was played out in the period from 1989 to 1991. First, debate about the etiology of AIDS invaded the International Conference on AIDS in San Francisco in 1990: [92] at a specially convened session, Luc Montagnier placed himself in the camp of Shyh-Ching Lo by announcing that he had found a mycoplasma in a significant percentage of AIDS patients (thirty-seven out of ninety-seven). Montagnier proposed that the mycoplasma might be a necessary cofactor that acts in conjunction with HIV to cause AIDS. The antibiotic tetracycline, by killing the mycoplasma, might therefore be of benefit to AIDS patients. [93] In particular, Montagnier thought that a cofactor such as mycoplasma could explain how HIV caused the destruction of the immune system, given that the virus was not found in many cells and given that the virus did not appear to kill cells directly. U.S. scientists were dismissive of Montagnier's new hypothesis. "Dr. Montagnier is out on a limb," said James Curran, director of the AIDS program at the CDC. Some scientists expressed the view that Montagnier was squandering his credibility; in the words of the *New York Times*, they "[wondered] aloud why Dr. Montagnier would risk his professional standing by backing such a theory without more evidence." [94]

Later, HIV dissenters would reap support by pointing to the way the "orthodox" had silenced one of their own when he dared to step out of line. Duesberg would indirectly benefit from Montagnier's intervention, effectively riding on the coattails of the French scientist in the mainstream media. At the 1990 conference, however, this San Francisco Bay Area resident was far from the action. At a hotel two blocks away from the official conference, Duesberg addressed a symposium on alternative treatments for AIDS. A dismissive report by a Reuters correspondent described the mix of alternative treatments proposed by the panelists as "a witch's cauldron of boiling blood, mushrooms and mistletoe," and associated Duesberg with this imagery by noting that "his contentious theory . . . has brought charges of 'quackery' against him." [95]

Duesberg fared better in a different arena, a British television documentary called "The AIDS Catch," produced by Joan Shenton and Meditel Productions, who had already featured Duesberg once, in 1988.[96] Shown on British television in June, just before the International Conference, the program ignited a firestorm in Britain by presenting the world of AIDS as seen through the eyes of the HIV dissenters. As the narrator declared: "Everything we currently accept about AIDS can be turned on its head." The narrator presented a range of questionable statistics, noting that in any one year in the United States, only a tiny fraction (1.5 percent) of HIV positives develop AIDS, but not indicating how many HIV positives develop AIDS over longer periods of time. In an argument against AZT, the show also claimed that "so far no one has lived longer than three years" on the drug, without explaining that AZT had not been in general use for much longer than that and that only the sickest patients had initially been prescribed it.

"The AIDS Catch" assembled in one place nearly all of the key dissenters. Duesberg was featured prominently on the show, along with Sonnabend and Callen. Lauritsen presented his observations on gay male culture, telling the interviewer: "They might take six different drugs in the course of an evening." British writer Jad Adams, whose pro-Duesberg book, *AIDS: The HIV Myth,* was published the previous year,[97] proposed psychological reasons for why "people *want* to believe in HIV." Gordon Stewart, an epidemiologist from Glasgow who supported the immune overload hypothesis, discussed poppers, which he described as "very toxic indeed." The program also featured Walter Gilbert, the Nobel Prize–winning Harvard molecular biologist who had criticized *PNAS* in the interview with Liversidge. Gilbert was persuaded by the substance of many of Duesberg's arguments, but he made his most forceful point with reference to what he called "democratic theory," arguing that scientific progress comes about through the clash of opposing ideas: "The great lesson of history is that knowledge develops through the conflict of viewpoints, that if you have simply a consensus view, it generally stultifies, it fails to see the problems of that consensus; and it depends on the existence of critics to break up that iceberg and to permit knowledge to develop. This is, in fact, one of the underpinnings of democratic theory; it's one of the basic reasons that we believe in notions of free speech; and it's one of the great forces in terms of intellectual development."[98]

THE HERITAGE FOUNDATION
AND THE "RISK-AIDS HYPOTHESIS"

The third crucial arena for dissenting views during this time period was a lengthy (8,900-word) cover story by Duesberg and Bryan J. Ellison published in the summer 1990 issue of *Policy Review*, a publication of the Heritage Foundation, the well-known, right-wing think tank.[99] The essay was actually written by Ellison, a politically conservative graduate student in Duesberg's department and self-appointed popularizer of Duesberg's views. "Scientists weren't going to listen to him. They couldn't afford to," Ellison explained. "So I realized he had to take his case to the general public."[100] The article became, in the editor's words, "one of the three or four most-talked-about articles in the history of the magazine, . . . [eliciting] more letters to the editor than any in *Policy Review*'s history."[101] The article also incorporated the first formal presentation by Duesberg of an alternative explanation for the etiology of AIDS, which Duesberg and Ellison dubbed the "risk-AIDS hypothesis."

The biographical note explained that Duesberg had published critiques of the accepted "virus-AIDS hypothesis" in a number of scientific journals, such as *Cancer Research* and the *Proceedings of the National Academy of Sciences*. In this way, Duesberg's accumulated scientific credibility was now converted into credibility in a different, more public forum. However, a chief strategy of the *Policy Review* article was to present the critique not as Duesberg's personal crusade, but as the clamor of a growing chorus, within which Duesberg was just one voice. The article therefore attributed dissenting views whenever possible to people like Walter Gilbert and Harvey Bialy. More generally, it described "an increasing number of medical scientists and physicians [who] have been questioning whether HIV actually does cause AIDS"; the article linked together those who said HIV could not play a role, those who said HIV had not conclusively been proven to play a role, and those who argued for cofactors. The reader might never have heard of this expanding group, the authors explained, because "most of these doubters prefer not to be quoted, out of fear of losing research funding or of disapproval by peers." Skepticism therefore remained a minority position "due largely to inadequate attention provided by media sources."[102]

In the article, Duesberg and Ellison reiterated their standard arguments but also presented in expanded form a criticism that Duesberg had not previously discussed in print in great detail: they argued that the notion that HIV caused AIDS was based fundamentally on a tautology. According to the CDC's 1987 update of its surveillance definition, AIDS was (usually) diagnosed by a positive HIV antibody test, in the presence of one or more diseases from a list: "The disease-list includes not only Kaposi's sarcoma and *P. carinii* pneumonia, but also tuberculosis, cytomegalovirus, herpes, diarrhea, candidiasis, lymphoma, dementia, and many other diseases. If any of these very different diseases is found alone, it is likely to be diagnosed under its classical name. If the same condition is found alongside antibodies against HIV, it is called AIDS. The correlation between AIDS and HIV is thus an artifact of the definition itself." [103] Perfectly ordinary illnesses got stuck with the label "AIDS" if the ill person happened to be HIV positive; then researchers would turn around and say that, since everyone with AIDS was HIV positive, HIV must be the cause. This was an interesting argument, one which threw into question not only the logic of the causal claim but also the very status of "AIDS" as a legitimate disease category. It was an argument that Duesberg would often repeat in subsequent years; but it was somewhat disingenuous as posed.

Although the CDC's 1987 definition listed a number of diseases that, in an HIV-infected person, would result in an AIDS diagnosis,[104] many of them—like *Pneumocystis carinii* pneumonia, toxoplasmosis, and cryptosporidiosis, diseases typical of AIDS patients—were relatively rare in general. Others, like CMV, herpes, and candidiasis, were indeed common, but in these cases the CDC's specifications went further, requiring that the conditions be present in parts of the body where these infections normally did not take root. Similarly, tuberculosis was on the list—but only if it involved at least one site *other than* the lungs. Diarrhea, of course, was not on the list; Duesberg and Ellison were referring casually to what the CDC called the "HIV wasting syndrome," defined as "profound involuntary weight loss >10% of baseline body weight plus either chronic diarrhea (at least two loose stools per day for >30 days) or chronic weakness and documented fever (for >30 days, intermittent or constant) in the absence of a concurrent illness or condition other than HIV infection that could explain the findings. . . ." [105] The diagnostic definition of AIDS-related dementia was similarly restrictive. Overall, clinical markers of AIDS were rare diseases and conditions generally not seen in people who were *not* HIV positive. By failing to explain these details of the CDC's diagnostic algorithm and by suggesting that ordinary diarrhea and tuberculosis were being taken as markers of AIDS, Duesberg and Ellison were misleading their lay audience.

But at the same time, Duesberg and Ellison presented arguments to counter the assumption that the rare AIDS diseases, like Kaposi's sarcoma and PCP, were in fact so rare. They maintained that "not only have all 25 of these AIDS conditions existed for decades at a low level in the population, but HIV-free instances of the same diseases are still being diagnosed."[106] They also described a recent letter to *Lancet* by Robert Root-Bernstein, an associate professor of physiology at Michigan State University and recipient of a MacArthur fellowship—one of the so-called "genius grants" provided, no-strings-attached, to individuals in a variety of fields who have been deemed unusually promising. Root-Bernstein's review of the medical literature had led him to conclude that perhaps 15 to 20 percent of all Kaposi's sarcoma cases before 1979 fit the pattern generally believed to have arisen only with the AIDS epidemic: young victims with a short survival time. Citing Sonnabend, Root-Bernstein had written: "Several hypotheses must be entertained—that AIDS is not new; that HIV is only one of several possible causes of AIDS; or that HIV is itself a new, opportunistic infection that takes advantage of previously immunosuppressed individuals."[107]

The existence of "AIDS" diseases in people who are not antibody positive, in Duesberg and Ellison's view, was evidence for their alternative hypothesis, the risk-AIDS hypothesis. They proposed "that the AIDS diseases are entirely separate conditions caused by a variety of factors, most of which have in common only that they involve risk behavior." But like Sonnabend and others who had trod this path before them, the authors recognized that "a risk hypothesis must explain the recent increases in the various AIDS diseases, and why these have all been concentrated in particular risk groups." So Duesberg and Ellison put forward a potpourri of potential causes of the AIDS marker illnesses, linking Kaposi's sarcoma with popper use by gay men; AIDS dementia with psychoactive drugs and syphilis; and the wasting syndrome, "found most heavily in African AIDS patients," with "the extremes of malnutrition and the lack of sanitation on most of that continent," compounded in recent years by "wars and totalitarian regimes."[108]

Many of these arguments were widely familiar from debates early in the epidemic: the claims about African health conditions, for example, mirror Sonnabend's speculations about Haitians in 1983. And indeed, to explain the systemic failure of immune response that is characteristic of AIDS, Duesberg and Ellison's article explicitly endorsed the immune overload hypothesis,[109] incorporating it within their risk-AIDS hypothesis: "Joseph Sonnabend, a New York physician who founded the journal *AIDS Research* in 1983, has pointed out that repeated, constant infections may eventually overload the immune system, causing its failure; still worse are simultaneous infections by two or more diseases."[110] Duesberg and Ellison also pointed to heavy drug use as a major cause of immunosuppression. They claimed that abuse of alcohol, heroin, cocaine, marijuana, Valium, and amphetamines "can all be found as part of the life histories of many AIDS patients"; "when combined with regular and prolonged malnutrition, as is done with many active homosexuals[111] and with heroin addicts, this can lead to complete immune collapse." To round out the picture, the authors noted the long-term immunosuppressive effects of antibiotics and claim that "active homosexuals . . . often [take] large amounts of tetracycline and other antibiotics each evening before entering the bath houses."[112]

Duesberg and Ellison didn't provide any sources for their ethnographic data, and in interviews both of them acknowledged having little direct knowledge of gay life despite its vibrant expression in San Francisco, only miles from the Berkeley campus. In part the authors were drawing on early medical claims about "how the gay lifestyle" was related to the epidemic of immune suppression, which in turn borrowed from earlier and contemporary medical literature on gay men who attended clinics for treatment of sexually transmitted diseases (see chapter 1). Communication with John Lauritsen may also have played its part in shaping their biased understandings of gay male behavior. In a letter to Duesberg written just a few months earlier, Lauritsen had characterized the Mineshaft, the Saint, and St. Mark's Baths—the most prominent New York City venues for uninhibited gay male sex in the years before the epidemic—as "hell-holes which were the arenas for truly psychopathic drug abuse as obligatory tribal ritual."[113]

Gay men and injection drug users had always been the focus of immune overload theories. But no one promoting such a perspective in 1990 could avoid discussion of the other "risk groups," and Duesberg and Ellison understood this. They explained (again echoing Sonnabend's claims from seven years earlier) that blood transfusion recipients were at risk of developing immunodeficiency because of pathogens present in transfused blood. Moreover, people receiving blood transfusions typically did so because they were already quite ill or had undergone surgery, and both the trauma of the surgical procedure and the anesthesia could have immunosuppressive effects. In fact, Duesberg and Ellison claimed, "with or without HIV infection, half of all [transfusion] recipients do not survive their first year after transfusion." Similarly they noted that "hemophilia has always been a fatal condition," and that the blood products received by its sufferers were immunosuppressive. Finally, cases of AIDS in infants could be traced to "combinations of most of the above risk factors"; 95 percent of these babies were born to mothers who either used drugs or were sex partners of drug users, or had received transfusions, or had hemophilia. According to Duesberg and Ellison: "The risk behavior of many of their mothers has reached these victims, but their conditions are renamed AIDS when in the presence of antibodies against HIV." [114]

In the conclusion to the article, Duesberg and Ellison turned to the policy implications of their argument. "The most urgent of these," they said, concerned the widespread administration of AZT. This powerful drug worked by inhibiting the replication of the virus, but "by doing this the drug also kills all actively growing cells in the patient," including immune system cells. If the virus was harmless, as the authors maintained, then "inhibiting HIV would accomplish nothing, while AZT actually produces the very immune suppression it is supposed to prevent." AZT, by this view, was just another harmful drug—like heroin, cocaine, and poppers—that contributed to immune overload. Second, the risk-AIDS hypothesis called into question the existing AIDS education strategies. Condoms and sterile needles were fine if the goal was to prevent hepatitis and other infectious diseases. But the hazard of these programs, Duesberg and Ellison maintained, was that they lulled the practitioners of risk behaviors into a false sense of security. By failing to "[emphasize] the danger of the risk behavior itself—particularly drug-taking—[these programs] may inadvertently encourage spread of the disease." [115]

The HIV hypothesis "has not yet saved a single life, despite federal spending of $3 billion per year," Duesberg and Ellison reminded their readers in closing.[116] Instead of sinking more money down the same hole, the government should begin funding "studies on the causes of the separate AIDS-diseases and their appropriate therapies." The rest of the $3 billion "might then be saved and returned to the taxpayers," wrote the authors in a suggestion that presumably did not clash with the conservative agenda of Policy Review.

The next issue of the magazine was devoted to letters in response to Duesberg and Ellison—the total length of the letter section was over 13,000 words, one and a half times the length of the original article. Both the establishment and the dissenters were well represented. Howard Temin stressed the "tragic" pediatric evidence: in one study, fifteen of sixteen HIV-infected children of infected mothers had AIDS or pre-AIDS symptoms, while none of thirty-nine uninfected children of infected mothers showed signs of illness. Wrote Temin: "Duesberg and Ellison state that 'the risk behavior of many of their mothers has reached these victims.' It is clear that what reached the children was HIV."[117] Warren Winkelstein, the Berkeley epidemiologist, wrote in with the most recent results from the ongoing San Francisco Men's Health Study. Out of 386 homosexual men who had been HIV positive when entering the study six years before, 140 (36 percent) had developed AIDS, and the majority of them had died. Forty homosexual men had become infected since entering the study, and 2 (5 percent) had developed AIDS. But of 370 homosexual men who had remained uninfected, none developed AIDS.[118]

An interesting letter came from Michael Fumento, who had written a popular book called *The Myth of Heterosexual AIDS*. Each of them a controversial figure, Duesberg and Fumento shared the belief that AIDS was a "risk group disease" and not a threat to the general population. But they were on opposite sides when it came to the etiological debate. Noting that his "initial reaction to anyone challenging the AIDS industry in any way is favorable," Fumento continued: "but in the case of Peter Duesberg and his co-author Bryan Ellison, I really must demur." After raising objections to Duesberg and Ellison's arguments, Fumento threw down the gauntlet: "What I would suggest, in perfect seriousness, is that before the authors write another article suggesting that it is perfectly okay for HIV-infected persons to have unprotected sex with uninfected persons or vice-versa, that they, in a public forum, inject themselves with HIV. Apparently Duesberg has hinted he may do it; I think he should go beyond that. Readers have a right to know just how much faith the authors have in their own theory."[119]

Duesberg and Ellison were given the last word, and they had plenty to say.[120] They began by expressing their pleasure that "the debate that should have occurred . . . years ago" was finally taking place. They then launched into a critique of the cohort studies that Winkelstein and other letter writers had cited as definitive. The existing studies proved nothing, in Duesberg and Ellison's view, because they failed to demonstrate that illness was the consequence of HIV, not risk behavior. A controlled study actually designed to distinguish between the two causal hypotheses would be set up quite differently. It would compare two large groups of people, HIV positives and HIV negatives. But the two groups would be carefully matched for "every health risk that might possibly be involved in the various AIDS diseases."

Duesberg and Ellison also responded to various arguments that letter writers had raised—about babies with AIDS, about wives of hemophiliacs, about needle-stick injuries. Only "media sensationalism," they argued, could convince people that wives of hemophiliacs were at great risk of AIDS if they had no other risk factors. Those cases that had occurred were quite explainable: "Since AIDS is merely, by definition, a list of old diseases that are renamed when in the presence of antibodies against HIV, one should not be surprised to find an occasional such wife who happens to contract HIV and, coincidentally, one of the many diseases on the AIDS list." A controlled study, they believed, would show that HIV-positive wives developed AIDS indicator diseases at the same rate as HIV-negative wives.

The real problem, in Duesberg and Ellison's view, was that the established AIDS researchers abandoned scientific principles when it suited their interests. Instead of controlled studies, these researchers invoked anecdotal evidence. When Koch's postulates failed them, they "casually try to abandon those timetested, commonsensical" rules of scientific method. And "when all else fails," they started "changing the rules," "rather than bringing the hypothesis into question," as real scientists were supposed to do. To explain why so few antibody-positive people had AIDS, "a latent period first had to be invented, then extended to its present, and still growing, total of 10 to 11 years." Duesberg and Ellison concluded by declaring themselves "quite willing to carry out the Fumento test." But their degree of interest in doing so depended on the attention it could attract to their cause: "If he will arrange for sufficient national publicity, if he would be convinced by our action, and if he will thereafter help us bring exposure to our viewpoint, we will indeed be quite happy to have ourselves publicly injected with HIV. Perhaps Fumento will also be willing to check on our health status in the year 2000, or after whatever additional time is eventually added to the virus' latent period."[121]

"THE IMPACT OF THE TRUCK"

The International AIDS Conferences, the documentary "The AIDS Catch," and the *Policy Review* article and ensuing debate were three arenas in which the causation controversy bubbled into clear public view in 1989, 1990, and 1991. Elsewhere, the controversy was not invisible, but it simmered more quietly. In scientific communities and gay communities, in the mainstream press and the alternative press, various players pushed their claims, seeking to establish their credibility or undercut that of others. In the process, dissenters who had been predicted to fade into oblivion instead demonstrated their staying power. This quiet jockeying for position would set the stage for a fierce resurgence of the causation controversy in 1992.

Formal scientific debate continued throughout this period. One exchange that was followed closely by insiders took place in the *Journal of Acquired Immune Deficiency Syndromes* between Duesberg and Alfred Evans of the Department of Epidemiology and Public Health of the Yale University School of Medicine.[122] Evans was an authority on Koch's postulates and had been writing about them since the 1970s; he emphasized that "the postulates of causation have changed and will continue to change with the new technology and new concepts of pathogenesis." Revealing his historical bent, Evans also noted that Duesberg's offer to be injected with HIV was reminiscent of a similar act by German researcher Max von Pettenkofer. In 1892 at the age of seventy-four, von Pettenkofer drank a milliliter of "a fresh culture of cholera vibrio derived from a fatal case" to attempt to prove his point that cofactors were required to cause the disease. Von Pettenkofer was lucky: he didn't develop serious cholera, although he did have gas and diarrhea for a week afterwards. Evans urged Duesberg not to follow in von Pettenkofer's footsteps.[123]

Duesberg also published articles and letters in *Science, Nature, The Scientist,* the *New England Journal of Medicine,* and the Pasteur Institute's *Research in Immunology,* among other places. In these publications Duesberg tended to restate his earlier views while responding to critics. Increasingly, he invoked other dissenters as allies in his writings, citing work by scientist and nonscientist alike—Jad Adams, Celia Farber, John Lauritsen, Harry Rubin, Joseph Sonnabend, Katie Leishman, Anthony Liversidge, and Gordon Stewart.[124] Robert Root-Bernstein, the young physiologist whose letter to *Lancet* had attracted Duesberg's notice, also kept busy. He expanded on his position in a

1990 article in a journal called *Perspectives in Biology and Medicine*. Although careful to maintain an official position of agnosticism, Root-Bernstein stressed the prevalence of risk factors among people with AIDS—chronic or repeated infectious diseases, drug use, anesthetics, antibiotics, semen exposure, blood exposure, and malnutrition.[125]

For the average layperson not inclined to peruse the pages of the medical and scientific journals, the easiest place to learn about the HIV dissidents during this time period was, ironically enough, the pages of Robert Gallo's *Virus Hunting,* a book for the general reader published in 1991.[126] Though in the past Gallo had declared himself "too busy" even to bother reading Duesberg's articles, this book included an entire chapter entitled "About Causes of Disease (and, in Particular, Why HIV Is the Cause of AIDS)"—a chapter that, amid discussion of Montagnier's mycoplasmas and Root-Bernstein's risk arguments, devoted a full ten pages to refuting Peter Duesberg.

"When are we ready to say that we know the cause of a disease?" asked Gallo, taking aim at the crux of the controversy. "To a greater extent than we might want to believe, there are few hard-and-fast rules [and] certainly no cookbook recipe to follow," he added, noting that Robert Koch "has been taken too literally and too seriously for too long." But most diseases did have a *sine qua non,* though other factors might contribute to the severity, speed of onset, or likelihood of development. Gallo offered the analogy of head injury in the case of a truck that crashes into a group of bicyclists, some of whom are wearing helmets, some of whom hit concrete, and some of whom are clad in red shirts: "We could argue that the cause of the head injury was concrete, the red shirts, the absence of a helmet, or the truck—but we don't. The impact of the truck is the *sine qua non,* the cause. The others are influential positive or negative factors or correlations with no influence at all, as in the case of the red shirts."[127] "Of course there are diseases where there is true multifactorial [causation]," Gallo later commented, reflecting on the etiology of some types of cancer. But "HIV causes AIDS, nothing else: you take it away, [AIDS] goes away."[128]

Gallo's book did not dispute the possibility of contributing causes—indeed, over the past few years, he had been proposing that a virus called HHV-6 (human herpes virus, number six) might speed up the process by which HIV destroyed T cells. But HIV could also do its work without HHV-6, while HHV-6 alone did not cause AIDS. HIV, in other words, was both a *necessary* and *sufficient* cause. Montagnier, by contrast, was now proposing that a mycoplasma might be a second *necessary* cause along with HIV—a claim that Gallo found "astonishing." Montagnier's cofactor theory provided "added longevity to confused and confusing . . . arguments that HIV is not the primary cause of AIDS," Gallo complained. What particularly irked him was that Montagnier had thereby "lent *some* support to Duesberg (who, interestingly enough, dismissed Montagnier's idea)." [129]

Gallo could hardly deny that Montagnier had impressive credentials for commenting on questions of medical science. But he was quick to observe that "the vast majority of people who have raised, re-raised, and re-re-raised objections to the conclusion of an HIV cause of AIDS"—here Gallo names Jad Adams, Katie Leishman, Anthony Liversidge, and Chuck Ortleb—"seem to have little or even no experience in science or medicine." What of Duesberg? Gallo acknowledged his colleague's indisputable scientific accomplishments, but stressed that they might not have prepared him to comment credibly on AIDS: "He made very significant contributions to our understanding of the molecular biology of animal (especially chicken) retroviruses many years ago and is a member of the National Academy of Sciences. On the other hand, he is not an epidemiologist, a physician, or a public health official. More important, to my knowledge Duesberg has never worked on any naturally occurring disease of animals or on any disease of humans, including AIDS. Nor, I believe, has he ever worked with HIV." [130]

During the 1989–1991 period, Duesberg also continued to receive publicity in the mass media, including a long and generally sympathetic feature article by Garry Abrams in the *Los Angeles Times* that asked whether the scientist was "Hero or Heretic." [131] Abrams noted that Duesberg was shocked to learn in fall 1990 that the NIH had declined to renew his five hundred thousand–dollar-a-year Outstanding Investigator Grant. While renewal of such grants is far from automatic, the review committee had written that Duesberg had become "less productive, perhaps reflecting a dilution of his efforts with nonscientific issues." This was a serious blow to Duesberg, and Abrams implied that it was direct punishment for heresy, with the phrase "nonscientific issues" serving as a euphemism for Duesberg's campaign against the orthodox position on AIDS.

One symptom of the thickening of debate was that the media began covering the media coverage. *USA Today* ran an article on *Spin* magazine, "the only general interest publication pushing [Duesberg's] theory."[132] Charles Trueheart reported on the *Policy Review* debate for the *Washington Post,* suggesting that the authors' emphasis on the role of personal behavior in the cause of AIDS "may explain why their article appears in this conservative journal."[133] *Lies of Our Times,* an alternative magazine dedicated to policing the writings of the *New York Times,* complained that the newspaper had never mentioned Duesberg since Philip Boffey's original article in 1988, and it claimed that "the silence of the *Times* kept Duesberg out of the major media for three years."[134]

Duesberg also was promoted in places like the *New York Native* by authors like Lauritsen.[135] Elsewhere in the gay press, the causation controversy was a marginal issue but one that provoked periodic heated exchanges. Writing in the *Bay Area Reporter,* a San Francisco gay newspaper, columnist and AIDS activist Michael Botkin described the "peculiar revival of interest" in Duesberg's theories.[136] Duesberg "continues to be shunned by virtually all serious AIDS activists," wrote Botkin, "but has sparked some interest from heterosexual, HIV-negative, radical-posing journalists." But while some commentators worried about the consequences of knee-jerk anti-expertism, others expressed the opposite concern—that gays were inexplicably naïve and were following the medical establishment like placid sheep. In a discussion of Duesberg's arguments and Montagnier's "startling admission," Ralph Garrett wrote to the *San Diego Gay Times:* "In the face of such a scandal, among the questions we in the gay community should be asking ourselves is how could we have credulously surrendered our lives and deferred our better judgement to an authority which has proved to be just as corruptible as any other? . . . What madness could have come over us?"[137]

FROM OUTSIDE TO INSIDE AND BACK AGAIN

Conventional views of science presume a top-down model of knowledge dissemination. True ideas originate within a select community of educated specialists; from there, they percolate "downward"; eventually, in watered-down or distorted form, they penetrate the consciousness of the masses. But as Stephen Hilgartner has argued, this model fails to capture the ways in which "popularized knowledge feeds back into the research process."[138] Duesberg's views on AIDS are an interesting example. Early in the epidemic, ideas about "immune overload" diffused from researchers to doctors and patients and were taken up by lay theorists such as Callen and Lauritsen. Many of these same ideas then reemerged in the scientific articles of Duesberg, who cited the lay publications in his footnotes and thanked their authors in his acknowledgments.[139] As Hilgartner noted, "when one looks carefully for the *precise location* of the boundary between genuine scientific knowledge and popularized representations, one runs into trouble. . . ."[140]

There is still another sense in which the pursuit of scientific credibility by Duesberg reveals the considerable permeability of boundaries between the "inside" and the "outside" of science in the case of AIDS. On one hand, Duesberg's success in promoting his views depended heavily on his status as an "insider." As of 1986, dissenting voices on the causation of AIDS were marginalized, and they might have remained so had someone with the scientific credibility of Peter Duesberg not entered the debate. On the other hand, Duesberg's capacity to sustain his critique then depended heavily on support from "outside." His article in *Cancer Research* might have gathered dust on library shelves, if not for the active promotion of his views by a group of lay supporters who succeeded in pushing the controversy into the mass media. This publicity led to Duesberg's presentation of his arguments in official forums, such as the AmFAR conference, *Science,* and *PNAS.* By extending his credibility from one arena to another—using his scientific credentials to buy him popular support, then using the popular support to push for recognition by his colleagues—Duesberg gained staying power. The next chapter describes how Duesberg sought to continue his battle and how the "AIDS establishment" responded.

CHAPTER 4

THE DEBATE THAT
WOULDN'T DIE

The Controversy Reignites (1991–1992)

FROM ISOLATION TO ORGANIZATION

In mid-1991, the struggle by Duesberg and other HIV dissenters to create credibility for their claims in both popular and professional arenas was given a significant boost by the founding of an organization. The impetus came from a molecular biologist named Charles Thomas Jr., a former Harvard professor and current director of a small biotechnology research institute in San Diego. Thomas later commented that he believed "it was a matter of civic duty" to get involved, saying, "I've worked on viruses and I can read and understand this literature. . . . I felt real fabrications were taking place." [1]

The group took form in a flurry of faxes between Thomas, Duesberg, Robert Root-Bernstein, Berkeley law professor Philip Johnson, and an actuary from Kansas City named Robert Maver. Thomas originally dubbed the organization "Friends of HIV," and, in a "Dear Colleague" form letter mailed to potential supporters, he asked them how they liked the title. [2] In the end, sobriety prevailed over facetiousness and the organization became the "Group for the Scientific Reappraisal of the HIV/AIDS Hypothesis." The group submitted a statement to both *Science* and *Nature* in June 1991 and asked that it be published as a letter to the editor. The full statement read: "It is widely believed by the general public that a retrovirus called HIV causes the group of diseases called AIDS. Many biomedical scientists now question this hypothesis. We propose that a thorough reappraisal of the existing evidence for and against this hypothesis be conducted by a suitable independent group. We further propose that critical epidemiological studies be devised and undertaken."[3]

The letter was notably restrained in tone and in content. By calling simply for reappraisal and by not advocating an alternative hypothesis or making any of the more controversial claims that had been advanced earlier by Duesberg and other dissenters, the letter was well suited to attract support. It went to *Nature* and *Science* with twenty-eight signatures, and by the following year Thomas had gathered a total of fifty-three. The signatories were mostly from the United States, but there were a few from Switzerland, Italy, Britain, Germany, and Australia. The list included familiar names, like Harvey Bialy, Gordon Stewart, and John Lauritsen. But others were new to the public controversy, and many of them came with respectable credentials. Of the fifty-three who had signed by June 1992, twelve had M.D.'s and twenty-five had Ph.D.'s. Twenty of the fifty-three gave academic affiliations with departments like physiology, biochemistry, medicine, pharmacology, toxicology, and physics.

Yet remarkably enough, the letter never saw publication, having been rejected not only by *Nature* and *Science,* but by *Lancet* and the *New England Journal of Medicine* as well.[4] While this gatekeeping may have kept a minority view out of the prestigious scientific and medical publications, it also guaranteed favorable publicity for the group in the mainstream media. One journalist with the San Diego County edition of the *Los Angeles Times* interviewed Thomas and wrote a story focusing on the suppression of dissent and the plague of "political correctness" in biomedicine.[5] The *Chronicle of Higher Education* also profiled the group in December 1991, in an article that described Duesberg's fight to recover his Outstanding Investigator Grant and noted that Duesberg's representative in Congress, Ron Dellums, had looked into the NIH's handling of the grant application.[6]

Meanwhile, backing for Duesberg arrived from an unlikely quarter. "Professor Peter Duesberg . . . is probably sleeping more easily at night," suggested John Maddox, the editor of *Nature,* in a September 1991 piece in the "News and Views" section called "AIDS Research Turned Upside Down." Maddox summarized two recent and perplexing studies that suggested the presence of autoimmune mechanisms in the development of AIDS. "None of this would imply that HIV is irrelevant to AIDS," Maddox concluded, "but that an immune response to foreign cells, most probably lymphocytes, is also necessary. Duesberg will be saying, 'I told you so.'" In the past, "Duesberg has been pilloried for his heterodox views . . . and faced with the threat that his research funds would be snatched away," wrote Maddox. "Now there [is] some evidence to support his long fight against the establishment (among which, sadly, he counts this journal)." [7]

"Pilloried Professor May Be Right about Aids," proclaimed London's *Daily Telegraph*. [8] "New Study Vindicates Duesberg, Calls AIDS an Autoimmune Disease" read an article in the *Bay Area Reporter*. [9] Others were more cautious in their conclusions. A reporter for *Science,* in an article called "Duesberg Vindicated? Not Yet," cited "numerous . . . researchers [who] failed to see any connection between [the two studies] and the stand taken by Duesberg." One of the researchers whose article had provoked the fuss told *Science:* "We have nothing in common with [Duesberg's] idea that HIV has nothing to do with AIDS." No fan of the autoimmune hypothesis himself, Duesberg agreed, saying "Those studies have nothing to do with [my position]." [10]

Joseph Palca, the reporter for *Science,* focused on Maddox's motives for endorsing Duesberg, given that Duesberg occupied such an extreme position in the debate. Maddox explained to Palca: "I'm not for a minute saying Duesberg is right in all points. But I feel sorry that *Nature* has not done more to give his view prominence. It would have hastened the process by which the scientific community is coming around to the view that the pathogenesis of AIDS is more complicated than the baby-talk stories we were all given a few years ago." [11] This was the real issue, Joseph Sonnabend commented in a column in the gay and lesbian magazine *NYQ*—the "vast gulf between the simplistic view of the pathogenesis of AIDS that has been presented by those who lead the AIDS research establishment . . . and the painful reality that we have almost no understanding of the pathogenesis of this disease." The "baby-talk story"—that HIV causes AIDS in all infected people by directly killing T cells and that the only cofactor is the passage of time—"was not arrived at as the result of years of intense and painstaking research," Sonnabend complained, "but was almost instantly discovered in 1984, and presented not as speculation but as established fact." [12]

THE "DRUG-AIDS HYPOTHESIS"

As the implications of Maddox's intervention were sorted out in various arenas, Duesberg scored another partial victory:

the publication in a professional journal of a formal statement of his own hypothesis as to the causes of AIDS. The article was published in *Biomedicine & Pharmacotherapy* after a yearlong, ultimately unsuccessful, campaign by Duesberg to publish once again in the far more prestigious *Proceedings of the National Academy of Sciences*. The *Proceedings* had published Duesberg's views on AIDS twice before but each time had sent the submissions out for peer review, breaking with its ordinarily relaxed procedures for academy members. Both times the reviews had been critical; both times editor Igor Dawid ultimately had relented. This time Dawid put his foot down, writing Duesberg in February 1991 that the article had been rejected. One referee had called the paper a "flight of ideas" and "grossly incomplete," while the second referee favored publication. The third referee acknowledged, "I am no expert in the fields concerned" and made a political argument: "In all likelihood the publication of this article in PNAS would be harmful to the reputation of the journal, and has a potential for being harmful to the HIV infected segment of the population." [13]

What was all the fuss about? In "The Role of Drugs in the Origin of AIDS," Duesberg presented what could be considered the fourth version in a sequence of publicly expressed views about the etiology of AIDS. Back in 1987, Duesberg had started out saying he didn't know what caused AIDS; all he was certain of was that it wasn't HIV. "The charge was then leveled that I was destructive, I was only negative, I was not contributing anything," Duesberg later recalled.[14] But very soon afterward, he began making statements consistent with the immune overload hypothesis. In 1990 his student Bryan Ellison's *Policy Review* article had expanded this hypothesis (as reworked by Root-Bernstein) and extended it to the other risk groups, formalizing it as the risk-AIDS hypothesis. But in the very course of discussions with Ellison as the article was being written, Duesberg had become increasingly uncomfortable with the generalized focus on any and all forms of risk behavior.[15]

In place of the risk-AIDS hypothesis, Duesberg began to formulate a more parsimonious explanation, the "drug-AIDS hypothesis," which emphasized toxicological causes of AIDS. In a move that signaled his disagreement with some of the other HIV dissidents, such as Sonnabend and Callen, Duesberg dismissed the significance of repeated infections. AIDS was not caused by an infectious agent—not HIV, not CMV, not Epstein-Barr virus, not any combination of the above. Drug consumption—not promiscuous sex—was the lifestyle practice associated with AIDS, Duesberg increasingly became convinced. Leaving aside the hemophilia and transfusion cases, which had their own explanations, nearly every case of AIDS in the United States and Europe could be attributed to drug abuse.

In his 1992 article in *Biomedicine & Pharmacotherapy,* Duesberg presented his case in more formal terms. The article included 132 references, mostly to scientific publications but also to popular works by Jad Adams and John Lauritsen. Ever since the turn of the century, Duesberg wrote, "evidence has accumulated that addiction to psychoactive drugs leads to immune suppression and clinical abnormalities similar to AIDS, including lymphopenia, lymphadenopathy, fever, weight loss, septicemia, and increased susceptibility to infections and neurological disorders." These clinical abnormalities became epidemic in the early 1980s as a result of "a massive escalation in the consumption of psychoactive drugs," Duesberg explained, with reference to Justice Department statistics. "Thus the American AIDS epidemic is a subset of the AIDS epidemic." Indeed, only half of the drug-induced immunodeficiency cases receive public notice, due to the hegemony of the HIV hypothesis: "Only the pneumonias, tuberculoses, and dementias of the 50% of American intravenous drug users with HIV are recorded as AIDS, while those of their HIV-negative counterparts are diagnosed by their old names." [16]

How would Duesberg prove a claim that AIDS is caused by drugs? Koch's postulates were not relevant in this case, since they applied only to infectious agents. Duesberg was arguing that the relation between drugs and AIDS was analogous to that between smoking and lung cancer: prolonged and repeated exposure to the toxic substance or substances eventually resulted in disease in some percentage of cases. The problem is that causal relationships of this sort are notoriously difficult to establish, and epidemiologists devote considerable energy to teasing out the various lifestyle risk factors that might confound the relationship (Is the smoker also overweight? Does the smoker drink alcohol?). But Duesberg was not an epidemiologist and had conducted no controlled studies. Nor did his proven expertise in molecular biology or retrovirology have much bearing in this case. Duesberg simply set out to construct a persuasive argument, relying on his background in chemistry and facts at his disposal from his scouring of the published literature.

After quickly reviewing his case for the implausibility of the reigning hypothesis, Duesberg began by noting the "chronological coincidences" between the AIDS and drug epidemics in the United States. Moreover, "drugs and AIDS appear to claim their victims from the same risk groups." Intravenous drug users comprised about a third of all AIDS patients, Duesberg explained. And about 60 percent of AIDS patients in the United States were male homosexuals, who, according to Duesberg, were disproportionate consumers of drugs. Duesberg reported on a number of studies, including a 1990 survey of "3,916 self-identified American homosexual men, the largest of its kind," which found that 83 percent had used one or more drugs—including poppers, cocaine, amphetamines, and LSD—during the previous six months. Finally, Duesberg turned to another "risk group," healthy antibody positives who had taken "cytocidal DNA chain terminators" such as AZT. "Thus an unknown, but possibly a high percentage of the 30,000 Americans that currently develop AIDS per year have used AZT prior to or after the onset of AIDS." [17]

Even if accepted at face value, these arguments about prevalence of drug use among AIDS risk groups were not particularly weighty in establishing the role of drugs in the causation of AIDS. Indeed, in his own attacks on the HIV hypothesis, Duesberg had frequently invoked the maxim that "correlation is not causation": just because HIV, or drug use, or anything else had been correlated with AIDS, researchers could not necessarily conclude that they had identified a cause. However, AZT presented Duesberg with a particularly convenient target, because by 1992 no one liked the drug very much despite its widespread administration. AZT did not cure AIDS, and it had substantial and potentially dangerous side effects. The initial study that showed it prolonged life in AIDS patients had been ended early when, for ethical reasons, the drug was supplied to study participants getting only a placebo, and some argued that, as a result, there was no clear evidence of the drug's long-term effects.[18] Since 1990 the drug had also been prescribed to asymptomatic HIV positives in hopes of preventing progression to AIDS. But recent studies had been equivocal, suggesting that while the drug might indeed delay the onset of opportunistic infections, it might have no ultimate effect on longevity. By this reading, HIV positives faced a Hobson's choice in the short term—refuse AZT and suffer minor opportunistic infections or take AZT and endure its adverse effects—but arrived at the same place in the end. Another often-criticized but much publicized study had suggested that AZT might be less effective in African-Americans and Latinos than in whites.[19]

To be sure, most doctors continued to prescribe AZT (or chemically related drugs), and public health authorities continued to promote it as the indicated treatment for HIV positives with abnormally low T-cell counts. But enthusiasm for the drug had waned appreciably. Over the years, particularly in New York, some in the AIDS movement had come out against AZT—including dissenters in the causation controversy, like Ortleb, Lauritsen, Sonnabend, and Callen, as well as some who accepted the HIV hypothesis.[20] Callen—who was well known for the accomplishment of being alive a decade after his AIDS diagnosis—attributed his survival, in large part, to his refusal to take AZT.[21]

In his critique, Duesberg emphasized the drug's side effects: anemia, nausea, muscle atrophy, hepatitis, insomnia, headaches, seizures, and vomiting, among others. Yet although none of these conditions would justify an AIDS diagnosis, Duesberg did not explain his claim (perhaps borrowed from the title of Lauritsen's book, *AZT: Poison by Prescription*) that AZT is "AIDS by prescription." Certainly if Duesberg were held to the same rigorous standards of proof that he proposed for the HIV orthodoxy, his argument would have to be found wanting. He had provided no conclusive evidence isolating long-term drug use as the cause of AIDS; he could point to no controlled longitudinal studies of the kind he insisted that the AIDS establishment must perform. And along the way he presented a number of arguments that can only be characterized as specious: "Within 48 weeks on AZT, 172 (56%) out of 308 Australian AIDS patients developed one or more new AIDS diseases, including pneumonia and candidiasis. This indicates that AZT induces AIDS disease within less than 1 year and thus much faster than the 10 years HIV is said to need to cause AIDS."[22] This was like arguing that if a flu sufferer took aspirin, and four hours later her fever returned, then aspirin must cause fever even more rapidly than the influenza virus. Perhaps comments such as these were intended only to goad his critics and were not meant to be taken too seriously. Or perhaps by this point, Duesberg was so embittered by the behavior of his scientific colleagues—who, he believed, had blackballed him, tried to silence him, and succeeded in cutting his funding—that he was willing to employ any rhetorical device at his disposal to cast doubt on the worth of their accomplishments.

By a different calculus, Duesberg might be said to have achieved his objectives with the article in *Biomedicine & Pharmacotherapy*: he had supplemented what, after all, was his main point—that HIV could not be the cause of AIDS—by proposing an alternative explanation in a legitimate scientific publication. In the past, experts had taunted Duesberg: "Perhaps he would be willing to tell us what, in his view, is the cause of AIDS and what he would do about it. . . . It would seem only fair for Professor Duesberg either to come up with an equally strong candidate or to lend his support to eradicating HIV and thus AIDS."[23] Now Duesberg could claim to have met that challenge, and he could return to exerting public pressure on the proponents of the AIDS orthodoxy to prove the official story of AIDS causation.

THE HIV HERETICS
AND THE "MURDOCH PRESS"

Suddenly, in spring 1992, the causation controversy exploded in the pages of the British press. Between April 26 and May 31, more than twenty articles or opinion pieces on the topic were published in the pages of the *Times*, the *Sunday Times*, the *Independent*, and the *Daily Telegraph*, or released over the wire by Reuters. The furor was kicked off by the *Sunday Times*, which—along with the technically separate daily *Times*, also owned by publishing mogul Rupert Murdoch—had been prone toward headline-grabbing coverage of AIDS. These newspapers had explored the controversial view that the AIDS epidemic might be the unintended by-product of vaccine trials in Africa in the 1950s, which may have exposed vaccine recipients to monkey viruses similar to HIV. They had also fiercely questioned the view that heterosexuals were at risk of AIDS. Now, in a front-page, headline story, accompanied by a much longer, forty-four hundred–word, double-page spread inside the newspaper as well as a sidebar on Montagnier, science writer Neville Hodgkinson described a "Startling Challenge to Aids Orthodoxy" mounted by "two of the world's experts on viruses," Montagnier and Duesberg.[24]

Both scientists, Hodgkinson reported, "are to challenge the orthodox view that HIV is the exclusive cause of Aids" at an alternative AIDS conference to be held in Amsterdam the following month. Hodgkinson emphasized the shift in Montagnier's position on causation over the years, quoting the French scientist as saying: "We were naive. . . . We thought this one virus was doing all the destruction. Now we have to understand the other factors in this." And he described the rude reception that Montagnier had received in 1990 when he tried to present his views on cofactors at the International Conference in San Francisco. Hodgkinson quoted one observer: "There was Montagnier, the Jesus of HIV, and they threw him out of the temple."[25]

One of several members of the group profiled by Hodgkinson was

Dr. Kary Mullis, a scientist who in 1983 had invented the technique called polymerase chain reaction that had transformed biotechnology research. (The *Financial Times* has called PCR "probably the most important development in genetics research since the discovery of gene-splicing in 1973," noting that the market for the technology is likely to be worth $1 billion a year by 1996.[26] In October 1993, Mullis received the Nobel Prize in chemistry for inventing PCR.) Mullis had no expertise in AIDS, but his dissent carried a certain weight, given that his invention had actually been employed to support the orthodox position. Before the invention and distribution of PCR, scientists had been able to find HIV in only one out of every ten thousand to one hundred thousand T cells, raising serious questions about how the virus could be destroying the immune system. But once the same researchers began using PCR, they were able to find the virus in about one percent of T cells—which didn't answer all the questions but at least came closer to doing so. Mullis, however, was not impressed; he told Hodgkinson: "I can't find a single virologist who will give me references which show that HIV is the probable cause of AIDS."[27]

The science editor of the daily *Times*, Nigel Hawkes, followed up with a shorter article the following day describing the alternative conference to be held in Amsterdam. "Professor Montagnier's presence is likely to give a higher profile to a campaign over AIDS which has been ignored or dismissed by mainstream medical opinion," wrote Hawkes.[28] Meanwhile, *Reuters Financial Report* noted the financial implication of the *Times*'s articles for Wellcome Foundation, the British-based parent of Burroughs Wellcome, manufacturer of AZT. Shares of Wellcome stock "took an initial tumble on the article," dropping fifty-two pence.[29] A few days later, the *Times*'s rival, the *Independent*, weighed in with a report from Steve Connor, a science correspondent who had coauthored a well-known book about AIDS. Connor quoted Dr. Kenneth Calman, Britain's chief medical officer, who had appeared on television to express his concern that the *Times* articles might encourage complacency in response to AIDS.[30]

Soon afterward, the *Independent* published an opposing commentary by William Leith, who compared resistance to Duesberg and Montagnier with the opposition that Darwin and Copernicus had encountered from scientists of their day. "Why do people react so badly to new scientific discoveries?" Leith asked rhetorically.[31] Connor responded with his own op-ed piece, which asked some pointed questions about what Leith had referred to as "the Duesberg-Montagnier theory." Montagnier's name brought credibility, and the dissenters were understandably anxious to "enroll" him by presenting him as a fellow traveler. But Connor was having none of it. "Readers of several British newspapers could be forgiven for forming the impression that Professor Duesberg has won over a powerful ally," wrote Connor. In fact, Connor explained, Montagnier would be attending the alternative conference in order to *oppose* Duesberg. He quoted Montagnier's current opinion of Duesberg: "He's wrong because he doesn't take all the data into account, whether deliberately or not. I will go to the conference to prove Duesberg is wrong." [32]

Connor argued that the *Times*'s misrepresentation of Montagnier's relationship to the HIV controversy was typical of an article that devoted two pages to Duesberg "but largely ignored the welter of evidence against his claim." Malcolm Dean, writing in the "News & Comment" section of the British medical journal *Lancet*, made a similar point in an article on "AIDS and the Murdoch Press." Decrying the *Times*'s "deep Conservative bias which the editor desperately tries to conceal by anti-establishment campaigns," Dean argued that "of course sceptics should be given space, but iconoclasts should be pushed as hard as establishment figures to justify their assertions." [33]

MAVERICKS AND HIGH-FLYERS

Darwin, Copernicus, Galileo—such names are often invoked to enhance the credibility of anti-establishment figures in science. These comparisons put a premium on challenge and innovation while equating "normal" science with dogma, superstition, and intellectual stagnation. In fact, the heroic imagery of revolutionary science appealed to many of the protagonists in the causation controversy, constituting an important dimension of what Pierre Bourdieu would call their scientific habitus—the particular set of dispositions and "generative schemes of perception, appreciation and action" that engender "the choice of objects, the solution of problems, and the evaluation of solutions." [34]

Duesberg himself was a good example—a brilliant high-achiever, with a history of swimming against the current, a researcher who disdained the mediocrity that he equated with establishment science. The peer review process that governed the scientific world punished the "Mozarts" while rewarding the "Salieris," Duesberg explained, leaving little doubt as to how he would classify himself. Peer review was "good for technicians, but not for innovation"; it constituted the "stabilization of mediocrity."[35]

For Root-Bernstein—at twenty-seven the second youngest to receive a MacArthur "genius grant" in the 1981 cohort of winners—the $144,000 award meant that he could abandon a "restricting" and "boring" postdoctoral fellowship and conduct a study of scientific creativity. One reviewer of Root-Bernstein's book *Discovering* noted its clear sympathies: "Root-Bernstein's characters venture the heretical notion that the clustered, prize-ridden, hierarchical culture of modern science may actually impede important discovery. . . . What do today's superstar academic-administrator-researchers really think of seminal investigators like Mendel, a monk who discovered the laws of heredity in a monastery garden without federal grants . . . ? Would establishment science even listen to such outside maverick voices today?"[36]

Kary Mullis, called by *Time* magazine the "hippie-holdout biochemist" and the "Last of the Great Tinkerers," says he conceived of the breakthrough technique of PCR "while winding through the mountains of Northern California" at midnight in his Honda Civic.[37] Claiming to read widely in cosmology, mysticism, mathematics, virology, chemistry, and artificial intelligence,[38] Mullis published an article in *Nature* on "The Cosmological Significance of Time Reversal" while a graduate student in biochemistry at the University of California at Berkeley.[39] "If you're too establishment-oriented, you're not likely to come up with something really original," Mullis told the *Los Angeles Times*.[40] In 1993, when he won the Nobel Prize, Mullis was pictured on the front page of the local *San Diego Union-Tribune* in a wetsuit, surfboard under one arm; reporters marveled at the collection of giant inflatable penguins that adorned his living room.[41]

Mavericks, innovators, individualists—these were people who were unafraid to cross disciplinary boundaries and venture outside of their areas of expertise. And they shared a critical view—call it a loathing—of contemporary "big science" and the way it squelched imaginative efforts. "When a new theory deviates from that held by the majority, it is labeled 'controversial' rather than 'original,'" Duesberg wrote in a commentary piece in *The Scientist,* with specific reference to Montagnier, Root-Bernstein, and himself; "and the 'controversial' label is tantamount to a death sentence, manifested by non-invitations to meetings, non-citations in the literature, non-nominations for awards, and non-funding of research grants."[42]

GATHERING OF THE TRIBES

Sponsored by a Dutch organization called the Foundation for Alternative AIDS Research, which stressed "freedom of information" and "freedom of thought," the alternative conference promised by the *Sunday Times* took place from May 14 to 16, 1992. Many of the key HIV dissenters were there: Michael Callen, Joseph Sonnabend, John Lauritsen, Joan McKenna, Gordon Stewart, Robert Root-Bernstein, Joan Shenton, Celia Farber, Jad Adams—along with, of course, the featured attractions, Duesberg and Montagnier. Other supporters of alternative positions came from a number of countries on the Continent, including Switzerland, Belgium, and the Netherlands. Representatives of the orthodox position were also in attendance, including three Dutch researchers, Roel Coutinho, Jaap Goudsmit, and Frank Miedema. In all, about two hundred people showed up for the event.

A Reuters report quoted the Secretary of Britain's Medical Research Council, who denounced the claims presented at the alternative conference as "a lethal cocktail of untruth and ignorance."[43] But Nigel Hawkes, writing from Amsterdam for the *Times* of London, framed the issue as one of freedom of belief versus the suppression of heresy. He led off with: "In an old church in Amsterdam once used by religious liberals escaping persecution, a group of free-thinkers yesterday met to denounce the authorised version of Aids. . . ."[44] Hawkes noted that "Montagnier insisted that the virus was a necessary part" of the spread of the epidemic, but he presented Montagnier as sympathetic to the dissenters: "'Dogmatism is a deadly sin in the process of science,' Professor Montagnier concluded. This was clear evidence, some might say, that he backed the efforts of the alternative Aids group to take a fresh look at a disease that has been spreading for a decade without a cure or a clear understanding of how it functions being found."

The considerable debate in the British press caused some Canadian publications to pick up the issue. The magazine *Macleans* published a long article on the Amsterdam conference,[45] and the *Toronto Star* ran a story describing what it called "The New AIDS Controversy."[46] But in the United States, home to most of the prominent HIV heretics, the alternative conference was almost entirely ignored by the mainstream press. National Public Radio's *Weekend Edition* ran a brief and not terribly illuminating report picked up from a correspondent for the

Canadian Broadcasting Corporation.[47] But only readers of the gay press would have been likely to know significant details or to have followed the specific controversy concerning the role of Montagnier.

Initially, writers in gay publications followed the lead of the *Sunday Times* in assuming that Montagnier had defected to the dissident camp. An article in the New York–based magazine *QW*, entitled "HIV Does Not Cause AIDS, Virus Discoverer Claims," commented: "Although the multifactorial approach is not new, it is surprising coming from someone who is considered relatively conservative and has championed the traditional 'HIV causes AIDS' theory."[48] Similarly, Neenyah Ostrom's article in the *Native* was headlined: "Montagnier: HIV Is Not the Cause,"[49] while the *San Francisco Sentinel* reported that "other respected AIDS experts have begun to agree with Duesberg, most notably, Luc Montagnier. . . ."[50]

Claims such as these apparently provoked consternation at San Francisco's Project Inform. One of the most authoritative voices on treatment issues within the AIDS movement, Project Inform had taken many anti-establishment stands. But on the question of causation, the organization stood squarely in the mainstream. Indeed, Executive Director Martin Delaney had become friends with Robert Gallo—initially out of the pragmatic position that it was more useful to the cause of AIDS research to have Gallo on board, but ultimately out of genuine respect for the researcher's talents and a belief that Gallo was being unfairly treated in the controversy surrounding the discovery of HIV.[51] Delaney immediately wrote to Montagnier at the Pasteur Institute to express concern about the *Times*'s implication of an alliance between Montagnier and Duesberg and to request clarification of his views. Just before leaving for the alternative conference, Montagnier sent off a letter in response, which Delaney released to the press.[52]

In the letter, Montagnier described the *Sunday Times* article as "misleading since it mixed a correct account of my interview with anti-HIV non scientific theories." However, "as you may recall from our meeting in 1990, my permanent position has been to keep an open mind and not to neglect any facts." Montagnier went on to reiterate his belief that mycoplasma may serve as cofactors, and that various indirect mechanisms—particularly one called "apoptosis" or "programmed cell death"—may be involved in T-cell depletion. But he stressed: "This is just opposite to the view that AIDS is not caused by HIV and is not a transmissible disease."[53]

PROJECT INFORM STAKES ITS CLAIMS

The seriousness with which Project Inform took the resurgence of interest in the causation controversy was indicated by the publication in early June of a six-page "Discussion Paper" devoted entirely to the topic. The report began by blasting the media for their irresponsibility and sensationalism. Why do reporters love the HIV dissenters? Why have they confused Montagnier's position with Duesberg's, despite Montagnier's own disavowals? "Apparently because it makes a good story—'Conventional Wisdom Is Wrong! Top Scientists in Error Ten Years! Secrets! Coverup! Big Business, Big Science Collusion!' . . . Such is the sorry state of AIDS reporting in some circles today." [54]

Focusing on four groups opposing the HIV hypothesis—the *New York Native, Spin* magazine, assorted journalists, and certain scientists—Project Inform was at pains to question the credibility of each and to uncover motivations for adopting heretical stances. Accusing the *Native* of a "supermarket tabloid" mentality, the report described the newspaper as "driven not by any scientific data but by a seething hatred of Dr. Robert Gallo. . . ." And for writers at *Spin,* as well as "a few journalists" writing for publications like the *Times* of London and the *Atlantic Monthly,* the apparent motivations were "a generic distrust of authority and government science." [55]

In considering the fourth, crucial group of HIV dissenters—the scientists—Project Inform's report similarly emphasized the issue of credibility. Root-Bernstein "works in a field not directly related to AIDS" and "has not conducted or published any AIDS research other than editorials," yet "Spin calls him 'one of the leading AIDS researchers in the US.'" Kary Mullis, while "obviously a serious scientist," was similarly "an outsider to AIDS research"; furthermore, his PCR test "has, if anything, helped to bolster the case for HIV." Of all the heretical scientists, only Sonnabend "is professionally involved with AIDS," but "primarily as a clinician": "While Dr. Sonnabend has earned respect in many ways, his arguments against HIV are no more valid than the others." [56]

The case against the credibility of Peter Duesberg was given more extended treatment. Project Inform explicitly posed the crucial question: "Is Peter Duesberg an 'AIDS expert'? That depends on the definition of 'expert.'" The report reviewed the evidence in terms that mirrored Gallo's characterization of his colleague: Duesberg had never conducted laboratory, clinical, or epidemiological research on AIDS or HIV. He was trained in chemistry, not the biological sciences. He had "no known professional expertise regarding the immune system, was not an expert in the study of human viruses or retroviruses, nor in human disease in general (except for cancer)." True, he once mapped the genetic code of a retrovirus, but that work "bears little direct connection to AIDS." [57]

In focusing on formal credentials, Project Inform walked a fine line. This, after all, was a grassroots organization staffed by self-educated AIDS experts; its executive director, before the epidemic came along, had been a business consultant. A big part of Project Inform's work involved disseminating highly technical knowledge about AIDS to laypeople in order to create what might be called a mass-based expertise. In its reckoning of the tokens of expertise, Project Inform was not about to argue that academic degrees or journal publications are everything. Lacking the right credentials, Peter Duesberg could still be considered an AIDS expert of sorts—but not in a way that would make him stand out from the crowd: "Perhaps his most relevant work is that he has studied the medical literature on AIDS (as have thousands of patients, physicians, and activists), and this qualifies as a form of expertise." But "Duesberg's supporters and the media spread misinformation when they present him as an 'AIDS researcher' in the sense that phrase is usually meant." His published writings on AIDS were "simply editorials." [58]

Project Inform noted that there was a "legitimate" scientific question that had been "lost in the fog" generated by media fascination with Duesberg and other dissenters: How does HIV cause AIDS? Following the lead of Gallo and others, the report emphasized that pathogenesis was separate from etiology; while part one of the report was entitled "Is HIV the Cause of AIDS?" part two was called "How Does HIV Cause AIDS?" Here Project Inform adopted an agnostic position, informing its readers about a variety of hypotheses, including "specific co-factors," "general infectious co-factors," "superantigens," "apoptosis" (Montagnier's position), "autoimmunity," "overactivation," and "antigen diversity threshold." Project Inform's point was that speculation about these pathogenetic mechanisms was an entirely mainstream endeavor and had been since the beginning. "Few if any researchers," the report argued, "ever claimed that AIDS was solely the result of HIV killing [helper T] cells. It was the media who spread that view, apparently to simplify AIDS for the public." [59]

While reviewing the various positions on etiology and pathogenesis, the report also took time to blast Duesberg's alternative causal hypothesis: "By linking AIDS to behavior, rather than a virus, Duesberg paints all but the 'innocent' victims of AIDS as promiscuous drug abusers.... When such views are expressed by fundamentalists and right wing politicians, they are routinely and correctly branded *as homophobia and racism*. Such well-known bigots as Congressman William Dannemeyer today quote Duesberg as the scientific source of their views." Against these charges, the report reminded readers of a "simple truth" known by "anyone in a community hard hit by AIDS"—that "some who have died did have histories of promiscuity and drug abuse, but many, many others did not." [60]

LEFT AND RIGHT

By labeling Duesberg homophobic, and by associating him with political enemies on the right, Project Inform sought to annul any credibility that Duesberg might enjoy in gay and lesbian communities. Duesberg himself, however, assiduously rejected any taint of homophobia: "In reality I've paid more ... to them than ... most of my fellow AIDS researchers, who're making millions of dollars by killing homosexuals by the hundreds of thousands with AZT.... It's actually absurd that I'm being labeled the homophobe, when I might in fact have found the real cause of their problem...." [61] Whatever Duesberg's beliefs, it is certainly the case that the political configurations in the Duesberg controversy have been more complex than simple labels could suggest. For example, some left-wing commentators have supported Duesberg out of a principled objection to monocausal disease models. "Ruling classes embraced modern medicine because the germ theory blamed disease on invisible microbes and not hazardous conditions," according to one pro-Duesberg magazine article from 1989. [62] Yet the appeal of Duesberg's views to conservatives—certainly including those with little sympathy for the gay movement—cannot be denied.

Charles Thomas, the organizer of the Group for the Scientific Reappraisal, has described himself as "libertarian" and claimed that he left Harvard in disgust because the universities had become "totally corrupted by affirmative action, political correctness, the whole nine yards." He criticized the AIDS activist movement as one of "victimology": by portraying AIDS as an "act of God," rather than the consequence of behavior, homosexuals generated sympathy and government funding.[63] Philip Johnson, the Berkeley law professor on the group's steering committee, has also been known for his conservative views. Bryan Ellison made no bones about why he sought to promote Duesberg in the Heritage Foundation's *Policy Review,* as well as in *California Political Review,* a journal that has also featured articles about "Hollywood's leftward tilt" and Republican California Governor Pete Wilson's "liberal surrender."[64] Tom Bethell, a columnist who has written in support of Duesberg in various publications, is well known for his right-wing positions, which have included endorsement of such political figures as Patrick Buchanan.[65] Bethell's columns in the *Los Angeles Times* include one entitled "We May Regret Going Along with This: The Gay-Rights Agenda Precludes Any Public Doubts."[66] Elsewhere he has expressed sympathy for homosexual "recovery" organizations (which encourage gays and lesbians to become straight).[67]

THE "VIETNAM SYNDROME"

Project Inform concluded its commentary with some speculation about Duesberg's motives for continuing to pursue the controversy. Portraying Duesberg as "a propagandist, not a reasoning scientist," Project Inform's report noted the incendiary quality of Duesberg's claims when he labeled AZT as "iatrogenic genocide": "He presses the hot buttons of genocide, distrust of authority, fear of doctors, and suspicion of business—all in two carefully chosen words." Why would Duesberg be doing this? What could he possibly stand to gain? And doesn't the fact that he is being silenced by the scientific establishment mean that the AIDS movement should support him? Project Inform had its analysis at the ready: "Having gone out on this limb, personally and professionally, he got stuck there and is hanging on with great tenacity. It is true that the scientific mainstream sometimes (but rarely) makes a giant error and clings stubbornly to it, it is far more common that individual scientists do so."[68]

Had Duesberg—along with other dissenters whose credibility was on the line, like Sonnabend and Root-Bernstein—simply gone too far to turn back? Had they become trapped by the nature of their prior investments? Even Bryan Ellison acknowledged, in describing his mentor's progress: "He slowly got more and more into it, and now, what's he going to do, back out?"[69] Yet such arguments cut both ways.

Thomas Ryan, a supporter of Duesberg writing in the gay magazine *Christopher Street,* used the metaphor of the U.S. government's pursuit of victory in Vietnam to describe the ongoing commitment of the establishment to the HIV hypothesis: they simply had invested too heavily to pull out. And this could be said not just of the scientists, whose professional reputations were at stake, but of the wider "AIDS community" that had fashioned its very identity in response to the ramifications of the HIV hypothesis. "If anything positive has resulted from the AIDS crisis, it is the solidarity it has inspired in the gay community, and nothing has so threatened that unity as the HIV debate," wrote Ryan.[70] Or as Drew Hopkins, another Duesberg sympathizer also writing in *Christopher Street,* observed: "If HIV is not the cause, the entire body of AIDS advocacy is undone from its foundation. Every issue must be re-examined from a new, uncertain perspective. Such a confusing period would also generate a dangerous vulnerability. As AIDS has become a more and more political issue, it would take very little for a Pat Robertson, Jesse Helms, or William Dannemeyer to seize the day, using the period of reassessment on the part of the AIDS community to conduct still more virulent campaigns of fear and hatred."[71]

"AIDS WITHOUT HIV"

The wave of publicity that seemed to propel Duesberg forward throughout 1992 picked up additional momentum in July, with the opening of the Eighth International AIDS Conference. Convening in Amsterdam like its "alternative" predecessor of a few months before, the conference was sidetracked by breathless reports in the mass media of an "epidemic" of cases of "AIDS" in people who tested negative for antibodies to both HIV-1 and HIV-2. "The patients are sick or dying, and most of them have risk factors," wrote *Newsweek,* describing a dozen such cases. "What they don't have is HIV."[72] Perhaps a new virus was at work, a possibility that seemed to gain credibility in the media due to the coincidental report by a southern California scientist of the isolation of an apparently new retrovirus in AIDS patients.[73] Or perhaps there were other routes that led to conditions like AIDS. *Newsweek*'s speculations must have inspired intense flashes of déjà vu in those familiar with the debates about causes of AIDS that had been enacted a long decade earlier: "Dr. Alvin Friedman-Kien of the New York University Medical Center notes that

gay men and IV drug users contract numerous infections, from gonorrhea to herpes and hepatitis. Some ostensible AIDS cases may simply
reflect the immune-suppressing effects of common germs or of poor
nutrition, he says." [74]

Besieged by reporters, scientists, and activists, James Curran, the
head of the CDC's AIDS office, was forced to address the new syndrome at a heated conference session. Curran acknowledged that the
CDC had been tracking such cases, but insisted, "These are not cases
of AIDS"; he then made the circular argument—which Duesberg must
have appreciated—that a definition of AIDS requires the presence of
HIV.[75] Duesberg wasted little time sending in a letter to *Science,* offering to provide to anyone who was interested "a list of references to
more than 800 HIV-free immunodeficiencies and AIDS-defining diseases in all major American and European risk groups," along with
references to "more than 2,200 HIV-free African AIDS cases." Rather
than rushing to conclusions about any new virus, Duesberg advised,
Science should focus attention on alternative explanations "that could
resolve the growing paradoxes of the virus-AIDS hypothesis." [76]

Only days after the first reports of the mysterious cases, this newest
controversy framed a debate in the pages of the *Los Angeles Times*
about the arguments of Peter Duesberg. Steve Heimoff wrote one of
the two, side-by-side, opposing op-ed pieces, leading off with the observation that reports of "AIDS without HIV" would "appear to signal at least partial, temporary vindication" of the Berkeley scientist.[77]
Describing Duesberg as "the unofficial leader of the revisionists," "an
international star of virology long before anyone heard of AIDS," and
"not just another conspiratorialist," Heimoff reported that many of
his arguments "have the ring of common sense." It would seem that
"there are now three legitimately contending theories regarding the
causes of AIDS," Heimoff said: the official CDC theory, Montagnier's
cofactor theory, and Duesberg's. Heimoff concluded: "If there is even
a remote chance that Duesberg is correct—and the latest reports increase that possibility—then the powers that be must leap into
action."

"Just because the Establishment has been wrong so often doesn't
necessarily make all of its critics right," Duesberg's old foe Michael
Fumento responded in the accompanying piece.[78] "Duesberg's methodology in determining that HIV doesn't cause AIDS is less science
than a game in which he tells his opponents to go into a round room
and sit in a corner." Turning to Duesberg's alternative hypothesis,

Fumento noted that the theory failed to explain AIDS in Africa, where neither AZT nor recreational drugs were in significant use. This prompted Duesberg and Ellison to respond, in a letter to the editor, that the official WHO statistics "reveal a tiny African AIDS epidemic" despite large numbers of HIV positives. They complained that Fumento also pointed to "media-publicized cases of ordinary people developing AIDS" but that he failed to mention that "Ali Gertz used cocaine, Ryan White suffered from fatal hemophilia, Paul Gann had traumatic heart surgery, Kimberly Bergalis used AZT, and Magic Johnson is symptom-free."[79]

In the gay and lesbian press, responses to the "AIDS without HIV" flap were generally dismissive. Many denounced the "media circus" or "media feeding frenzies" that seemed predictably to ensue when too many reporters knowing too little about AIDS found themselves together in one place with too little hard news to write about.[80] Martin Delaney, writing in his regular column in the *Advocate,* insisted on the "clear point" that "these events have nothing to do with the so-called Duesberg theory," and he warned that Duesberg's "supporters will no doubt seize on the new information as an assault on the role of HIV."[81]

On the far end of the spectrum, Chuck Ortleb penned an editorial for the *New York Native,* entitled "Honey, I Blew Up the HIV Paradigm." Attacking the CDC for "promoting the religious belief that HIV is the cause of AIDS," Ortleb pushed the *Native*'s current theory, that AIDS and the chronic fatigue syndrome were "variants of the same disease": "If the C.D.C. wants to know all cases of HIV-negative AIDS, we hereby report to them 13 million cases: the estimate of the number of people in the U.S. with Chronic Fatigue Syndrome [CFS]."[82] While the CDC was unlikely to have been impressed by Ortleb's statistics, indirect support for the *Native*'s publisher arrived from an unlikely source, when *Newsweek* published a follow-up story on "AIDS without HIV" that played up the chronic fatigue angle. "As more cases come to light, it's becoming clear that the newly defined syndrome has as much in common with CFS as it does with AIDS," said the *Newsweek* reporter, Geoffrey Cowley.[83]

Following on *Newsweek*'s lead, *Time* magazine published a cover story entitled "Invincible AIDS," which suggested that the global fight against the epidemic was in disarray.[84] But over the next few months, the AIDS establishment struggled to put its house back in order. In August the CDC convened a special panel to review all cases of "AIDS without HIV" that had been reported or that investigators had been able to dig out of medical records.[85] The panel dismissed as flawed the reports describing a new virus. But they agreed that a syndrome did exist—the CDC had dubbed it "idiopathic CD4+ T-lymphocytopenia" (ICL) to describe the depletion of helper T cells by an unknown cause[86]—though only thirty confirmed cases could be found in the United States. Moreover, in contrast to the earliest reports, it now appeared that more than half the ICL patients reported none of the AIDS risk factors. As compared with AIDS cases, people with ICL were more likely to be older than fifty, more likely to be white, and more likely to be female.

The consensus of panel members was that different patients were immune-suppressed for different reasons. Most likely there had always been small numbers of such cases, but they had never before come to national attention because there was little medical emphasis on T-cell testing. "Only in the last three to four years has CD4 [helper T-cell] testing become a mass industry," commented Martin Hirsch of Harvard Medical School.[87] The following month, the WHO reported similar findings based on a review of cases of ICL from around the world.[88]

The Dynamics of Closure: Whither the Controversy? (1992–1995)

THE DEFINITIVE STUDY?

Overshadowed by the news about "AIDS without HIV" were other research findings that augured less favorably for the future success of the HIV dissenters, particularly Duesberg. First, over the summer of 1992, two groups of researchers reported on the latest advances in isolating HIV from T cells using PCR technology. Instead of finding the virus in one out of every ten thousand or one hundred thousand cells, scientists were now succeeding in finding the virus in one out of every forty to two hundred cells.[89] The following January, Dr. Ashley Haase of the University of Minnesota and other researchers reported on their refinement of PCR called "PCR in situ," which allowed them to discover HIV in 10 to 30 percent of T cells and in high percentages of other cells as well. These findings, the authors explained, were "consistent with the emerging view that HIV infection *per se* could contribute substantially to depletion of immune cells in AIDS."[90]

Further relevant data were published in March, when two groups of researchers, one led by Haase and the other by Anthony Fauci, described finding "massive covert infection" of lymphoid cells in the spleen, tonsils, adenoids, and lymph nodes during the early stages of HIV infection—ten times more virus than could be detected in blood samples at that stage of illness.[91] "These developments," wrote *Nature* editor John Maddox in the *Times* of London, "convincingly give the lie to Duesberg's only cogent criticism of the conventional view that it is difficult to recover virus from the helper T-cells circulating in the blood." Maddox continued: "Now it seems probable that these vital components of the immune system are damaged and perhaps killed off in the relative obscurity of the lymph nodes and the other organs of the immune system."[92]

Another piece of news (which received little notice beyond a brief report in a *New York Times* article devoted mainly to other topics)[93] arrived in a presentation at the International AIDS Conference that was designed specifically to prove Duesberg wrong. The report was by Kevin Craib and other researchers with the Vancouver Lymph-adenopathy-AIDS Study, one of the principal cohort studies that had been tracking HIV-negative and HIV-positive gay men for nearly a decade. The study's authors noted Duesberg's argument that no controlled study had been conducted that could truly distinguish between lifestyle risk factors and HIV infection as possible causes of AIDS. "The purpose of this analysis," wrote Craib and his associates, "was to conduct just such a controlled analysis within a cohort of homosexual men."[94]

Looking back over their accumulated data, Craib and his coauthors investigated the incidence of AIDS-defining illnesses and changes in T-cell counts over time and tried to relate those clinical developments to HIV status, to exposure to psychoactive drugs, and to sexual behavior. They found that half of the 350 HIV-negative men in the study reported using psychoactive drugs. And about a quarter of them reported having been the receptive partner in anal intercourse with "casual partners." But despite these high incidences of (hypothesized) risk behavior, there were *no* signs of immune dysfunction in the seronegative group— no AIDS-defining illnesses and no drop in T-cell counts. Of 134 AIDS-defining illnesses in the full cohort, "every single one occurred in men with pre-existing evidence of HIV infection." Cofactors might determine which HIV positives contract which (if any) opportunistic infections, the authors concluded; "but claims that AIDS is caused by other exposures and not by HIV are clearly not borne out by these data."

The Berkeley epidemiologist Warren Winkelstein had already shown Duesberg unpublished figures, derived from the San Francisco Men's Health Study, that supported similar conclusions. Duesberg, however, insisted that unpublished data simply didn't count in the world of science, and he refused to acknowledge Winkelstein's findings unless they appeared in a peer-reviewed journal. Winkelstein maintained, in response, that these were really nonfindings and that scientists weren't generally in the business of publishing nonassociations.[95] But in the end Winkelstein was induced to answer to his nemesis; and in March 1993, an immunologist named Michael Ascher, along with Winkelstein and other colleagues, published a commentary in *Nature* entitled "Does Drug Use Cause AIDS?"[96] The article appeared the same week as the formal publication of Craib's study in *Lancet*—a double whammy that attracted the media attention that Craib's conference presentation had failed to elicit.[97]

Ascher and his colleagues assembled a point-by-point argument that seemed intent on addressing every objection that Duesberg had ever voiced or might conceivably muster in the future. It was a strong piece of science and very much a political document, one which acknowledged as its motivation "the wide publicity attracted by [Duesberg's] assertion."[98] Ascher and his colleagues reviewed the San Francisco Men's Health Study data for 1,027 study subjects over ninety-six months. According to interviews performed at the beginning of the study back in 1984, the 812 gay or bisexual men and the 215 straight men had used cocaine, marijuana, and amphetamines in roughly the same percentages during the two years prior to recruitment for the study. (For example, 36 percent of homosexuals/bisexuals and 39 percent of heterosexuals had reported using marijuana once a week or more.) Since 26 percent of the gay or bisexual men had been diagnosed with AIDS indicator diseases over the course of the study, one would therefore expect that roughly the same percentage of the heterosexuals would also have AIDS diseases, if drug use were indeed the cause. But in fact, there were *no* cases of AIDS indicator diseases in the heterosexual group.

Noting that "the clinical case definition of AIDS has been criticized as having subjective features and low specificity," the authors also presented data examining the relationship between T-cell counts over time, drug use, and one's status as antibody positive or negative. T-cell counts, after all, were "the primary pathognomonic feature of AIDS"; they were the best indicator of the health or impairment of the immune system in people at risk of AIDS. The results were striking: The average numbers of T cells (per cubic millimeter) for the seropositives declined steadily from about seven hundred in 1984 to about four hundred in 1992, regardless of extent of drug use. But the average numbers for the seronegatives stayed the same, at one thousand to twelve hundred T cells—although ironically, the heavy and moderate drug-using seronegatives actually had slightly *higher* T-cell counts than the seronegative abstainers. This was a surprising finding, but it hardly helped Duesberg's case. The researchers concluded with their own challenge for their adversary: "The energies of Duesberg and his followers could better be applied to unraveling the enigmatic mechanism of the HIV pathogenesis of AIDS."

THE TERMS OF THE DEBATE

One of the dissenters' strongest arguments, which made an appearance in practically every published statement that any of them had made over the course of more than eight years, was that closure had been reached prematurely in 1984. A "probable cause" had been identified that was soon taken to be "the cause," yet no one bothered to prove it definitively. Instead, the world simply acted on what it took to be the truth. By the mid-1990s, however—particularly as a result of data from long-running cohort studies—the state of the evidence looked rather different. Indeed, one might even argue that the dissenters' challenge and the ensuing controversy had served to *promote* clearer argumentation on behalf of the HIV hypothesis. In that sense, ironically, the dissenters may have helped to reinforce the dominance of the position they opposed.

Does this mean that the end of the controversy was in sight? That would have been an overly hasty conclusion, and one that ignored recognized pitfalls along the path to closure in scientific controversies. In their consideration of the question of how scientific controversies end, H. Tristram Engelhardt and Arthur L. Caplan have noted the danger in assuming that complex disputes can be adjudicated through straightforward, rational means. The notion that a controversy can be "settled" presupposes prior agreement on "(1) how to acquire evidence relevant to the dispute and (2) how to reason with the evidence in order to reach a rationally defensible conclusion that will resolve the controversy." In fact, differing perceptions of what "the controversy" is and what sort of evidence might "settle" it are *themselves* often stakes in a controversy. This is all the more likely to be true,

Engelhardt and Caplan have observed, when "stakeholders in the debate belong to . . . different communities with different appreciations of the evidence at stake" or to "competing social groups" with opposing political and ethical agendas.[99]

How does one prove disease causation? Without agreement on this basic question, there was little chance of consensus about the relation of HIV to AIDS. In the early 1980s, many researchers, including even Gallo, seemed to have Koch's postulates at least generally in mind as they sought to isolate the virus, to induce the syndrome in primates, and to trace transmission of AIDS through infected blood products (see chapter 2). But when challenged by Duesberg, researchers argued that Koch's postulates were rarely satisfied in practice, especially for viruses; and they pointed to well-known examples.

As Duesberg pressed his case, both sides moved toward the position that specific epidemiological evidence—especially controlled longitudinal data—is what could settle the question.[100] But where epidemiologists such as Winkelstein insisted that the existing data from cohort studies already provided a definitive answer, Duesberg maintained that a meaningful cohort study had not yet been performed: The existing studies were created with the goal of studying the progression of "HIV disease." They were not set up to determine what causes AIDS, let alone to study drugs as a possible cause, and, Duesberg claimed, the data that had been collected about participants' drug use were superficial and inadequate. Neither Winkelstein nor the Vancouver group asked about drug use occurring as far back as ten years prior to entry into the study; nor had any of the cohort studies included blood tests for drugs, which Duesberg claimed were necessary to verify if the study participants were answering truthfully.[101] From the perspective of Duesberg and his allies, these aspects of data collection rendered the cohort studies worthless in adjudicating between causal hypotheses. Duesberg's deconstruction of the cohort studies demonstrated clearly what science studies scholars have repeatedly argued: in situations of controversy, experiments alone cannot be expected to "settle" the dispute. "The problem with experiments," according to Harry Collins and Trevor Pinch, "is that they tell you nothing unless they are competently done, but in controversial science no-one can agree on a criterion of competence."[102] Moreover, any experiment is—admittedly—an artificial stand-in for real-world conditions. Does the experimental situation adequately represent and capture reality? Nothing inherent in the experiment itself forces the observer to accept it as such.[103]

Both sides remained convinced of the validity of their claims; each side saw the other as dogmatically defending its position by means of a constant renegotiation of the rules. From Duesberg's standpoint, the defenders of orthodoxy were always "moving the goalposts" whenever its predictions were proved false; from the vantage point of the dominant position, the dissenters were forever cooking up newer and stricter criteria of proof that their opponents were then expected to meet. "Like a child who questions every answer with another 'why,' he plays a game which will never end until he says it is over," was how Martin Delaney characterized Duesberg's methodology in late 1992.[104] But perhaps the real mistake was to imagine that there is one "scientific method" or set of "rules of evidence" upon which everyone could unproblematically agree.[105] Indeed, if the controversy has demonstrated anything, it is that scientific "rules of the road" like Koch's postulates or epidemiological cohort data, far from being unchallengeable benchmarks, may be as subject to interpretation and debate as the empirical phenomena they are invoked to explain.

Most likely there is no scientific test that would settle the causation controversy to the satisfaction of all sides. A different sort of proof probably would spell the end of the controversy, however: if the AIDS establishment were to succeed in finding an impressively successful antiviral drug or vaccine, it is unlikely that anyone would continue to pay much attention to the dissidents. They would simply fade from the scene. This, however, is not entirely logical, for, as René Dubos has argued, it can be dangerous to infer medical etiology "backwards" from treatment effectiveness: "While drenching with water may help in putting out a blaze, few are the cases in which fire has its origin in a lack of water."[106] Yet at its root the support for the dissenters stems precisely from disappointment with the establishment's lack of therapeutic success, as the dissenters themselves have been acutely aware. Michael Callen told a Canadian television program in 1989: "It seems to me that if . . . you've got a chemical that is anti-retroviral . . . and you give it to people who have a disease that you claim is caused by a retrovirus and they don't get better, that would tend to suggest—at a minimum—that something a lot more complicated than having or not having HIV is going on."[107] The more time that has passed without a cure being discovered, the more persuasive has been the argument that the AIDS establishment has "produced nothing" and—by extension—their etiological hypothesis must be bankrupt. From a logical standpoint, this, of course, follows even less obviously than the converse claim that the *existence* of a successful treatment would *verify* the causal hypothesis. But the argument has a rhetorical power that cannot be denied. "As long as there's no cure, this will lurk," Robert Gallo reflected in 1994.[108]

Meanwhile, the struggle has gone on, and the HIV dissenters have continued to make the news. By now several of the principals have told their stories in book-length detail. Root-Bernstein's *Rethinking AIDS: The Tragic Cost of Premature Consensus,* published by Free Press, weighed in at 512 pages and included 100 pages of notes. It reviewed the anomalies in the HIV hypothesis, discussed a range of multifactorial theories of AIDS, and delved deeply into theories of autoimmune mechanisms.[109] Lauritsen's *The AIDS War: Propaganda, Profiteering and Genocide from the Medical-Industrial Complex,* a reprinting of many of his articles, likewise ran nearly 500 pages.[110] Ellison and Duesberg encountered more obstacles with their book, which was accepted but then dropped by two different publishers. By 1994 the book fell victim to a bitter feud that erupted between the two authors and led to a parting of the ways. Working alone, Duesberg finally published the book *Inventing the AIDS Virus* in 1996. In addition to 463 pages of new text, the book included reprints of several of Duesberg's scientific articles; it also featured a foreword by Kary Mullis. In this extensive review for the general reader, Duesberg summarized the views he had been putting forward for nearly a decade—not only on the HIV hypothesis and the drug-AIDS hypothesis, but on the status of the field of virology and the politics of science in general.[111]

The ranks of the dissenters were depleted in December 1993 by the death of Michael Callen, who had lived with AIDS for nearly twelve years and played a central role in a range of activist projects.[112] Other dissenters have continued to engage public attention. Notable occasions have included the appearances by Duesberg, Kary Mullis, and Philip Johnson at a special panel of the annual meeting of the Pacific Division of the American Academy for the Advancement of Science; a Florida physician's public self-injection with apparently HIV-infected blood to draw attention to "the greatest scam ever perpetrated"; and a freshman Republican Congressman's attempt to force government scientists at the NIH and CDC to consider the view that HIV does not cause AIDS.[113]

Perhaps most noteworthy, however, was a high-profile "Special News Report" called "The Duesberg Phenomenon," published in *Science* in late 1994 and taking up an extraordinary eight pages of the premier journal.[114] "Because the Duesberg phenomenon has not gone away and may be growing," wrote Jon Cohen, the AIDS reporter for *Science* and the author of the news report, "*Science* has decided this was a good time to examine Duesberg's main claims." Cohen's strategy was to tackle Duesberg's arguments head-on; in a series of sidebars, he considered each of the critical test cases. Although scrupulous in presenting Duesberg's views, the article suggested that Duesberg was wrong on all counts: being HIV positive was the key variable associated with HIV-related illness for hemophiliacs; Koch's third postulate had been satisfied by the accidental infection of three laboratory workers, all of whom developed symptoms of immune suppression prior to taking any antiviral drugs; and large, recent studies of extended AZT use showed no evidence that the drug caused AIDS.[115] Not surprisingly, this intervention ignited yet another wave of publicity: though Cohen may have intended exactly otherwise, his article propelled the Duesberg phenomenon onward. Indeed, a long article in *The Scientist* published in March 1995, which led off with the special report in *Science,* was entitled "A Controversy That Will Not Die: The Role of HIV in Causing AIDS."[116]

Years after the publication of his article in *Cancer Research,* Peter Duesberg has settled in for the long haul. The HIV controversy has become his life; his office on the Berkeley campus is the war room of a campaign waged simultaneously on multiple fronts. Duesberg maintains a frenetic pace, juggling reporters and visitors between poring over the latest AIDS publications and preparing his latest rebuttals. Though he might not agree with much that Anthony Fauci has to say, he would doubtless concur with one prediction that the NIH scientist made back in 1989: "I am probably going to be answering Peter Duesberg for the rest of my life."[117]

Causation and Credibility

The story told in part one—the story of the early search for the cause of AIDS, the initial consolidation of the HIV hypothesis, and the challenges subsequently posed to that hypothesis—has important implications for the study of scientific fact-making in politicized environments. The construction of belief about the causes of AIDS, and the dynamics of controversy, cannot be understood through an analysis of the "scientific field" as traditionally understood—as a self-contained arena in which credentialed researchers are the only important actors. Rather, a highly public and somewhat "open" field has been the site of incessant struggle, negotiation, cooperation, and interaction among a variety of individuals, institutions, and organizations. What are the tactics by which credibility is advanced or attacked in this field? What are the distinctive characteristics of the attempts to resolve controversy in this case?

CREDIBILITY TACTICS

In an analysis of scientific controversy, Collins and Pinch have suggested that it can be useful to distinguish between struggles waged in what they call the "constitutive forum" and those that are enacted in the "contingent forum." The constitutive forum is the world in which scientific knowledge-production is traditionally believed to unfold—the world of "scientific theorising and experiment and corresponding publication and criticism in the learned journals." The contingent forum, by contrast, includes everything that is supposedly "external" to real science: "popular and semi-popular journals, discussion and gossip, fund raising and publicity seeking, the setting up and joining of professional organisations, the corralling of student followers," and so forth. Collins and Pinch's point is emphatically not that one domain is "scientific" while the other is "extra-scientific." Rather, they seek to show how scientific debates are advanced through recourse to different types of arguments, some of which seek to create the appearance of being "based on universalisable non-contingent premises," while others do not.[118]

Clearly, the AIDS causation controversy has heavily depended on both modes of argumentation. Working within the constitutive forum, AIDS dissenters such as Duesberg have highlighted inconsistencies in the orthodox position, enumerated predictions that have not been fulfilled, pointed to violations of "classical methods" such as Koch's postulates, and made use of medical analogies that compare the conventional wisdom about AIDS to that of other diseases "mistakenly" thought to be caused by microbes. In response, the proponents of the orthodox position have spelled out specific lines of rebuttal, defended the mainstream position through "clarifications" and auxiliary hypotheses, and invoked their own medical analogies that compared AIDS to other conditions where Koch's postulates have not been satisfied. In Susan Leigh Star's terms, both sides have manipulated "hierarchies of credibility" through "claims that one procedure or approach is more scientifically viable, or technically astute, than another." [119]

At the same time, scientists and medical doctors, not to mention lay participants in the controversy, have been quick to employ the contingent forum to assail the credibility of their opponents. Their mechanisms for doing so have been surprisingly familiar, as revealed by a comparison with the controversy in the 1970s and 1980s over fluoridating public water supplies. In that controversy, as Brian Martin's analysis makes clear, the mainstream position has enjoyed a near-monopoly of scientific credibility, but dissenters have found ways to undercut the credibility of their opponents. [120]

Certainly the most obvious tactic available to the dominant group in such controversies is to try to ignore their opponents—as scientists successfully did with Sonnabend but had more trouble doing with Duesberg. When this tactic fails, the dominant group is typically confronted with the question of whether or not to engage in public debate. Defenders of fluoridation expressed the same sorts of concerns that Fauci and others did about debating Duesberg. One fluoridation enthusiast wrote in the *American Journal of Public Health*: "A debate simply serves to give more credibility to fluoridation opponents." As Martin has observed, experts who refuse to debate risk being perceived as arrogant, yet simply by engaging in debate they risk undercutting their own expert status by being viewed as partisans. Scientists supporting the dominant position walk a tightrope in trying to retain both their scientific credibility and their moral authority. [121]

In the AIDS causation controversy, as in that over fluoridation, actors on all sides have sought to undermine claims by venting ad hominem attacks against their opponents. In doing so, they have attempted to tarnish their opponents' credibility by challenging either their expert status or their motivations or both. As Martin has noted, supporters of the mainstream position tend to work especially hard to attack the credibility of those opponents who have the most legitimate credentials; [122] and the intensity and range of criticism directed at Duesberg—that he's just a chemist, that he's never worked on human diseases, that it's all a "game" with him and "he has to know he's wrong" [123]—would seem to bear out the general point. Although "more than one can play the game of attacking the credentials, motivations, and honesty of those with opposite views," Martin has said in reference to fluoridation, the majority position tends to win this "battle over reputation in an overwhelming fashion because they have the preponderance of professional support and especially the backing of professional societies." [124]

In the case of AIDS, defenders of the HIV hypothesis could point not only to all the prominent national and international organizations that agreed that HIV causes AIDS (as Gallo, for example, was apt to do), but could even invoke the general consensus among grassroots activists, who were themselves typically critical of established authority. As ACT UP member Michael Botkin wrote in his column in the *Bay Area Reporter,* what "bugged" him about the fans of Duesberg was "the way they completely ignore the opinion of the AIDS movement." Noted Botkin: "ACT UP is no dupe of either the federal government or the medical mainstream. Everyone loves a good conspiracy theory, and certainly it's easy to believe that the government is blind, incompetent and corrupt. But if Duesberg's theory has some substance to it, why hasn't it garnered some interest, if not support, in the savvy, skeptical AIDS movement?" [125] This move on Botkin's part might be described as the "monopolization of oppositional credibility."

Some of the most powerful weapons available to the defenders of the dominant position in scientific controversies are the sanctions they can exercise against dissenters. Through control over professional organizations, funding institutions, and journals, they can suppress heretical views and even punish those who dare voice them. Martin has recorded a variety of examples in the case of fluoridation. When a Minnesota dentist spoke out against fluoridation, his local dental society suspended him for one year without giving him a chance to speak in his own defense. In 1964, when a U.S. sociology student conducted a survey of a group of doctors and discovered that only half the respondents favored fluoridation, the student reportedly was chewed out by an assistant dean "for abusing the good name of her school." An Australian chemistry professor claimed in 1973 that "his staff and equipment had been taken away because of his public opposition to fluoridation." When an article critical of fluoridation was submitted to an Australian journal, it was rejected over the telephone by an editor who claimed "it might encourage the antifluoridationists." [126]

Arguably, these examples are reminiscent of the experiences of Duesberg. The Berkeley scientist has indeed had increasing difficulty getting his views represented in prominent scientific journals, while some of the comments by reviewers and editors have suggested that political considerations (such as protecting the journal's reputation)

have been one factor in the process. He has seen his funding terminated in circumstances that invited suspicion. And he has reported
being ostracized by his colleagues and former friends. At the same
time, as Martin has pointed out, dissenters in scientific controversies
can use such experiences of "unjustifiable" scientific behavior as "a
resource in their struggle": "Opponents of fluoridation frequently
raise these cases of 'suppression' as showing the political rather than
the scientific basis for the promotion of fluoridation." [127]

Criticizing instances of suppression and gatekeeping is one example
of a more general tactic that both sides in the causation controversy
have employed—what Martin has described as "highlighting discrep-
ancies between the stated norms of scientific behavior and the actual
behavior of certain scientists." [128] Duesberg has made frequent reference to the charges of fraud that have been brought against Gallo,
while opponents of Duesberg have argued that, by speaking to a lay
audience, he has sacrificed his scientific integrity. And each side has
accused the other of a dogmatism that is antithetical to the true spirit
of scientific inquiry: their predictions have been falsified, their arguments have holes in them, yet they refuse to forswear their beliefs. "A
powerful hypothesis has to explain and predict," dissenter Harvey Bialy has told *Spin:* "I ask you, what kind of scientist continues to support a hypothesis that fails to explain and fails to predict?" [129] Writing
in the *San Francisco Chronicle,* Martin Delaney has turned the argument back against Duesberg: "Duesberg is well aware of [contrary]
evidence, having been briefed regularly by his faculty peers. Yet he
clings to his views, in spite of any and all data, while presenting no
original AIDS-related data of his own, a puzzling pattern for someone
who claims devotion to science." [130]

MAINSTREAM AND ALTERNATIVE MEDIA

The extensive participation of the media has had important consequences for how credibility struggles have been waged
in the AIDS causation controversy. Of course, the media are not
monolithic, and different sorts of media have played different kinds
of roles. The gay press has been far more receptive to giving space
to nonmainstream positions and to citing the noncredentialed as legitimate experts. Alternative news vehicles like *Spin,* the *New York
Native,* and the Meditel television programs have themselves become
important actors in the controversy, intent on advancing certain

positions and demoting others. But as a general rule, the media, by their very presence, have transformed the collective assessment of credibility.

According to Anthony Fauci, "the media are great equalizers in science, which is most disturbing to us scientists"; "any scientist quoted in the media becomes an 'expert.'" Because Duesberg was presented by the media as credible, many people became concerned that the HIV hypothesis is a hoax, Fauci explained, adding that his own sister had called him repeatedly to ask: "Are you sure he's wrong?" [131] Journalistic norms of "balance" impelled reporters to present the controversy as having "two sides"; media consumers, unable to judge for themselves the relative solidity of consensus among AIDS researchers, assumed controversy was rampant. [132]

Martin Delaney, along with other defenders of the established position, has emphasized the penchant for sensationalism and sympathy for anti-establishment views found among at least some journalists and publishers. Yet to dissenters like Duesberg and Jad Adams, the problem is precisely the opposite: the media are the obedient lapdogs of government science. As Duesberg put it: "The press has been functioning like *this* [taps tape recorder] for the AIDS establishment. They have been Sonys. . . . Fauci calls the press and there it goes in the *New York Times* and the *Los Angeles Times*. Front page. No Fumento balancing it, no second guy writing what you have said. [They] speak directly to the American public. Immediately. That's the difference." [133] Duesberg's critics complain vehemently about the amount of ink that the media have devoted to him, but Duesberg's perspective is completely the reverse: "I mean, measure it against the . . . 1,000 [articles] on the virus hypothesis that the *New York Times* alone publishes a year. . . . You will have a factor of like 1,000 . . . to one . . . in their favor. And that's how it works in the propaganda business. That's why Goebbels and others were so successful." In Britain, Duesberg has acknowledged, the media have been more critical, as have been some alternative reporters in the United States like Farber and Lauritsen. But in general the United States "is actually extremely conformist in many ways," Duesberg has complained. [134]

Various analysts have claimed that reporters covering science and medicine—who often fail to have a thorough grasp of the scientific principles at stake—can become especially dependent on their contacts. [135] "Such symbiosis between journalist and source is common in the American media," according to an analysis by Rae Goodell, "but especially intense in science reporting." [136] One study of U.S. media coverage of the potential swine flu epidemic found that "in spite of the many hundreds of experts who might have been contacted for comment, the same group of medical spokespeople from government authorities was quoted to the virtual exclusion of anyone else." [137] Duesberg has claimed that the same phenomenon is at work in AIDS reporting. Because journalists are so dependent on their official sources, they decline to cover nonmajority views out of fear of being "frozen out": "They won't get further information on the subject from the mainstream. . . . And then they're out." After all, he has said, "without AIDS, you can't be a science reporter these days." [138]

"My regard for science reporters is very, very low," Duesberg has concluded; and that's one thing that he, Gallo, and Fauci would all seem to agree on.[139] Yet everyone in the AIDS causation controversy also recognizes the singular importance of playing to the media. In explaining why most people accept the orthodox position, Duesberg told *California Monthly*: "Science is really now a popularity contest, made by newspapers. You hype something in the press, and people take it from there." [140] Duesberg was being critical, but of course, he has played the same game; and he had little choice but to do so if he wanted to advance his claims in the controversy.

DEMOCRACY AS RHETORIC AND REALITY

Perhaps the most important factor altering the grounds for credibility in the AIDS causation controversy is the deeply embedded concern with "democracy"—understood in various ways. The most obvious examples of this preoccupation relate to questions of "academic freedom" or "freedom of thought." Duesberg's supporters routinely insisted upon his "right to speak the truth"; a *San Francisco Examiner* editorial blasting Duesberg nonetheless acknowledged his "right to air his view even in the face of nearly unanimous scientific disapproval." [141] A more profound democratizing claim, also pushed by some of the HIV dissenters, is that the scientific marketplace must be opened up to *all* those who seek to compete within it. "The 'AIDS establishment' is under the impression that it has a right to govern all discourse on AIDS," complained Celia Farber in *Spin*. "It feels no one has any business disrupting its conclusions and treatment strategies. But don't all those AIDS posters remind us, 'AIDS is everybody's disease'? Doesn't that include the people who question those who made the posters? Isn't it everyone's debate, too?" [142]

This is a very different kind of claim, one which proposes that science ought to be opened up to anyone who seeks to present knowledge as credible or evaluate the credibility of others. Ironically, even Duesberg has had his doubts about such a project and would reserve science for the scientists. "I'm not *excluding* anybody else," Duesberg has hastened to add. "It would be great if others would participate too, but they're too easily misled or bought. I mean, [scientists] give them a slide . . . and it shows something with T-cells . . . and people say, 'Oh my god, these guys must know everything.' And so you can easily impact a gay activist or counteractivist by this type of information without telling them anything. . . ." [143] There may indeed be limits to the extent that lay activists can contribute to answering questions such as what causes AIDS. At the same time, there is no avoiding the astonishingly public and contested nature of biomedical science in the late twentieth century, particularly in the AIDS epidemic. Like many of his mainstream critics, Duesberg would have us return to a mythical golden age when researchers did their work in peace, protected from the play of "politics." Yet his own interventions have helped to open the gates to the citadel—and the ordinary people who have gotten the chance to step inside are not likely to surrender that prerogative.

FROM CAUSATION TO TREATMENT

The democratizing claims of laypeople, while surfacing regularly in the causation controversies, have been even more pronounced in the evolution of debates about treatments for AIDS. These debates, the topic of part two, have been enacted concurrently with the causation controversies, and they involve some of the same protagonists; indeed, references in past chapters to topics such as AZT, which feature prominently in part two, suggest a certain overlap. More profoundly, the intervention of laypeople, particularly within gay communities, in debates about the nature and causation of AIDS from 1981 onward helped construct "knowledge-empowered" communities that could then participate in even more radical ways in debates about treatments.

Yet in certain respects, research into treatment is different from the sort of research involved in determining the cause of AIDS. Since drugs cannot be tested without patients willing to participate in clinical trials, laypeople occupy a central position in the very process of knowledge-making. And since the approval of drugs is often a highly politicized process involving government agencies, pharmaceutical companies, and other players, debates about the safety and efficacy of treatments travel with particular ease between the pages of scientific publications, the mass media, and—in the case of AIDS—activist publications and the gay and lesbian press. The chapters that follow track the history of research into antiviral AIDS drugs and explore the crucial role of AIDS activists in transforming themselves into experts who could speak credibly about treatments. The interventions of the AIDS movement have had profound implications for the social construction of belief—for what we come to think is true about the safety and efficacy of antiviral drugs.

PART 2

THE POLITICS
OF TREATMENT

CHAPTER 5

POINTS OF
DEPARTURE

Targeting a Retrovirus (1984–1986)

April 24, 1984: A triumphant Margaret Heckler, secretary of health and human services, announced to the expectant reporters assembled at a Washington, D.C., press conference that the cause of AIDS had been found. This report of a virus linked to AIDS ushered in a new wave of debates—about who should receive credit for the discovery of the putative causal agent, which practices were most responsible for its transmission, and whether a retroviral causation was indeed sufficiently proven. But the general acceptance of the retroviral hypothesis of AIDS causation had still other implications that were both immediate and far reaching. Up until that point, medical treatment of people with AIDS had been aimed at controlling, as well as possible, the opportunistic infections and cancers that progressively devastated the bodies of immune-suppressed individuals. These were stopgap measures, at best—not only because many of the opportunistic diseases were difficult to treat, but also because each infection that subsided would generally be replaced by yet another. Lacking an understanding of the fundamental causes of immunosuppression, biomedical science had little hope of reversing the downward course of illness.

The discovery of Luc Montagnier's "LAV," Robert Gallo's "HTLV-III," and Jay Levy's "ARV" instantly changed the scientific agenda for AIDS research. Suddenly it became possible to use a new vocabulary, one with words like "cure" and "vaccine." Perhaps the most extreme reactions came from politicians with a vested interest in promoting a triumphalist (and nationalist) account of scientific progress. A blood test for the virus would be available in a few months and a vaccine to prevent AIDS would be developed and ready for testing in about two years, announced Secretary Heckler, to the visible discomfort of some of the prominent scientists with her on the podium.[1]

In fact, there were no insurmountable obstacles to the development of the blood test for antibodies to HTLV-III, which was licensed by the Food and Drug Administration (FDA) in just under a year. But those more familiar with the inherent difficulties of vaccine research knew that scientists had succeeded in designing reasonably effective prophylactic vaccines against only a dozen viral illnesses. The most recent such vaccine, against hepatitis B, had taken most of a decade to bring to market. Dr. Anthony Fauci, head of the National Institute of Allergy and Infectious Diseases (NIAID) of the National Institutes of Health (NIH), quickly sought to dispel illusions and dampen inflated expectations. "To be perfectly honest," he told the New York Times a few days after the press conference, "we don't have any idea how long it's going to take to develop a vaccine, if indeed we will be able to develop a vaccine."[2]

A similar degree of uncertainty combined with high hopes surrounded the investigation of treatments for those already suffering from AIDS. The public and the media spoke of "cures," a term which conjured up images of a penicillin-like drug that would quickly and efficiently rid the body of the invading microorganism. But unlike the bacteria and fungi that antibiotics treat, viruses—from the common ones, like the cold virus, to the rare and deadly ones, like Ebola—have seldom proven amenable to medical intervention. Viruses insinuate themselves into cellular DNA—the genetic code in the cell's nucleus— transforming infected body cells into factories for the production of more virus. To rid the body of a virus, therefore, requires eliminating every infected body cell without killing uninfected body cells—and scientists in 1984 had little to no idea about how such a task might be accomplished with HTLV-III. Indeed, at the time that the virus was discovered, only *three* antiviral agents of any kind were licensed for use in the United States, and none of them was entirely effective: amantadine, a drug used against influenza A; vidarabine, which was used against various viral infections of the eye; and acyclovir, a drug used for treating the herpes simplex virus.[3]

THE LOGIC OF TREATMENT

The search for a treatment against an infectious agent can proceed according to a clear theoretical logic or a hit-and-miss pragmatism. At one extreme, researchers may use their knowledge of the pathogen and the disease process to synthesize a novel compound that will target the pathogen or interrupt the pathogenesis (the development of disease). If the newly synthesized drug acts against the infectious agent in vitro and proves to be not too toxic in animal testing, then it can be tried in humans to see if the theoretically predicted effect is observable in practice. At the other extreme, researchers may simply "see what works" by taking existing drugs whose potential efficacy seems plausible (for example, drugs with known antiviral activity) and adding them to a test tube containing the infectious agent. Such evidence of activity of a drug against a pathogen in vitro is no guarantee, to be sure, that the drug will have any effect on a disease process inside of a living human being or that the human being will be able to tolerate the drug. But it is a good way of screening for promising therapeutic agents.

Since it takes time to synthesize new compounds, and since biomedical researchers knew little about the structure, properties, or life cycle of what would come to be called the human immunodeficiency virus (HIV), hit-and-miss pragmatism was the more likely pathway to quick results. But researchers did possess one crucial fact from the outset that could guide them in the selection of likely agents for testing: they believed they were dealing with a *retro*virus, composed not of DNA, like most viruses, but RNA. An ordinary DNA virus enters the nucleus of an infected cell and causes the cell to carry out the genetic instructions encoded in the virus's DNA; it transcribes its DNA into RNA, which is then assembled into proteins that form a new virus. But before a retrovirus can integrate itself into the nucleus of an infected cell and replicate, it first has to convert its RNA into DNA—to rewrite its own genetic code "backwards" in a process called reverse transcription.[4] To complete that process, the virus relies on an enzyme it produces, called *reverse transcriptase;* this enzyme, in other words, is absolutely essential to the process of viral replication. Inhibit the reverse transcriptase and you inhibit the viral spread: You don't "cure" the patient in the sense of ridding the body of already infected cells and restoring a functioning immune system, but you do—at least in theory—prevent the virus from going on to infect new cells. This treatment strategy made particular sense if you assumed, as many researchers did, a straightforward model of how HIV caused immune system damage: if AIDS was the long-term result of HIV's *direct cytopathic* (cell-killing) effects on helper T cells (also called CD4 cells), then stopping the virus in its tracks should prevent the virus from killing more such cells, thereby keeping the immune system from deteriorating further.[5]

It didn't take long for both National Cancer Institute (NCI) scientists and those connected with the Pasteur Institute in France to pursue this promising lead. In October 1984, a group of NCI researchers including Gallo and Samuel Broder, the director of the NCI, published an article in *Science* describing their in vitro studies with a drug called suramin, which was "known to inhibit the reverse transcriptase of a number of retroviruses."[6] Suramin had been developed by the Bayer Company in Germany more than half a century ago, and, though never licensed in the United States, it had been used extensively in Africa and South America for the treatment of certain parasitic diseases. The NCI researchers found that when suramin was added to HTLV-III in the test tube, the virus became incapable of infecting and killing helper T cells.

Meanwhile, collaborators of Montagnier in France, having made similar assumptions about the logic of treating AIDS, began giving a compound directly to patients—antimoniotungstate, or HPA-23, which was known to incapacitate the reverse transcriptase of certain retroviruses that infect mice.[7] By February 1985, they could offer a brief report in *Lancet* on a fifteen-day course of treatment with four patients. Comparing the before-and-after assays showed that the drug regimen appeared successful in curtailing the replication of LAV.

But the French researchers also had some words of caution against assuming any easy successes in the fight against AIDS. Even though "infection with LAV seems to be an essential step in the pathogenesis of AIDS," nonetheless a drug that acted against the virus "may not be able to cure the disease." This might be because antiviral therapy came too late, after the virus had already done irreparable damage to the immune system. Or it might be that the pathways from infection to development of AIDS involved more than just direct cell-killing. Perhaps LAV infection instigated "autoimmune mechanisms"—failures of the immune system to distinguish between body cells and invaders, leading the immune system to turn on itself and target other immune cells. In that case, "AIDS could prove to be self-perpetuating even in the face of inhibition of LAV multiplication."[8] Even if a compound like HPA-23 were eventually proven to be a safe and effective antiviral agent—even if it could be administered to humans in a clinically effective dose, even if its side effects proved tolerable, and even if the initial, promising results could be confirmed in controlled clinical trials with large numbers of patients—it still might not be sufficient to keep AIDS patients alive. "An antiviral won't be the miracle, but it will be absolutely obligatory," Jean Claude Chermann, one of the study coauthors and one of the discoverers of LAV, told *Newsweek* in April.[9]

That month, more than two thousand researchers from thirty countries converged on Atlanta to attend the first of what would become an annual milestone: the International Conference on AIDS.[10] Researchers in the United States and Europe reported at the conference that testing had begun, or was about to begin, with six drugs in small numbers of patients. These drugs, all of which had been found to have some inhibitory effect on the virus in the test tube, included suramin and HPA-23, as well as ribavirin, an antiviral drug made by a small Southern California pharmaceutical company.

Such studies were just the initial step on the long, uphill path to the marketing of a new drug in the United States.[11] With the passage of the Pure Food and Drug Act in 1906 and the Food, Drug, and Cosmetic Act in 1938, the FDA had been empowered to require that drug manufacturers submit evidence from "adequate tests" showing that a drug was safe, before it could be licensed for sale. Since safety was a relative term, the FDA was expected to assess risk and benefits, which implied making some additional determination of whether the drug was indeed effective. In 1962, in response to public uproar after the drug thalidomide was found to cause birth defects, Congress passed an amendment to the Food, Drug, and Cosmetic Act called the Kefauver-Harris amendment. (Thalidomide had never been licensed in the United States, but some pregnant women participating in studies had received it.) Although the issue with thalidomide was one of safety, the effect of the Kefauver-Harris amendment was to shift the emphasis of drug regulation more heavily in the direction of requiring formal, scientific proof of efficacy.[12]

As Harry Marks has described, by the early 1970s, "with the growth in influence of the National Institutes of Health and the rise of biostatistics as a distinct discipline . . . , the nature and methods of drug evaluation had achieved a form of scientific and bureaucratic orthodoxy."[13] Usually, the FDA asked for evidence from at least three "phases" of randomized clinical trials in human subjects performed sequentially: a small Phase I trial to study the drug's toxicity and determine a good dosage for drug absorption; a larger, longer Phase II trial to test the drug's efficacy; and a still larger Phase III trial to bolster the evidence of efficacy in comparison with other treatments for the condition. Each of these studies required planning, recruiting of subjects, careful monitoring, and interpretation and write-up; and the FDA often took its own good time to reach its conclusions, which it made on the basis of recommendations from expert advisory panels. Typically, it might take a drug six or eight years to leap the regulatory hurdles. Critics pointed to the paltry number of drugs that made it to market in the post-Kefauver-Harris environment and argued that U.S. standards were unjustifiably higher than those of other countries. Consumer protectionists responded that U.S. standards were appropriately high, since many countries around the world couldn't afford to perform elaborate drug tests and therefore relied on the FDA to determine what was safe and effective.

Just like medications, any potential vaccine against AIDS would have to pass through extensive testing that included various phases of clinical trials, before the FDA licensed its use. But as reports at the International Conference made clear, even Phase I trials were still a long way off. Researchers had, however, begun identifying "subunits" of the virus that might serve to generate a protective immune response. Using parts of the virus, it was generally assumed, was a safer strategy than using the whole virus: researchers could induce an immune response without having to worry about the risk of accidentally infecting the healthy vaccine recipient. One problem, however, was the recent discovery—Gallo called it "worrisome"—of considerable genetic variation among different strains of the virus.[14] This raised the question of whether any particular subunit could generate protection against every strain. "We have a long way to go before AIDS is preventable or treatable," Dr. Martin Hirsch of Massachusetts General Hospital concluded in reviewing the conference, "but the first steps have been taken, and we are on our way."[15]

THE GENESIS OF TREATMENT ACTIVISM

Observers in gay and lesbian communities had other, more critical perceptions of the International Conference and the depth of the scientific and political commitment to finding treatments for AIDS. Secretary Heckler's statement at the conference regarding the nation's priorities was widely reported—that AIDS must be stopped "before it spreads to the heterosexual community." Commentators familiar with other scientific conferences observed some distinctive aspects of this one: "The meeting was unusual for the remarkable mixture of participants—doctors and scientists of almost every discipline rubbing elbows with gay activists and media personalities," said the newsletter of the Bay Area Physicians for Human Rights, the gay doctors' group: "The unlikely combinations led to comments about 'strange bedfellows,' but there is no proof of the reality of that phrase."[16]

Moments of levity notwithstanding, this was a threatening time for gay communities. With the availability of the HTLV-III antibody test, many would soon be learning for the first time that they were infected with the virus and faced with an uncertain future. At the same time, as the epidemic became more of a mainstream issue in the United States following reports of actor Rock Hudson's AIDS illness, fears of contagion on the part of the mass public multiplied, leading in many instances to stigmatization of homosexuals, whether healthy or ill. Gay rights and AIDS advocacy organizations feared that those testing positive for viral antibodies would be subject to discrimination, including loss of their jobs, housing, health insurance, and anonymity. In March 1985, the conservative commentator William F. Buckley Jr. proposed, in a notorious *New York Times* op-ed piece, that "everyone detected with AIDS should be tattooed in the upper forearm to protect common-needle users, and on the buttocks, to prevent the victimization of other homosexuals. . . ."[17]

The activist response to AIDS by gays and lesbians dated to the earliest days of the epidemic (see chapter 1). It rested on the firm base of gay rights activism constructed in the previous decade, with its sex-positive ethic and its suspicious take on medical claims.[18] Now, in response to the new wave of provocations, many who had kept themselves at arm's length from such activism suddenly found themselves drawn into the fray. For a generation of relatively privileged, middle-class gay men, government had been something to restrict, to keep out of their "private" lives. As the boundary between private illness and public health exploded, these same men sought active governmental involvement to fund emergency AIDS research and to protect people with AIDS against discriminatory treatment.[19] However, such assistance was far from the top of the agenda of the Reagan administration, which consistently requested modest funds for AIDS research only to see Congress boost the amounts on its own initiative. Lesbians, often radicalized by feminism in general and influenced by the feminist health movement of the 1970s in particular, also mobilized in increasing numbers, frequently assuming leadership roles in AIDS struggles.[20]

While the mainstream national gay rights organizations focused on issues of discrimination and budget appropriations, new voices emerged on the horizon. People with AIDS and their supporters discovered in early 1985 that ribavirin, one of the experimental drugs reported to inhibit reverse transcriptase, was available for two dollars a box in the *farmacias* of Mexico's border towns. Soon a steady stream of couriers were running shipments of ribavirin, along with an unapproved immune-boosting drug called isoprinosine, past U.S. customs and from there to AIDS patients all over the United States.[21]

Elsewhere, wealthy gay men with connections found other pathways to therapies reported to have potential benefit. "There are some Americans in Paris these days who are not so much interested in abstract art or avant-garde literature as they are in saving their own lives," wrote *Newsweek* in August, a week after Rock Hudson became the most prominent "AIDS exile" to seek treatment with HPA-23.[22] Embarrassed by stories of the "AIDS exiles," the FDA announced that it would permit the administration of HPA-23, along with the other antiviral AIDS drugs that had entered testing, on a "compassionate use" basis—a long-standing FDA mechanism for releasing experimental drugs on a case-by-case basis when requested by physicians for their terminally ill patients, in situations where no standard therapy is available. But the FDA spokesperson struggled to explain that the decision to permit compassionate use was in no way meant to suggest that HPA-23 actually *worked*. "There is no proven treatment for AIDS yet," he emphasized. "Everyone is assuming that this is a panacea, and there is none."[23] The French, meanwhile, had been forced to discontinue HPA-23 in some patients because of its toxic effects on the blood and the liver.[24]

The availability of drugs in other countries, however, only inclined the new AIDS activists to press for easier access by U.S. patients to a range of experimental compounds. Martin Delaney, at this time a Bay Area business consultant, former seminary student, and current ribavirin "smuggler," emerged as a key voice in these debates. "We don't know for sure how these drugs will work," Delaney told a community forum in the Castro district, the heart of San Francisco's gay community. "But it makes more sense than the next best thing, which is dying without trying anything." In October, Delaney held a press conference to announce the opening of a new organization, Project Inform, which would conduct studies to determine the benefits of experimental drugs being used in the community, like ribavirin and isoprinosine. "No matter what the medical authorities say, people are using these drugs," Delaney told reporters skeptical of the idea of community-based research. "What we want to do is provide a safe, monitored environment to learn what effects they are having."[25]

Some years back, Delaney himself had participated in an experimental trial of a drug to treat chronic hepatitis. The drug had cured his hepatitis but left him with permanent damage to the nerves in his feet. Delaney considered it a fair bargain; but the drug was thought too toxic, the trial was terminated, and the treatment never approved. It was an experience that would color Delaney's response to the AIDS epidemic.[26] Who should decide what risks a patient can assume—the doctor or the patient?

RIGHTS, RISKS, AND ETHICS

The extensive literature on the ethics of clinical research[27] reflects considerable emphasis on protection of human subjects in biomedical experimentation. This, however, is a rather recent development that has paralleled the rise in importance of the randomized clinical trial both in biomedical fact-making and in regulatory decision making.[28] As historian David Rothman has described, the pivotal moment occurred in 1966 with the *New England Journal of Medicine*'s publication of a whistle-blowing review article by Henry Beecher, replete with disturbing, recent examples of unethical and potentially harmful experimental research. Beecher catalogued incidents of "investigators who had risked 'the health or the life of their subjects' without informing them of the dangers or obtaining their permission"—for example, withholding penicillin from servicemen with streptococcal infections as part of a study of an alternative therapy.[29] These revelations were followed a few years later by public outrage and congressional hearings in response to news media disclosures about the Tuskegee syphilis study, conducted openly for decades under the auspices of the U.S. Public Health Service, in which hundreds of poor, black sharecroppers were denied existing treatment so that researchers could study the "natural history" of the disease.[30] In 1974 Congress created the National Commission for the Protection of Human Subjects, which issued guidelines on research. In addition, the

NIH began requiring that each research center seeking federal funds for biomedical research on human subjects establish an "institutional review board" to evaluate the ethics of each proposed research "protocol" (the plan for the study).[31]

As Rothman and Harold Edgar have noted, the irony in these protective measures and in the new regulatory regime at the FDA was that they ran counter to the egalitarian and libertarian trends of the 1960s and 1970s in general and to the critique of paternalistic medicine in particular. "Just when patients secured greater autonomy—the right to know a diagnosis, to accept or refuse treatment—the experts at the FDA and review boards controlled the right to regulate new drugs and research protocols."[32] Soon AIDS patients and their advocates began rebelling against what they saw as well-intentioned but deadly paternalism. Activists like Delaney would exert a demand for greater patient autonomy by challenging medical authority from two directions at once. On one hand, they would insist that patients interested in trying experimental drugs should have the right to assume risks rather than endure the benevolent protection of the authorities. On the other hand, they would criticize certain approved and accepted research methods, like trials in which some patients received placebos, characterizing them as unethical for subjecting patients to unfair risks that the patients *did not* want to assume.

THE STATE OF THE ART, 1985

As virologists and molecular biologists learned more about the life cycle of the virus, researchers began to speculate about other ways of halting its replication, besides interfering with reverse transcription. NCI researchers analyzed the different points of attack in an article published in September in *Cancer Research.*[33] First, in order to infect a cell and begin replicating, the outer proteins of the virus (called the "envelope") had to bind to the surface of the cell. Perhaps this binding could be blocked through the use of antibodies; but since most AIDS patients produced antibodies to HTLV-III and became ill nonetheless, it might be that such antibodies were insufficiently protective. Second, after binding to the cell surface, the virus "enters the target cell by an as yet unknown mechanism." If this mechanism could be identified, perhaps entry could be blocked. Third, after reverse transcription and integration of the viral DNA into the nucleus of the host cell, the virus proceeded to manufacture new viral proteins. The authors noted that this transcription process appeared to be boosted by a protein, the product of a recently discovered viral gene called *tat* (for "transactivation"), a gene not found in other known retroviruses. A drug that interfered with this protein might also be an effective antiviral agent. Finally, the new viral proteins were processed and assembled into a fully formed new virus, which was released from the cell by budding. "Our knowledge of these steps is rudimentary at best," the NCI researchers acknowledged, though "interferons have been shown to inhibit the release of other retroviruses. . . ."

While this was all very nice in theory, the NCI researchers concluded that the best immediate bet remained the reverse transcriptase inhibitors, like suramin. Unfortunately, the early reports on suramin, based on a small Phase I toxicity study by NCI and NIAID, were proving to be mixed at best. The drug did seem to reduce viral replication in vivo as it had in vitro. But "it did not produce clinical or immunological improvement with the regimen used."[34] A larger, Phase II trial would be needed to find out more about the efficacy of the drug. But the concerns about suramin were quickly confirmed a few months into the Phase II study. The drug was far too toxic: it appeared to have caused adrenal failure in several patients and may have hastened some patients' deaths.[35] Later, some treatment activists would claim that the study had been poorly monitored and had subjected its participants to needless risk.[36] The principal investigators, on the other hand, would offer the suramin study both as a cautionary tale and "as an example of how a clinical trial should be conducted": "Trials such as this one . . . prevent potentially harmful drugs from being distributed to large numbers of patients in the community."[37]

Those skeptical about the viral hypothesis (see part one) interpreted the ongoing difficulties with treatment research as evidence of the inadequacies of the reigning causal models. "If we have agents that effectively inhibit the replication of this virus," said New York physician Dr. Joseph Sonnabend in a *New York Native* interview in October 1985, "but [those agents] make no impact on the course of this disease, I think it will make apparent, for some people, the actual role of HTLV-III in causing this disease."[38] But research and media attention continued to focus on antiretroviral agents, and in early 1986, NCI researchers found themselves with a potential success on their hands.

"WAITING FOR THE RIGHT DISEASE"

Samuel Broder, the head of the NCI, had not been putting all his eggs in the suramin basket. In late 1984 he had put out the word to the big pharmaceutical companies (the ones he considered capable of quickly bringing a drug to market): Send us anything you have on the shelf that might inhibit a retrovirus, and we'll do the assay to see if it halts replication of HTLV-III.[39] Burroughs Wellcome, the North Carolina–based subsidiary of a large British firm called Wellcome PLC, submitted ten compounds, and in February 1985 one of Broder's researchers, Hiroaki Mitsuya, found that one of the compounds was a reverse transcriptase inhibitor with strong antiviral activity: azidothymidine, called 3'-Azido-3'-Deoxythymidine in full or just AZT for short.

AZT had a peculiar history. In the early 1960s, a researcher named Jerome Horwitz at the Michigan Cancer Foundation decided to design a drug that would keep cancer cells from duplicating. With funding from the NCI, and working with such unlikely ingredients as herring sperm, Horwitz and his coworkers synthesized a group of compounds called dideoxythymidines that were designed to look like nucleosides, the building blocks of DNA. In theory, these "nucleoside analogues" would substitute themselves for real nucleosides, thereby interfering with formation of DNA molecules. Without more DNA, the cancer cells would simply stop duplicating. In practice, the treatment was a complete failure. Horwitz gave AZT and the other dideoxythymidines to mice with leukemia, but the drugs showed no effect. "My colleagues and I said that we had a very interesting set of compounds that were waiting for the right disease."[40]

Burroughs Wellcome had tested AZT against animal viruses but had dropped this line of inquiry since it was unrewarding. Now, after getting the good news about AZT from Broder, Burroughs Wellcome filed an "IND" (investigational new drug application) with the FDA. Phase I trials began in July 1985 with nineteen U.S. AIDS patients, under the auspices of the NCI and in collaboration with Duke University. Mitsuya announced the results of the six-week study on the last day of an AIDS conference the following January: AZT kept the virus from replicating in fifteen of the nineteen research subjects, boosting their immune systems (as measured by their T-cell counts) and relieving some of their symptoms. "It's not a dream drug," Mitsuya explained in a television interview, stressing the need for additional testing.[41]

The formal publication of the study in *Lancet* in March 1986 spelled out more of the details.[42] Researchers recently had discovered that AIDS was frequently accompanied by neurological impairments, which indicated that the virus was also affecting cells in the brain. An effective therapy, therefore, would have to be capable of crossing a circulatory system defense called the "blood-brain barrier," a feat that many drugs could not accomplish. Fortunately, AZT did appear to cross the blood-brain barrier. In addition, though some subjects had experienced headaches or had developed low white cell counts, the drug could be tolerated relatively well. This was a relief, because AZT "might have been expected to produce intolerable side effects" (in the words of Jean Marx, the reporter for *Science* who described the trial), given the mechanism of drug action.[43] AZT "fooled" the reverse transcriptase enzyme into using it, in place of the nucleoside it imitated, when transcribing the virus's RNA to DNA. Then, once AZT was added to the growing DNA chain, AZT's structure prevented any additional nucleosides from being added on: reverse transcription simply came to a halt at that point, and the virus stopped replicating. But the problem was that since AZT terminated DNA synthesis, one might logically anticipate that it would have harmful effects on the DNA in *healthy* cells.

Having shown initial evidence of relative drug *safety,* the researchers had accomplished the formal objectives of a Phase I trial. But there was nothing to prevent them from reporting the apparent good news about *efficacy*—the news that attracted media attention. "The results also suggest that at least some immunological reconstitution occurred in most of the patients . . . , and that a clinical response was obtained in some." However, these findings had to be treated cautiously, since simply being in a trial "may have a strong placebo effect in influencing such factors as appetite and sense of well-being, and it is even possible that improved nutrition may then induce changes in immune function." Only the next step—a so-called "placebo-controlled" Phase II study, conducted in "double-blind" fashion so that neither the subjects nor the researchers would know who was receiving AZT and who was receiving a placebo (a look-alike dummy pill)—could determine whether the observed clinical improvements were truly due to the drug. (This study would be funded by Burroughs Wellcome and conducted at a number of academic centers, including the University of Miami, where it was under the direction of Dr. Margaret Fischl, and the University of California at San Diego, under Dr. Douglas Richman.) The NCI researchers concluded with a summary of the questions that remained to be answered: "We cannot say whether AZT can be tolerated over a long time, whether viral drug resistance will develop, or ultimately whether AZT will affect disease progression or survival in patients with HTLV-III-induced disease. These are issues which can be resolved only by appropriately controlled long-term studies."[44]

Clinical Trials Take Center Stage (1986–1987)

BECOMING EXPERTS

"The general public, and even most AIDS organizations and activists, do not yet realize that we already have an effective, inexpensive, and probably safe treatment for AIDS." This was the characterization of AZT offered by John James, editor and publisher of a San Francisco–based newsletter called *AIDS Treatment News* (*ATN*), in its third issue, published May 1986. Yet large-scale studies of AZT, James reported, were still several months away from starting, and "if all goes well, your doctor might be able to get AZT in about two years." This was hardly an acceptable time frame in James's view, and he offered a simple justification for his position: "We should point out that ten thousand people are expected to die of AIDS in the next year. And with deaths doubling every year, a little math shows that a two-year delay between when a treatment is known to work and when it becomes available means that three quarters of the deaths which ever occur from the epidemic will have been preventable."[45]

Of course, James's grim logic hinged on the meaning of the deceptively straightforward phrase "when a treatment is known to work": what do we mean by "known," and what do we mean by "work"? As far as James was concerned, though the effects of long-term use indeed remained unknown, it was clear that AZT did *something*. But from the standpoint of researchers—at least when speaking in their official capacities—it was precisely the point of the next round of testing to determine whether AZT in fact worked. Furthermore, as James himself fully realized, the sort of evidence that impressed him would not get Burroughs Wellcome past the front door of the FDA.

A former computer programmer with no formal medical or scientific training, James had just launched what would become the most prominent grassroots AIDS treatment publication in the United States.[46] *ATN* rapidly emerged as a crucial resource for doctors and patients alike; within a year, it had a circulation of thirty-five hundred.[47] The newsletter provided the latest inside word on the up-and-coming drugs as well as the alternative therapies that didn't make it into formal clinical trials. It would go on to engage as well in a sweeping and detailed critique of the federal drug-testing and regulatory enterprise. As Debbie Indyk and David Rier have noted in a study of grassroots AIDS publications like *ATN,* such organs of communication effectively "[circumvent] the assessment of gatekeepers such as [medical journal] reviewers and editors. . . ." The result has been not only that more, and more varied, material has made it "through the net," but that "researchers, clinicians, and patients often confront new data almost simultaneously—sometimes, patients even see it first. . . ."[48]

In those early days, James had another pressing goal—to convince other activists and AIDS organizations that a new task confronted them. Already they had become experts about prevention strategies, antibody testing, antidiscrimination legislation, and the health care delivery system. Now it was time to learn a new set of tricks. "So far, community-based AIDS organizations have been uninvolved in treatment issues, and have seldom followed what is going on," wrote James in a call to arms in that same May 1986 issue. "With independent information and analysis, we can bring specific pressure to bear to get experimental treatments handled properly. So far, there has been little pressure because *we have relied on experts* to interpret for us what is going on. They tell us what will not rock the boat. The companies who want their profits, the bureaucrats who want their turf, and the doctors who want to avoid making waves have all been at the table. The persons with AIDS who want their lives must be there, too [emphasis added]." To "rely solely on official institutions for our information," James bluntly advised, "is a form of group suicide."[49]

Over the following months, James elaborated this strategy for engagement with clinical research. It wasn't that the researchers conducting AIDS clinical trials were evil or incompetent, but that they were "too close to their own specialties and overly dependent on the continued good graces of funding sources" to be capable of generating or publicly communicating an objective assessment of treatment research issues. On the other hand, these researchers were crucial sources of data: "Physicians and scientists already have pieces of the information, and they need someone they can talk to who can put the pieces together and let people know what is going on." There was nothing pie-in-the-sky, James insisted, about proposing that lay activists could become experts themselves: "Non-scientists can fairly easily grasp treatment-research issues; these don't require an extensive background in biology or medicine." [50]

It was the right time to pay attention to the organization of clinical trials. With $100 million in federal funding, the NIH was in the process of setting up a nationwide network of fourteen research centers, dubbed AIDS Treatment Evaluation Units (ATEUs), which sought to enroll an additional one thousand of the nation's ten thousand living AIDS patients in government-sponsored Phase II trials of a select group of drugs, including AZT, foscarnet, HPA-23, and ribavirin. [51] Following the standard NIH procedure for "extramural research" (so called to distinguish it from the NIH's own in-house or "intramural" research), NIH would farm out the work to researchers, mostly at academic centers, who had designed and submitted the study protocols and would serve as the principal investigators for the studies.

But the process of setting up the ATEUs was slow and chaotic. Since HIV was an infectious agent, the National Institute of Allergy and Infectious Diseases, under the leadership of Anthony Fauci, had claimed ownership of AIDS treatment research. NIAID, however, had never organized clinical trials on this scale, and Fauci would soon be subjected to intense criticism by activists for what appeared to be incompetence. If Fauci were less intent on amassing power within the federal health bureaucracy, some suggested, he would have left AIDS treatment research with the NCI, where it began, relying on that institute's proven expertise in organizing large, multisite clinical trials for cancer therapies. [52]

THE GOLD STANDARD

Practically unknown before the Second World War, randomized clinical trials had rapidly, recently, and incontrovertibly become established as the "gold standard" in biomedicine. Such trials are presumed capable of establishing the risks and benefits of new drugs or of weeding out ineffective or dangerous drugs that doctors have prescribed on the basis of anecdotal evidence. Of course, sometimes anecdotal evidence is perfectly adequate: When an antibiotic brings about rapid miracle cures of diseases that are otherwise often fatal, doctors can safely trust the "evidence of their own eyes." But drugs with more marginal, or less rapid, effects are often harder to evaluate. If a patient gets *somewhat* better over the course of a few months, is it the drug that is responsible or some other factor in the patient's life? Randomized clinical trials claimed to take the guesswork out of medical judgments.

These trials, many commentators have noted, are also crucial to the "scientization" of modern medicine—the legitimation of medicine as a fully scientific practice resting not just on the basic biological sciences but on the knowledge base generated by its own, distinct laboratory method.[53] Studies that proceed through the right steps—beginning with the random assignment of patients to either the treatment arm or the control arm—are presumed to generate true knowledge, while those with procedural failings are not. This reification of method, Harry Marks has said in an analysis of the history of such trials, has tended to bracket the *political* judgments that the use of the method necessarily entails: "On what basis do we choose a significance level?" "On what basis do we integrate the findings from a given experiment with the relevant body of theoretical or empirical literature?" And insofar as the use of such trials has encouraged researchers to privilege "trustworthy answers to a simply put question" over "a contestable reply to a more complex inquiry," it has remained unclear whether the *type* of knowledge generated is useful—whether the trials provide meaningful guidance to the doctors, patients, and officials who would use them. In this sense, as Marks has argued, reliance on randomized clinical trial may beg the fundamental policy question: What is the problem to which they are the solution?[54]

By 1986, as many as four hundred thousand to eight hundred thousand U.S. patients were enrolled in such trials every year.[55] The number of clinical trials reported in the scientific literature had grown by 30 percent in the first half of the decade alone, from 3,414 in 1980 to 4,372 in 1985. The practical impact, as Dr. Sidney Wolfe of Ralph Nader's Health Research Group commented in 1986, was that "patients have much greater access to new treatments now than they did a decade ago."[56] But a more subtle consequence of this steady expansion of clinical research was that it had shifted the social meaning of the trials.

To the study investigators and the research establishment, the trials were simply scientific experiments; but in the eyes of those suffering from serious illnesses, controlled clinical trials were an important *means of access* to otherwise unavailable drugs—drugs endowed with the glimmer of scientific promise by simple virtue of their novelty and the fact that they were being studied. So, for example, in December

1985, when the NCI announced a small study of a new experimental cancer treatment using interleukin-2, two thousand people telephoned within two days to find out how to get into the trial.[57] The differing perceptions of the essential purpose of clinical trials would soon put people with AIDS and their representatives on a collision course with the FDA and medical researchers.

"GREAT PROMISE FOR PROLONGING LIFE"

The announcement came on September 20, 1986, after several days of rumors and speculation, and it made front-page news around the country: Margaret Fischl's Phase II trial of AZT had been ended early, after the NIH's Data and Safety Monitoring Board—whose job it was to take periodic "peeks" at trials in progress[58]—concluded that the drug was so effective that it would be unethical to keep the control group on placebos any longer. AZT "holds great promise for prolonging life for certain patients with AIDS," Dr. Robert Windom, the assistant secretary for health, told reporters, adding that he had asked the FDA to consider AZT for licensing as expeditiously as possible.[59] But AZT, Windom also made clear, "is not a cure for AIDS."[60]

The study had been conducted in double-blind fashion with 145 subjects getting AZT and 137 a sugar pill identical in appearance, according to the formal write-up, which appeared in the *New England Journal of Medicine* the following July.[61] All the patients had AIDS or AIDS symptoms, and there was a similar range of T-cell counts in the two arms of the study. At the time the study was terminated, 19 patients in the placebo arm had died. Only 1 patient receiving AZT had died, and this was a remarkable difference. (It was also a *statistically significant* difference: the probability that these results might have occurred by chance was well beneath the accepted statistical threshold of one in twenty.) There had been a total of 45 new opportunistic infections in the placebo arm of the study, versus only 24 in the treatment arm. More problematically, "severe adverse reactions," particularly bone marrow suppression, had been observed in the study: a full 24 percent of the AZT recipients had experienced anemia, and 21 percent required blood transfusions. AZT use also caused nausea, myalgia, insomnia, and severe headaches.[62]

With the support of the NIH and FDA, Burroughs Wellcome announced that it would supply AZT free of charge to any AIDS patient who had suffered an attack of *Pneumocystis carinii* pneumonia, the most deadly of the opportunistic infections, during the past 120 days, pending the drug's formal approval. It would be distributed on a case-by-case basis only through physicians who submitted requests and agreed to supply data to Burroughs Wellcome; and the NIH set up a toll-free number for doctors to call to request the forms to file. Within weeks, after many doctors and people with AIDS protested that these criteria were arbitrary, Burroughs Wellcome agreed to expand the program to include any of the 7,000 people with AIDS who had suffered pneumocystis at any point.[63]

On March 20, 1987, less than three years after the Heckler press conference announcing the discovery of HTLV-III, the FDA approved AZT for use in the 33,000 Americans diagnosed with AIDS, on the basis of a positive recommendation by the panel of experts on the FDA's Anti-Infective Advisory Committee.[64] The drug had proceeded from in vitro studies to full approval in just two years and had been approved without a Phase III study. The United Kingdom, France, and Norway had also licensed AZT in the preceding weeks.

Burroughs Wellcome announced that it would sell its product under the brand name "Retrovir" at a price that would amount to eight thousand to ten thousand dollars per patient each year. The company refused to disclose its profit margins for AZT—a drug that, after all, had been invented by a federally funded cancer researcher in Detroit a quarter-century earlier, had been sitting on Burroughs Wellcome's shelves for years, and then had been shown effective against HIV in vitro by scientists at NCI and Duke University. One pharmaceutical industry analyst quoted in the *New York Times* estimated the profit at up to 40 percent and predicted that Retrovir would soon be "the company's largest contributor to revenue and earnings."[65] It was widely assumed that the price reflected the company's assessment—shared by researchers and conveyed to patients by the media—that the life span of the drug was limited since new and better antiviral drugs would be available soon. In practice the price meant that only rich countries could afford to subsidize it. AZT was—and is—essentially unavailable to all those outside of the so-called first world.

The pricing of AZT was not the only point of controversy. "At least half of all AIDS patients that should be eligible to take the drug either cannot take it at all or must take a lower dose to prevent toxicity," reported a news article in *Science*. (It would later become apparent that the originally prescribed dosage of twelve hundred milligrams per day was unnecessarily high.) "We found it nearly impossible to keep patients on the drug," said Jerome Groopman, a prominent researcher and clinician who tried giving AZT to fourteen patients on a compassionate use basis.[66] "AZT may be a genie that we are letting out of the bottle," Dr. Itzak Brook of the FDA's Anti-Infective Advisory Committee told *Time* magazine in February.[67] Brook had been both the chair of the committee and the sole dissenting vote on the recommendation to license the drug.

In a more formal commentary published in the *Journal of the American Medical Association* (*JAMA*), Brook explained that the committee "recognized that the benefit in very sick patients outweighed the serious toxic effects, but it was concerned by the fact that the long-term efficacy and toxicity are, to date, unknown and require further studies." Moreover, many committee members, according to Brook, were concerned that once the drug was approved, HIV-infected people with mild symptoms or none at all might gain access to the drug (since once a drug is licensed, any physician can prescribe it to a patient, whether or not the patient fits the official "indications"). For mildly symptomatic and asymptomatic patients, there were as yet no data from which to conclude either that the drug had benefits or that the benefits exceeded the risks.[68]

As *Time* suggested, halting the test early and offering the drug to patients in the placebo arm "robbed researchers of the chance to judge, under controlled conditions, any long-range effects of AZT, which might be as dangerous as the treated disease."[69] In fact, as the *Washington Post* had reported, the days before the announcement of the study's outcome had been marked by serious, behind-the-scenes soul searching: some government officials and researchers had been so concerned about the impact that releasing the drug might have on the capacity to conduct future research that they had implored the media not to carry the story about the trial's findings until a policy decision had been reached, lest the publicity itself create irresistible pressure for the release of the drug.[70] But research ethics, political realities, and the prevailing construction of belief precluded any alternative course of action. "I don't see how you can have a placebo group," said Dr. Charles Schable of the Centers for Disease Control (CDC), "because if you're pretty sure it's going to work, why should you not give it to people?"[71]

THE POLITICS OF "INDIFFERENCE"

To use the language preferred by those who are experts on clinical trials, the AZT study was no longer at an "indifference point" (or, it no longer maintained a state of "equipoise"). In order to conduct an ethical experiment on human beings in which one group receives Treatment A and the other receives Treatment B, "the clinical investigator [must] be in a state of genuine uncertainty regarding the comparative merits of treatments A and B." [72] If this precariously balanced state does not hold—if the researcher has good reason to believe that one treatment is superior—then it would be considered unethical to subject either group to the putatively inferior treatment. When the Phase II AZT study began, it was technically at the indifference point: John James's belief that the drug was "known to work" notwithstanding, investigators like Fischl and Richman believed that there were no hard data supporting AZT's efficacy, since the suggestive results from the uncontrolled Phase I trial may simply have been due to a placebo effect and since that trial had lasted for only a few weeks. But once the Data and Safety Monitoring Board had "unblinded" the study to see the results so far, equipoise no longer held: clear statistical evidence showed a treatment difference between the AZT recipients and those given placebos.

The requirement that a trial could be conducted only when a state of equipoise existed was intended to protect the rights of human subjects by imposing an objective standard on the design of medical experimentation. In practice, like many such rules of scientific practice, this one was subject to negotiation and interpretation. After all, any time researchers test a drug, they do so because they have *some* reason to think it might work; indeed, probably few investigators take upon themselves the arduous task of designing and conducting a clinical trial unless, on some "gut level," they believe the study might succeed. At what point, therefore, do reasoned guesswork and personal belief come to violate a state of "genuine uncertainty"? Clearly, there is no firm, universally apparent, dividing line separating equipoise from its absence. So certain was Jonas Salk of the efficacy of his polio vaccine that he opposed conducting a double-blind, placebo-controlled trial, arguing that such a "fetish of orthodoxy" would unnecessarily doom some of those in the placebo group to contracting polio. Other researchers countered that in the absence of such a study, the vaccine would never achieve broad credibility among doctors and scientists. [73]

Inevitably, the assessment of equipoise becomes a *social* and often *political* process, embedded in the complex interactions and negotiations that establish the credibility of treatments in different quarters.[74]

More problematically still, there is no reason to assume that researchers and research subjects will be equally "indifferent" about the potential merits of therapies, or will be indifferent in quite the same way. "It is clear that research subjects may rationally prefer one treatment arm of a randomized clinical trial . . . rather than another even if there is no medical reason for the choice," commented medical ethicist Robert Veatch, pointing to patients' complex evaluations of side effects of drugs and quality-of-life concerns. "Only in the rarest of circumstances will active subjects really be indifferent to the two treatment options if indeed they really understand what these options are."[75]

PLACEBOS UNDER ATTACK

The fact that researchers and research subjects could differ in their understandings of equipoise was unlikely to lead to controversy in comparisons between two active treatments, one old and one new. But comparisons between a potentially active drug and an inert placebo were far more capable of sparking an uproar among patients with a life-threatening disease. The use of placebos in the Phase II AZT trial was one of the first such cases to be criticized by AIDS treatment activists. In blunt terms, in order to be successful the study required that a sufficient number of patients die: only by pointing to deaths in the placebo group could researchers establish that those receiving the active treatment did comparatively better. Furthermore, to avoid introducing confounding variables into the study, the protocol forbade participants to receive other medication during the study. All this made a certain sense from the standpoint of experimental design, but it was difficult to justify to those people occupying the dual social roles of "patient" and "research subject"—people who began with the assumption that the purpose of medicine was to *help* them. Researchers insisted that clinical trials should not be confused with treatment— that being a research subject is not the same as being a patient. But this was a difficult distinction to put across in the best of circumstances, and it did not resonate with people with AIDS who were fighting to stay alive. In essence, the same practices and procedures that gave biomedicine its credibility as a science were threatening the credibility of medicine as a healing profession.

Mathilde Krim, a New York cancer researcher who had become the co-chair of the American Foundation for AIDS Research (AmFAR), argued at a New York demonstration in summer 1986 that "the double-blind clinical trial on AZT is an insult to morality."[76] But defenders of placebo-controlled trials characterized them as the quickest route to the truth and pointed to their track record in weeding out ineffective drugs that practicing physicians had believed in. Without the science of clinical trials in general, and without double-blind, placebo-controlled trials in particular, physicians were left with nothing but anecdotes and hunches. Douglas Richman, the AZT researcher at the University of California at San Diego, argued in 1988: "In the field of antiviral therapy alone, numerous anecdotal claims were made for the benefits of corticosteroids for chronic hepatitis B, of iododeoxyuridine for herpes simplex encephalitis, and cytosine arabinoside for disseminated herpes zoster. These clinical observations made by concerned physicians were proved to be erroneous in randomized, double-blind, placebo-controlled studies. In fact, the study drug in each case did more harm than the placebo."[77]

The opposite error—erroneously rejecting an effective therapy—was also possible in the absence of placebo-controlled trials. Indeed, said Richman, if there had been no double-blind, placebo-controlled trials, AZT probably would have been discarded. Since AZT showed no impact on the rate of opportunistic infections for the first six weeks of the study and no impact on survival for an even longer period, it would have been easy to conclude from an uncontrolled study that AZT was toxic and ineffective.[78] In response, some, such as Krim, argued that placebo controls weren't the only option for a controlled study. Data obtained from treatment groups could be compared with the medical records of matched cohorts of other AIDS patients who had been followed in the past in studies of the natural history of AIDS (a method called "historical controls"). Or patients in treatment groups could be compared against their own medical records from the weeks prior to their entry into the study. Similar methods had been employed successfully in research with cancer drugs.[79]

Beyond the questions about whether double-blind, placebo-controlled trials were ethical, there began to emerge, in response to the Phase II AZT study, a growing concern about whether such trials were in practical terms *possible*. The essence of a double-blind trial is that neither the subject nor the investigator knows whether the subject is receiving the drug or the placebo. But how can such information be disguised in the case of a relatively toxic drug that produces symptoms like nausea and headaches? And how do researchers anticipate the actions of patients understandably anxious about the possibility that they were squandering their remaining days swallowing sugar pills? Even before the trial had ended, rumors began to trickle in from various quarters: some patients were seeking to lessen their risk of getting the placebo by pooling their pills with other research subjects. In Miami, patients had learned to open up the capsules and taste the contents to distinguish the bitter-tasting AZT from the sweet-tasting placebo. Dr. David Barry, the director of research at Burroughs Wellcome, complaining implausibly that never before in the company's history had any research subject ever opened up a capsule in a placebo-controlled trial, quickly instructed his chemists to make the placebo as bitter as AZT. But patients in both Miami and San Francisco were then reported to be bringing their pills in to local chemists for analysis.[80]

Presumably such practices were not invented by AIDS patients. But the prevalence of AIDS within relatively well-defined communities, and the growing sophistication of the emergent treatment underground, made it likely that strategies for "beating the system" diffused more rapidly and more extensively among AIDS patients than among, say, research subjects in cancer trials. (Ironically, such behavior also risked extending the length of the trial, by increasing the time required to show a statistically significant difference between the AZT group and the placebo group—an example of the clash between the individual and social good that makes such trials so vexing.)[81]

Researchers insisted that their own monitoring methods revealed little abuse: blood tests identified few patients in the placebo arms of studies who had obtained the active drug. Still, reports of "noncompliance" raised serious questions about just how "objective" the much-vaunted double-blind trials really were. Those seeing only the tidy graphs and reading only the crisp prose in the *New England Journal of Medicine* might conceive of such trials as the essence of scientific rigor and, hence, the most solid basis for forming clinical and regulatory judgments. Those observing the conduct of a trial "from the inside" might conclude that knowledge was resting on something rather less solid than bedrock, and they might wonder why the research establishment chose to fetishize this mechanism for establishing biomedical truth.[82]

THE REPUDIATION OF VICTIMHOOD

So-called noncompliance—of patients who don't take their medicine, as well as research subjects who don't follow the protocols—is a long-standing concern among medical professionals. But preoccupation with the issue has skyrocketed in recent years. In one study of the medical literature, Ivan Emke was able to find only 22 articles published in English on the topic of compliance before 1960. But "by 1978, 850 more had been published. Between 1979 and 1985, another 3,200 articles on compliance were published."[83] Noncompliance has become a catchall category for things patients do that health providers find undesirable—a term that casts as much light on doctors' expectations as it does on patients' behavior.[84]

As Emke has noted, doctors tend to discuss what they call the "problem of noncompliance" as if it were purely an individual issue involving specific troublesome patients. But as far back as the Popular Health Movement of the 1830s and 1840s, noncompliance has also appeared in "organized" forms. The feminist health movement of the 1970s and 1980s is, in Emke's words, "the clearest modern example": "It represents more than simply a questioning of the medical orthodoxy, but also involves the setting up of alternative clinics, the support of unique therapies, and the democratization of medical knowledge."[85] The consequences of organized noncompliance for professional authority are suggested indirectly by an observation made by Eliot Freidson, the influential sociologist of medicine and the professions, who, writing in the 1960s, assumed there was a general absence of such organization among medical patients. Professional authority cannot function as such, said Freidson, unless "its clientele is a large, unorganized aggregate of individuals, leaving little possibility for the exertion of lay pressure to compromise occupationally preferred standards."[86]

"Noncompliance" is a vague term, emphasizing what patients *don't* do, rather than what they do. It also suggests a zero-sum game, as if AIDS patients and their doctors had no interests in common. In practice, the relationship between patients with AIDS or HIV infection and community doctors has often been a close one—particularly in gay communities where the doctors themselves are sometimes gay and, in not a few cases, are also infected with HIV. Rather than speaking of noncompliance, it might be more accurate to describe a series of shifts in the nature of the doctor-patient relationship, accompanied and often fueled by an unusual medical sophistication on the part of the patients.

As the extensive literature on the "doctor-patient relationship" suggests, there are many different models of such relationships. The doctor might be conceived as omnipotent or as simply an adviser to the patient. The patient might be imagined to be an inert object (as in surgery) or a competent decision maker (as in many chronic illnesses).[87] But as professional ethics have changed in recent years, and as the balance of power in the doctor-patient relationship has shifted, doctors have been increasingly inclined to acknowledge the full subjectivity of their patients.

AIDS patients have encouraged this cultural shift. Like their feminist predecessors, people with AIDS practiced "self-help with a vengeance," as Indyk and Rier have nicely characterized it[88]—an outright rejection of medical paternalism and an insistence that neither the medical establishment nor the government nor any other suspect authority would speak on behalf of people with AIDS or HIV. In 1985, groups of patients issued a "Founding Statement of People with AIDS/ARC" and a "Patient's Bill of Rights," which have been widely reprinted. The "Founding Statement" asserted: "We condemn attempts to label us as 'victims,' which implies defeat, and we are only occasionally 'patients,' which implies passivity, helplessness, and dependence upon others. We are 'people with AIDS.'"[89] People with AIDS insisted not only on their right to self-representation but also on the right to full explanations from health professionals, the right to anonymity and confidentiality, and the right to refuse specific treatments.[90] Decision-making power, ultimately, had to reside with the person whose life was on the line. This was not an assumption to which doctors necessarily were averse, but the ingrained culture of professional practice often tended to militate against it. At a 1988 conference on AIDS held in London, an anthropologist held up two books side by side to illustrate the gap in perceptions: one was called *AIDS: A Guide for Survival,* the other, *The Management of AIDS Patients.*[91] (Only two years later, as the balance of power and knowledge between doctors and patients shifted, *AIDS Treatment News* would publish an article for patients advising them how to go about "Managing Your Doctor."[92])

In explaining the medically "noncompliant" tendencies of groups like gay men and injection drug users with AIDS, some have emphasized their alienation from society: outcasts can be expected to rebel.[93]

Others have stressed the desperation of those confronted with imminent death. Yet for many people with AIDS, having the capacity to challenge their doctors over the terms of their medical treatment may stem less from their oppression or desperation than from their relative social advantages. Barrie R. Cassileth and Helene Brown have made a similar point about cancer patients who pursue alternative therapies: "Contrary to the stereotype, . . . patients who seek unproven methods include the educated, the middle to upper class, and those who are not necessarily terminal or even beyond hope of cure or remission by conventional treatments." Such patients are overrepresented because "several features of these [alternative] cures require time, financial resources, and an educated, questioning approach to illness. . . ."[94]

Similarly, many people with AIDS and their friends, lovers, and families are often equipped with the financial and cultural resources that permit them to reverse the unidirectional flow of power in the traditional doctor-patient relationship. Many are highly educated (though very often *not* in the hard sciences), highly motivated, and willing to work to learn the foreign language of biomedicine. "An offensive strategy began to emerge on the island of [hospital room] 1028," reported Paul Monette, in a memoir describing his lover's death, "especially as I took an increasingly hands-on role, pestering all the doctors: No explanation was too technical for me to follow, even if it took a string of phone calls to every connection I had. In school I'd never scored higher than a C in any science, falling headlong into literature, but now that I was locked in the lab I became as obsessed with A's as a premed student. Day by day the hard knowledge and raw data evolved into a language of discourse."[95]

One New York doctor described the results of such autodidactic strategies as he witnessed them with his patients: "You'd tell some young guy you were going to put a drip in his chest and he'd answer: 'No, Doc, I don't want a perfusion inserted in my subclavian artery,' which is the correct term for what you proposed doing."[96] In the eyes of some doctors, these were "bad" patients—troublesome know-it-alls who presumed to tell the doctor what to do. But others appreciated patients who took such an energetic interest in their own treatment.[97] The emerging partnerships between patients and health practitioners—and more generally, the expanding expertise residing in gay communities—would hold profound consequences for the politics of knowledge-making in the coming years.

CHAPTER 6

"DRUGS INTO BODIES"

Gaining Access (1987–1988)

"IT'S NOT THAT EASY"

With the steady continuation of basic research on HIV, researchers learned an increasing amount about the life cycle of the virus and its genetic structure. Montagnier's discovery in 1986 of a second, distinct HIV virus—named HIV-2—also believed capable of causing AIDS, produced complications for therapeutic strategies, since there was no reason to believe that a treatment against HIV-1 would necessarily prove efficacious against HIV-2. In practice, treatment strategies focused simply on HIV-1, the virus associated with AIDS around the world; relatively little treatment-oriented research was devoted to HIV-2, found almost exclusively in West African countries.

In contrast to the rapid accumulation of knowledge about the properties and life cycle of HIV-1, researchers lacked a clear understanding of the pathogenesis of AIDS—the steps by which HIV directly or indirectly brought about the decline in the numbers of helper T cells and the destruction of immune functioning. Since the virus could be detected in only a tiny fraction of T cells, it began to seem unlikely that the direct cytopathic effect of HIV could adequately account for the observed T-cell decline. This anomaly was one of the factors that prompted one prominent retrovirologist, Dr. Peter Duesberg of the University of California at Berkeley, to argue in March 1987 that HIV *could not* be the cause of AIDS (see chapter 3).

A number of research findings in the period from 1986 to 1988 shed some light on the mysteries of pathogenesis, with implications for therapeutic strategies. Gallo and coauthors noted in 1987 that infection with the virus could cause T cells to clump together, forming "multinucleated giant cells" called syncytia. "As these giant cells cannot divide appropriately," wrote Gallo, "cell death results." [1] Another clue to the question of how HIV could be so deadly when so few T cells were infected came with the discovery that HIV also infected the macrophages (from the Greek words for "big eater"), immune system scavenger cells present in the blood and other body tissues that surround and ingest foreign particles such as bacteria and protozoa. Since HIV could infect macrophages without killing them, macrophages could serve as reservoirs of infection within the body—"like beanbags, filled with hundreds of viral particles," in the words of Dr. Monte S. Meltzer of Walter Reed Army Institute of Research in Washington, D.C.[2] An important implication was that a truly effective antiviral would presumably have to function within macrophages as well as in helper T cells.

Vaccine development also continued at a rudimentary stage, since researchers lacked basic information about what type of immune response a vaccine should stimulate and what type of viral preparation could most safely and effectively generate such a response.[3] Was the goal to stimulate the "humoral" (antibody) arm of the immune system to generate an effective "neutralizing antibody" that could defend against HIV? Or was it to stimulate the "cell-mediated" arm (the arm that HIV itself attacks) to produce "killer T cells" that would be programmed to destroy an invading viral particle? Could either or both of these goals best be accomplished with whole virus or protein subunits, and should these be natural or genetically engineered? And once a candidate vaccine existed, how could it be tested to see if it worked? Chimpanzees were the only other species capable of being infected with HIV, but since they didn't develop AIDS, were they really a good "animal model" for AIDS research? Should researchers bypass animal testing and proceed directly to trials in humans? If so, the question of establishing efficacy became peculiarly tricky. One public health official admitted in 1986: "People have been talking vaccine, vaccine, vaccine for public consumption, and I have said it, too. But I always scratch my head and say this is not the kind of situation where it is going to be easy to do the testing."[4]

After all, in order to prove that a vaccine is effective, researchers have to show a difference in infection rates, in a double-blind trial, between those who received the vaccine and those who received a placebo. But in order to pass an ethics review, such a trial would have to include a "prevention component": each participant would have to be counseled on how to reduce the risk of HIV infection, and each would have to be strongly advised to practice these risk reduction techniques on the logic that he or she might be in the placebo group or might have received an ineffective trial vaccine. The difficulty, however, is that to the extent that the research subjects heed this counseling, there might be less of a difference in infection rates between the placebo group and the vaccine recipients. "The dilemma you might get into is that unless the volunteers continued with the practices that put them at risk, there would be nothing to study," commented Harold Jaffe of the CDC's AIDS program.[5] It was a telling instance of the clash between the "scientific method" and the "real world": once the controlled experiment moved beyond the bounds of the laboratory walls, the iron logic that gave the experiment its scientific credibility proved difficult, if not impossible, to comply with—at least without threatening the moral credibility on which science, as a public institution, depends.

Meanwhile, NIAID's ATEU program for clinical trials of AIDS drugs, announced with some fanfare in 1986, had barely gotten off the ground—"delayed for months by technical, ethical and financial problems, bureaucratic sluggishness and lack of cooperation from [Burroughs Wellcome]," according to the lead of a front-page *New York Times* article. By April 1987 only 350 patients were enrolled in trials, as compared to the 1,000 that Fauci had promised would be enrolled by the first of the year. Activists chalked the delays up to NIAID's incompetence: unlike, say, the National Cancer Institute, NIAID simply didn't have the experience with running large, multicenter clinical trials. But some researchers insisted that clinical trials necessarily take time to design properly and that "there are no short cuts to the truth."[6]

Fauci, paradoxically, put the blame on scientific progress: The licensing of AZT, in one fell swoop, had invalidated every existing protocol for tests of new antiviral drugs in AIDS patients. Now that AZT had become the standard of care for patients with advanced AIDS, it was no longer ethically acceptable to conduct placebo-controlled trials with such patients. Every protocol had to be rewritten to compare a group receiving the experimental drug with an "active control group" taking AZT. This was no minor substitution, since active-control trials raised different methodological questions and demanded different statistical interpretation. "Months of work suddenly required complete revision," explained Fauci. The scientist also had sharp words for Burroughs Wellcome, expressing his "frustration" that the company "literally has complete control over what does or does not get done" in NIAID trials involving AZT. Burroughs Wellcome had been quick to supply the AZT when ATEU researchers wanted to try administering the drug in combination with acyclovir, another Wellcome product. But it took six months to get the company's permission to test AZT in combination with alpha interferon, a drug produced by a competing pharmaceutical company.[7]

In 1987, Fauci took steps to put his own house in order. He abolished the ill-fated ATEU program for testing AIDS drugs and set up in its place a new network of researchers and research sites, called the AIDS Clinical Trials Group, or ACTG. And he hired away some of NCI's experts on clinical trials, including Dr. Daniel Hoth, an oncologist who was previously the chief of the investigational drug branch at NCI and who would run the ACTG program, and Dr. Susan Ellenberg, a biostatistician who would give expert advice on how to design the trials.[8] "It was really like trying to build a space shuttle in Bangladesh," recalled Hoth some years later, after his departure from NIAID: "We were trying to do two things at once. One was to build the infrastructure and the second was to actually do the research. It was like being out in the Persian Gulf and you had scaffolding over the aircraft carriers at night and in the day [you were flying] missions."[9]

From Hoth's perspective, part of the problem lay in the particular orientations of infectious-disease researchers and in how they differed from the oncologists with whom Hoth had worked in the past. Cancer researchers were used to running large, cooperative research projects; indeed, the average oncologist had at least a passing familiarity with such research since so many cancer patients were enrolled in trials. By contrast, many of the infectious-disease researchers who would run the government-funded trials at the various ACTG research sites around the country had little of this expertise. "So we were teaching people how to write protocols, how to deal with the FDA, how to think about strategic issues," Hoth recalled. Furthermore, it was obvious to oncologists "that you couldn't answer the most important questions by yourself because most of the important questions require very large trials"; cooperation, therefore, was the name of the game. But Hoth found the infectious-disease researchers to be resistant, at least initially, to this fundamental truth. "They live in a publish or perish mode," said Hoth. "That drove them towards individual protocols rather than cooperation. So it was very hard for them to 'get' the concept of a cooperative group." [10]

Criticism of the pace of drug testing continued throughout 1987 as patients pressed for studies of drugs ignored by the research establishment. Fauci complained to the press about the "misperception" that "if we're not testing every conceivable drug in a trial, we're falling short of our responsibility." As soon as any compound was reported to act against the virus in vitro, "everybody in New York and San Francisco is saying 'Why aren't you studying this? Thousands of people are dying in the streets, and this at least offers some hope. Why not try it?'" But "it's not that easy," Fauci insisted; most of these compounds proved to be of dubious value. In the words of Frank Young at the FDA, "the real problem is, where do you get the ideas and where do you get the compounds from?" [11]

According to the Nobel Prize–winning molecular biologist David Baltimore, advances in AIDS drug treatment would come not through "random screening" of potential agents but rather through a more directed process of "rational drug development." [12] As an example, many pointed to the biotechnology industry's latest contribution to AIDS research, a genetically engineered substance called soluble CD4, developed by the Genentech corporation in San Francisco. Soluble CD4 was designed to act as a "decoy" by imitating the CD4 molecule, the site on the immune system cells to which the virus binds. In theory, the virus would latch onto the soluble CD4 rather than attach itself to T cells; the effect of the drug on the virus, according to an enthusiastic NCI spokesperson, would be like "putting putty all over a porcupine." Samuel Broder was enthusiastic enough to tell the press: "It is one of the most important steps we have ever been able to take." [13] Unfortunately, a good result in the test tube with a "rationally engineered" drug proved to be just as poor a predictor of in vivo success as the results of many drugs stumbled upon by chance. Soluble CD4 bombed out in clinical trials, proving completely ineffective in controlling HIV infection.

SACRIFICIAL LAMBS

The NIAID-sponsored trials pursued scientifically safer and more predictable strategies. Since AZT had been shown to have efficacy, investigators focused attention on other dideoxynucleosides, the family of nucleoside analogues to which AZT belongs. Two drugs in particular showed promise: dideoxycytidine (ddC) and dideoxy-inosine (ddI). And since AZT's effect had been shown only in advanced cases of AIDS, it made sense to study the drug in less sick patients to see if it was beneficial to begin prescribing the drug earlier in the course of illness. Two large trials were begun: one, labeled "Protocol 016," studied AZT in mildly symptomatic HIV-infected patients; the other, "Protocol 019," focused on AZT use in asymptomatic patients. No one knew how many of such patients, if left untreated, would go on to develop AIDS. But whereas earlier in the epidemic authorities had suggested that perhaps 5, 10, or 20 percent of those infected would eventually develop AIDS, the experts increasingly were predicting that nearly every infected person might eventually do so. "Early intervention"—before the immune system had been severely compromised by the course of HIV infection—seemed therefore to make good intuitive sense. In fact, community-based treatment advocacy organizations like Project Inform had begun to stake their very identity on the notion of intervening early.

Ellen Cooper, the head of the FDA's Antiviral Drug Division, recalled that "there were a lot of people who would say to me at the agency, 'Well why are we even bothering to do studies in asymptomatics? . . . We know it's an antiviral, we know it works in more advanced patients. [Why not just] open up the indications to early patients?'"[14] And in practice, some doctors had already begun prescribing AZT to HIV-infected patients who did not have AIDS, prompting bitter controversy between advocates and critics of the practice. "I know you don't get better by yourself," commented one Los Angeles doctor with a large AIDS practice, in a pithy expression of the practicing physician's interventionist orientation. Itzak Brook, the FDA advisory committee chair who had voted against approving the drug, was quick to say "I told you so": "This is just what I was afraid of," he commented to the *New York Times*. Samuel Broder of the NCI suggested that doctors and patients should simply sit back and wait: "The best thing to do now is to let the scientific community work this out."[15] But Mathilde Krim, writing in a public policy journal, put the blame back on the NCI for having helped create the predicament in the first place: as far back as late 1985, NCI researchers had been discussing AZT in hopeful terms on national television, thereby enhancing the public's belief in the drug and raising the expectations of the patient community.[16]

With HIV-infected people clamoring for AZT, the 016 (mildly

symptomatic patients) and 019 (asymptomatic patients) trials became more important than ever. They also became ever more difficult to conduct. Since there was no approved treatment for patients in these categories, AZT still had to be measured against a placebo. But compared to the original Phase II AZT trial with AIDS patients, these were larger and longer studies—necessarily so, since otherwise there would be "too few" deaths in the placebo arm to prove anything, given the relative health of the patients. Fischl's AZT trial had involved only 137 patients on placebos, and they were kept on it for twenty-four weeks at most. By contrast, the 019 study, conducted by Dr. Paul Volberding of the University of California at San Francisco, had 428 people in the placebo arm, and it was expected to run for several years.

Soon articles in the gay press were publicizing the plight of the "sacrificial lambs" in the AZT studies, sentenced by the research establishment to "death by placebo." [17] Experts on clinical trials sought to emphasize the difference between the 016 and 019 studies and the earlier Phase II AZT study conducted with much sicker AIDS patients. That the patient community might find placebos difficult to countenance in trials of those facing "imminent death" was "entirely understandable," said Thomas Chalmers of the Harvard School of Public Health. But, he argued, "it is more difficult to understand that philosophy when one is dealing with asymptomatic patients . . . who may never develop AIDS and face a chance of being [made] sicker by a toxic and ineffective drug." [18]

However, the trial participants—who had tested positive, who had gleaned from numerous newspaper accounts that they had a "time bomb" ticking away inside of them, and who, in their day-to-day lives, could see the presumed end results reflected in the bodies of the friends and lovers they visited in hospitals, reflected in the obituaries they read, and reflected in the funerals they attended—quite simply drew different conclusions. One subject in the 019 trial who had discovered he was in the placebo arm commented, "Fuck them. I didn't agree to donate my body to science, if that is what they are doing, just sitting back doing nothing with me waiting until I get PCP [*Pneumocystis carinii* pneumonia] or something." He told a reporter for the gay press that he had covertly begun taking dextran sulfate, an unapproved drug available through the treatment underground. Some community physicians expressed their incredulity on learning that participants in these studies were not permitted to take prophylactic medication to ward off pneumocystis pneumonia. One doctor described an experience with one of his patients: "I said hello, and he handed me this lab slip from UCSF and started crying. He said they won't let me have aerosol pentamidine. . . . I looked at it, looked at him, and said, 'I don't believe you. Nobody would do that!' It drove me nuts!"[19]

DUAL ROLES AND "DOUBLE AGENTS"

The fundamental problem was that it was becoming more and more difficult for people with AIDS and HIV to occupy the dual roles of "patient" and "research subject." That these distinct roles might overlap without tension was always a convenient fiction. But in the cases of other illnesses such as cancer, the problem had been given more extended consideration. Most clinical research in cancer takes place on the "front lines" of patient care: a patient's own oncologist routinely enrolls him or her in research protocols that are integrated into the overall treatment plan. At least in theory, these oncologists are self-reflective about their role as what ethicist Robert Levine calls "double agents": they wear the hats of both "doctor" and "researcher" and must be responsible, simultaneously, to the abstract goal of knowledge and the concrete needs of their patients.[20] Researchers in infectious disease also saw patients, but they were far less likely than oncologists to have extended experience with patients suffering from chronic, life-threatening illnesses. Until AIDS, as David Rothman and Harold Edgar have explained, "most the research in infectious diseases, although certainly not all, did not involve desperately ill patients willing to take high risks for the slimmest possibility of a gain. Inevitably, in the realm of infectious diseases, the commitment to placebo-based random trials did not have to come up against agonizing questions."[21]

As these "agonizing questions" surfaced in trials like 016 and 019, community physicians not involved directly in clinical research (like the astonished doctor quoted above) found themselves caught smack in the middle between their own patients and the respected academic researchers conducting the trials. In more typical circumstances, these practitioners would likely have deferred to the academics, who enjoy high status within the broader medical community. (As Andrew Abbott has described it, such professionals reside closest to the profession's "pure" knowledge base and bask in its reflected glow.[22]) But the physicians on the front lines of the AIDS epidemic—the ones who saw hundreds of people with AIDS and HIV in their practices, who in some

cases were gay themselves and in some cases were HIV positive—
found their loyalties sharply divided. Many of them reacted with sympathy as activists began to propose ways of easing the tension between
the roles of "patient" and "subject"—ways of conducting research
that might serve the ends of both science and ethics.

A Knowledge-Empowered Movement

A LAB OF ONE'S OWN

By the mid-1980s, some groups of community physicians had banded together with patient groups to pioneer new forms
of knowledge-making. Instead of waiting for NIAID to test drugs in
its lengthy, cumbersome clinical trials at academic centers, primary-
care physicians and people with AIDS decided to go about designing
such trials themselves.[23] "By integrating scientific trials with normal
medical practice, community-based trials allow credible testing of
treatment options with far less administrative delay than usually involved, and at far less cost," said John James in *AIDS Treatment
News*.[24] As Mary-Rose Mueller has detailed in an analysis of
community-based research, this endeavor served as "a form of professional resistance [by community physicians] to academic medicine"
and an opportunity for them to stake out a new jurisdiction within
professional practice.[25] At the same time, community-based research
promised to bring scientific knowledge-production closer to popular
control. Scientists' power, as Bruno Latour has emphasized, stems at
least in some measure from their possession of laboratories; now the
AIDS movement sought to build its own.[26]

As John James explained in 1988, two very different models of
community-based research had arisen.[27] In San Francisco in 1985, researchers such as Donald Abrams, associated with the University of
California at San Francisco and San Francisco General Hospital, had
formed the County Community Consortium (CCC), a coalition of San
Francisco physicians with AIDS practices. The original purpose had
been to improve communication between researchers and doctors and
disseminate information about treatments more rapidly. Over time, as
some of the primary-care doctors became interested in participating
in research, the CCC evolved into a mechanism for organizing
community-based trials. The idea was that physicians would distribute
drugs, monitor patients, and collect data as an integral part of their

regular clinical work with patients. And it wasn't a new idea: in many ways it resembled the community-based cancer research effort sponsored by the NCI, called the Community Clinical Oncology Program.[28] "We have a distinct advantage in being able to follow up patients, because the research is being done where the patients are getting their primary care," commented Abrams, the head of the CCC. "So even if the patient stops participating in the study, we still know . . . what sort of outcomes they have. . . ."[29]

The second model was pioneered by people with AIDS in New York City, who worked together with a number of activist doctors, including the maverick Joseph Sonnabend. Frustrated by the slow pace of federally sponsored treatment research, they founded an organization called the Community Research Initiative (CRI), which opened its doors in May 1987 under the sponsorship of the local PWA Coalition, the advocacy group run by people with AIDS. From the start, people with AIDS or HIV infection participated in decision making about what trials CRI should conduct and even how they should be organized, "[setting] policies on placebo use, and [insisting] that trials under [CRI] sponsorship be effectively open to women and minorities, not only to gay men." The effect of such community participation, argued James, was to ensure smoother trials and higher levels of "compliance" with the protocols: "Such prior community involvement in policy issues around the selection and conduct of trials makes recruitment easier and increases patient-experimenter cooperation, for example by greatly reducing any need to 'cheat' in the study by taking other drugs without telling the researchers."[30] Community-based research was not suited for high-tech trials requiring sophisticated lab tests that the average primary-care physician did not have the equipment to perform. But other trials, involving minimal data collection, could easily be conducted out of doctors' offices. Drug companies, also impatient with the NIAID trials system, proved interested in the concept as well, and soon CRI had a number of contracts to conduct studies for different companies, both large and small.[31]

Still, community-based research invited skepticism. "Traditional researchers thought that community doctors would not be sophisticated enough to run trials," said Mathilde Krim, whose organization, AmFAR, would later become a chief funder of community-based research. "But actually they were highly sophisticated. . . . After all, they had been managing the disease for years."[32] This sort of "hands-on" expertise did not, in itself, establish community-based research as credible in the eyes of mainstream researchers or government health officials, who were more invested in a conception of medicine as "science," not "art." Rather, public demonstration of the credibility and viability of community-based AIDS research came with the testing of aerosolized pentamidine, a form of prevention against deadly pneumocystis pneumonia. It was a therapy that community-based research at the CCC and CRI effectively rescued after NIAID bungled its own efforts to test it.

In February 1987 researchers recruited by NIAID to participate in its clinical trials program rated research into prophylactic aerosolized pentamidine as a high priority: preventing pneumocystis pneumonia was a much better therapeutic strategy than simply treating people once they contracted the disease. But it wasn't until June the following year that researchers actually began to recruit patients into the NIAID trials, after more than a year of writing and rewriting the protocols and negotiating with Lyphomed, the manufacturer of the product. Meanwhile, in May 1987, a group of activists including Michael Callen, the well-known dissenter on the HIV hypothesis who was also on the board of CRI, had met with Anthony Fauci and pleaded for him to issue federal guidelines recommending pentamidine use to prevent PCP. When Fauci refused, citing the lack of data on efficacy, Callen returned to New York to tell his fellow board members: "We're going to have to test it ourselves." [33] In San Francisco, the CCC had also launched its own study, a three-armed trial where patients received different doses of pentamidine but no one received a placebo. Denied funding by NIAID, the CCC received money for the trial from Lyphomed and the University of California.

In 1989, after examining study data from both the CCC and CRI, the FDA approved aerosolized pentamidine for prophylactic use against PCP—the first time in its history that the agency approved a drug based solely on data from community-based research. [34] Before accepting the CRI's data, FDA representatives had visited the CRI's offices in New York and gone over their methods and their paperwork. They came away satisfied that "good science" was being done. This was essential for the legitimation of CRI, according to Dr. Bernard Bihari, a member of the board of directors: "Doing good science allowed us to establish our credibility." [35]

Plaudits soon arrived from all quarters. "The Community Research Initiative . . . offers the possibility to combine the technical expertise of the research community with the outreach potential of community health clinics and physicians in community practice," wrote the Presidential Commission on the HIV Epidemic in its 1988 report, urging direct federal funding of the community-based research programs.[36] One member of the commission described CRI as "one of the best things to have come out of the AIDS effort."[37] Said Anthony Fauci the following year: "What I see in the community programs is totally compatible with the mission of the NIH."[38]

ACTING UP

The successes of community-based research notwithstanding, those who cared about the overall progress of AIDS research could hardly afford to ignore the federal agencies that coordinated the bulk of the effort. In early 1987, deep concerns about NIAID's clinical trials and the FDA's regulatory requirements—not to mention the drug companies' obedience to the profit motive, the religious right's intolerance, and the Reagan administration's general indifference—combined to push AIDS activism into a new level of energy and organization. On the East Coast, the gay playwright and all-around rabble-rouser Larry Kramer, who had helped found the Gay Men's Health Crisis at an earlier juncture in the epidemic, was one of the initiators of a new group in New York City, a radical activist organization called the AIDS Coalition to Unleash Power—better known by its acronym, "ACT UP." On the West Coast, a group of San Franciscans who called themselves the Citizens for Medical Justice began organizing a series of demonstrations against Burroughs Wellcome at its Bay Area offices, protesting the price of AZT.[39] Citizens for Medical Justice then transformed itself into the AIDS Action Pledge,[40] which in turn became the San Francisco chapter of ACT UP.

Soon there was an ACT UP/Chicago and an ACT UP/Houston, an ACT UP/New Orleans and an ACT UP/Seattle. Although AIDS activism has remained significantly stronger in the United States than elsewhere, most likely due to the greater strength of the gay and lesbian movement and the greater salience of identity politics in general in the United States, ACT UP eventually developed international dimensions. By the early 1990s there were also ACT UP chapters in Sydney, London, Paris, Berlin, Amsterdam, and Montreal. Each chapter was autonomous, though informal links connected them.[41]

A magnet for radical, young gay men and women, ACT UP practiced an in-your-face politics of "no business as usual." Adopting styles of political and cultural practice deriving from sources as diverse as anarchism, the peace movement, the punk subculture, the feminist health movement, and gay liberation "zaps" of the 1970s, ACT UP became famous for its imaginative street theater, its skill at attracting news cameras, and its well-communicated sense of urgency.[42] "Silence = Death" read its characteristic slogan, set against the pink-triangle symbol of gay liberation (itself a symbolic appropriation of the patch worn by homosexuals in the Nazi death camps). ACT UP chapters typically had no formal leaders; in many cities, meetings operated by the consensus process.

As Joshua Gamson described in a participant-observation study of the San Francisco chapter, ACT UP shared the basic characteristics of so-called new social movements—"a (broadly) middle-class membership and a mix of instrumental, expressive, and identity-oriented activities." By "staging events and by carefully constructing and publicizing symbols," ACT UP "attacks the dominant representations of AIDS and of people with AIDS and makes attempts to replace them with alternative representations."[43] Though the New Yorkers were particularly well connected to the art world and the communications media, ACT UP in general quickly perfected a highly dramaturgical style of activism and an abiding concern with techniques of expression.[44]

On the national scene, the New York City chapter dominated, with more than 150 members at regular weekly meetings and a three hundred thousand–dollar budget by the end of 1988.[45] But chapters in San Francisco, Los Angeles, and Boston were also prominent within the movement. Activists came from all walks of life. Yet as results from a survey of ACT UP/New York members conducted by Gilbert Elbaz suggest, "the group was predominantly gay, white male [with ages] between 26 and 35." Members were also "predominantly seronegative, highly educated, and part of the new middle class." In Elbaz's sample of 413 activists, 80 percent were men and 78 percent were white. Thirty-five percent had done at least some postgraduate study. It was also a highly politicized group: More than half of Elbaz's respondents had participated in demonstrations before joining ACT UP; a good number had been involved in movements such as the peace movement and the feminist movement. Many of the women, in particular, had had experience with civil disobedience leading to arrest.[46]

For some, radical AIDS activism provided a "home" within the gay and lesbian movement. Commented New York activist David Barr, a lawyer by training: "I can't tell you how many gay men . . . that I know who said, 'ACT UP was the first time I've ever felt a part of a gay community.' That was certainly the case for me. I mean, the 'gay community' before that was always more alienating to me than anything else. . . ."[47] For others, like Michelle Roland, whose father had been jailed with Martin Luther King and who grew up reading United Farmworkers literature in her Berkeley home, joining the San Francisco chapter of ACT UP was a natural outgrowth of radical politics.[48] But many, including Roland, have pointed to the deaths of close friends as the immediate, mobilizing incidents that provoked them to become involved. And they have recalled their frustration with the prevalent notion that since AIDS was inevitably fatal, all that could be done for people with AIDS was to provide palliative care.[49]

THE DISCOURSE OF GENOCIDE

Especially in the early years of the epidemic, some had speculated openly that AIDS had emerged as an act of genocide—as a deliberate attempt, perhaps by government scientists, to eliminate "undesirable" populations by spreading an infectious agent among them. Now, with the rise of groups such as ACT UP, a new conception of genocide gained currency in activist rhetoric: genocide described the consequences of the failure of governmental and medical authorities to respond to the epidemic adequately. Genocide was not the product of anyone's action but the by-product of *in*action or willful neglect. As AIDS activists mobilized to focus public attention on the epidemic and convince a Republican administration to fund prevention, treatment, research, and social services, the new conception of genocide proved a useful framing device.

One of the prime enunciators of the charge of genocide-by-neglect was Larry Kramer, the New York activist. In a book entitled *Reports from the Holocaust,* Kramer argued that "a holocaust does not require a Hitler to be effective. . . . Holocausts can occur, and probably most often do occur, because of *inaction.* This inaction can be unintentional or deliberate." Kramer's sidestepping of the question of intentions in no way inclined him to be charitable toward those he considered perpetrators of genocide. Writing about Ronald Reagan and various government health officials, Kramer declared them all "equal to Hitler and his Nazi doctors performing their murderous experiments in the camps— not because of similar intentions, but because of similar results."[50]

Genocide by neglect became one of the key frames employed by

ACT UP in its formative years of mobilization. If, by this logic, government officials were murderers, then people with AIDS were to be understood as casualties of state-sponsored violence. In this context, the Nazi-era pink triangle in the ACT UP logo took on additional resonance. Soon the stark image of a bloody palm print could be seen stickered to the backs of black leather jackets from New York to San Francisco, with the caption reading: "The U.S. government has blood on its hands."

THE FDA UNDER FIRE

Though its targets were always multiple, throughout 1987 and 1988, ACT UP trained its attention particularly on the FDA, perceived to be the roadblock in the way of access to AIDS drugs.[51] In March 1987, the FDA commissioner announced a new plan to create a special category of unapproved drugs called Treatment Investigational New Drugs (Treatment INDs), to be available on a compassionate use basis to patients with terminal illnesses whose doctors contacted the FDA.[52] But in essence this was nothing more than a codification of existing, case-by-case compassionate use policies. AIDS activists were not mollified; "Drugs into bodies" was their war cry.

"Many of us who live in daily terror of the AIDS epidemic cannot understand why the Food and Drug Administration has been so intransigent in the face of this monstrous tidal wave of death," wrote Larry Kramer in an opinion piece published in the *New York Times*.[53] "There is no question on the part of anyone fighting AIDS that the F.D.A. constitutes the single most incomprehensible bottleneck in American bureaucratic history. . . ." "In addition to ribavirin, why is the F.D.A. withholding Ampligen; Glucan; DTC; DDC; AS 101; MTP-PE and AL 721?" he asked in reference to some of the many experimental drugs that were rumored to be efficacious. Patients had no interest in paternalism, Kramer insisted: "AIDS sufferers, who have nothing to lose, are more than willing to be guinea pigs." Similarly, Martin Delaney, executive director of the San Francisco–based Project Inform, struck a chord that resonated deeply with U.S. political culture by painting the FDA as a would-be "Big Brother" and insisting on the individual's basic right to choose.[54] In public debates and private meetings with AIDS clinical researchers and FDA officials, Delaney sought to reframe the very purpose of the FDA: rather than seek only to protect the public from ineffective or dangerous therapies, the FDA should take an active stance to promote the nation's health.

AIDS activists were not the only voices challenging the FDA. For years, conservatives from places ranging from the Heritage Foundation to the offices of the *Wall Street Journal* to—most recently—the corridors of the White House had been seeking to roll the "deregulation" bandwagon onward in order to focus on the pharmaceutical industry. The FDA was killing the drug companies and preventing useful products from getting to market, the argument ran; the best solution would be to repeal the Kefauver-Harris amendment, which had granted the FDA the authority to assess the safety and efficacy of drugs. "Especially considering who was the president, we had concern" about adding fuel to the deregulatory movement, recalled David Barr of ACT UP/New York: "But it wasn't enough concern that it would stop us from doing what we were doing." [55] Soon an unlikely alliance had developed—usually tacit, but sometimes explicit—between AIDS treatment activists and conservatives, leaving consumer protection groups and traditional liberals on the other side.

When cancer treatment advocates connected to the ultraconservative John Birch Society had used similar grounds to press for access to laetrile in the 1970s, a confluence of interest with pro-market forces was perhaps less surprising. [56] But when *AIDS Treatment News* plugged a Heritage Foundation report called "Red Tape for the Dying," describing it as proposing "a workable, politically possible change which could solve part of the AIDS 'drugjam,'" [57] or when Project Inform began collaborating on a regulatory proposal with the Competitive Policy Institute, a conservative policy group, [58] everything started to seem upside down, and liberal politicians might have been forgiven their bewilderment at becoming the target of criticism by their usual allies. Henry Waxman, the liberal chair of the health subcommittee of the House of Representatives, found himself in a peculiar plight when he raised objections to the Treatment IND proposal. The *Wall Street Journal,* suggesting that Waxman "has been to new-drug development in this country what the troll under the bridge was to forward progress in the Billy Goats Gruff," noted with evident glee: "If he opposes the administration initiative, it will be interesting to hear him explain it to AIDS victims in his West Hollywood constituency." [59]

The FDA was being pressured from all sides, particularly by the increasingly flagrant flouting of the law by the AIDS treatment underground. Importing unapproved drugs had become an organized and global operation, with regular couriers flying in treatments such as dextran sulfate from places like Japan and then distributing them at bargain prices to individuals all around the United States.[60] Organizations called "buyers clubs" (sometimes also called "guerrilla clinics"), operating in a gray zone of legality, had sprung up in major cities around the United States, swapping information about treatments and selling a range of unapproved compounds and alternative therapies.[61] By October 1987, Project Inform's newsletter reported ten such organizations in the United States, plus one in Vancouver and one in London.[62] These organizations had benevolent motivations and, indeed, protected their customers from less scrupulous entrepreneurs seeking to profit from "quack" remedies. But the FDA was far from convinced of the wisdom of tolerating their operations. "This is a very fine line we're walking," said Frank Young, the FDA commissioner, acknowledging the practical limits of pursuing a strict enforcement policy against the buyers clubs: "Since there's nothing else available except AZT, we are trying to make available the opportunity for patients to get other drugs and treat themselves." [63]

When Young appeared in Boston at the Lesbian and Gay Health Conference in July 1988, he confronted a hostile audience of one thousand; the first three rows were filled with ACT UP demonstrators holding signs saying "FDA, YOU'RE KILLING ME." While some demonstrators conducted a mock "die-in," others held up their watches with alarms ringing: for people with AIDS, time was running out. But to the surprise of the audience, Young had come to announce that the FDA would now permit the importing of unapproved AIDS drugs in small quantities for personal use.[64] In a remark to a reporter after his talk, Young described his motivations: "There is such a degree of desperation, and people are going to die. . . . I'm not going to be the Commissioner that robs them of hope." [65] But according to a reporter for *Science*, the change in policy "stunned" many in the research community: "One official in the federal government's AIDS Program went so far as to suggest that the FDA commissioner had gone 'temporarily insane.'" [66]

AIDS activists, however, had no intention of letting up the pressure on the FDA—certainly not in response to the limited new policy of importation for personal use. Plans began in New York City, San Francisco, and elsewhere for a demonstration that would "shut down" the FDA. In an early example of what would prove to be periodic position papers on the state of AIDS research, ACT UP/New York distributed a thirty-five-page, closely argued document entitled the "FDA Action Handbook," designed to explain to the mass membership the medical and political justification for the action. "Many Federal agencies, not to mention local and state ones, have been derelict in the fight on AIDS," wrote Jim Eigo and Mark Harrington, two of the authors: "Yet only *one* agency, the FDA, is actively blocking the delivery of promising drugs to PWAs and people with HIV infection."[67] Sections of the handbook included discussion of topics such as "What Is the FDA?" "A Brief History of the FDA," "The Standard Drug Approval Process," "Drug Horror Stories," and "Exclusion of Women, People of Color, Poor People, People in Rural Areas, IV Drug Users, Hemophiliacs, Prisoners & Children from Experimental Drug Trials." The document is noteworthy for its use of "atrocity tales" and for its construction of an antagonist identity:[68] "Like corporations, [government bureaucracies] consider the data of lives as raw material and grist for a perpetual-motion paper mill. Human need, suffering and death count for very little when compared to the imperatives of orderly process and well-maintained policies."[69]

On October 11, 1988, following a national display of the Names Project AIDS Quilt on the Capitol Mall in Washington, D.C., more than a thousand demonstrators from around the country converged on FDA headquarters in Rockville, Maryland, to "seize control" of what some labeled the "Federal Death Administration." Protesters fell to the ground holding mock tombstones with caustic inscriptions: "I got the placebo. R.I.P."; "As a person of color I was exempt from drug trials." Two hundred demonstrators were arrested by police, who wore rubber gloves to protect themselves from the supposed risk of HIV infection.[70]

It was a protest that, in the words of two chroniclers, "represented . . . a culmination of our early efforts. . . ." It also marked "a turning point in both recognition by the government of the seriousness and legitimacy of our demands and national awareness of the AIDS activist movement."[71] The ACT UP/New York Media Committee had "distilled" the message of the "FDA Action Handbook" to explain it to the press in simple terms: Protesters demanded immediate access to drugs proven safe and theoretically effective in Phase I trials. Double-blind, placebo-controlled trials should be declared unethical and replaced with alternative trial designs. The FDA should make it clear that it would not tolerate trials that prohibited its participants from taking simultaneous prophylaxis against opportunistic infections. People from all affected populations—gays, injection drug users, and people with hemophilia; women and men; whites and people of color—must be given access to trials. Medicaid and private health insurance should cover experimental drug therapies.[72]

"The meeting at the FDA two weeks later was very different," recalled David Barr, "because, not only had we been able to show our firepower out on the street, but when we sat down at the table we had a list of issues that we understood—we were very knowledgeable about them by that time. . . ." Significantly, activist strategies and tactics in negotiation with FDA officials differed considerably from the colorful display outside the building. That "was theater and we knew it was theater," explained Barr. "It was a much smaller group of people who were actually inside at the table, and we wouldn't go in there saying, 'Okay, we want to go through these forty demands with you.' We were savvy enough to say [ahead of time], 'What are our issues at this meeting with this group of people? Let's talk about these five things, and what is our priority'—and we learned how to do a meeting. . . ."[73]

The simultaneous use of insider and outsider tactics meant, however, that activists needed to establish working relationships with the same people they had vilified in public statements and demonstrations. Similarly, activists needed to engage with the nuts and bolts of policies and research practices whose defects they had heretofore been content to paint with a broad brush. Though activists continued their bitter criticisms of government agencies and individual scientists, they resisted the notion—found, for example, in the animal rights movement[74]—that the scientific establishment was "the enemy" in some absolutist sense. "I wouldn't exaggerate how polite we were," reflected Mark Harrington. "At the same time, I would just say that it was clear from the very beginning [that we recognized that], as Maggie Thatcher said when she met Gorbachev, 'We can do business.' We wanted to make some moral points, but we didn't want to wallow in being victims, or powerless, or oppressed, or always right. We wanted to engage and find out if there was common ground."[75]

BEYOND THE FDA

The *Wall Street Journal* made effective literary use of the iconography of the protest in its editorial two days afterward, which described the "battle between people who have all the time in the world and people who have little time left in their lives."[76] But what the *Journal* may have failed to observe was how the activists themselves had already set their sights well beyond the walls of the FDA building. Though the main goal, to be sure, was access to treatments, in pursuit of that goal activists had to engage with the researchers and the health professionals, the pharmaceutical houses and the insurance companies, NIAID and the NCI and the Department of Health and Human Services. For all its importance as a symbolic target, the FDA was just one player; and the demonstration in Rockville, for all its significance in the construction and legitimation of a nationwide movement, in a sense represented the end of an era. Arguments about competing philosophies of drug regulation would continue. But the more activists learned about the FDA's drug approval policies, the more they became enmeshed in debating the details of what counted, in the agency's eyes, as "good science." And the more they became concerned with the science of clinical trials, the more the focus of their energy shifted from the FDA to NIAID. "While the question of a person's freedom to use a treatment whether or not it works is indeed an important issue," commented *AIDS Treatment News* in 1988, heralding this new turn, "the more important question is what treatments do in fact work, and how can the evidence be collected, evaluated, and applied quickly and effectively."[77]

Of course, these two issues—the ethics of access to therapies and the methodology of clinical trials—often came together in concrete ways. For example, some worried about the potential conflict between access and research: would unrestricted access to experimental treatments hamper researchers' abilities to conduct trials? After all, if every person with AIDS could obtain an experimental drug with a minimum of hassle, why would anyone enroll in a clinical trial? In effect, the capacity to conduct clinical trials presupposed coercion through control of the supply of the drugs. Researchers and health officials took this point for granted; for example, Ellen Cooper, the head of the FDA's Antiviral Drug Division, argued in *JAMA* that "a national policy of early widespread availability of unproved experimental agents would slow or even halt the completion of controlled clinical trials through which therapeutic advances are established and then improved on. . . ."[78] Recalled Cooper: "I really understood, or empathized with, where they were coming from, which is . . . the individual patient with a life-threatening disease."[79] But in her view, it was a simple question of the greatest good for the greatest number; and the individual's right to treatment would have to take a back seat to research that could benefit the public at large.[80]

AIDS activists protested the implicit coercion, suggesting, in Martin Delaney's words, that it was "morally offensive [to] use access to treatment as a lever to force subjects into studies. The fact that such an argument is openly made demonstrates how detached the regulators' mindset has become." [81] But to the extent that activists succeeded in swaying researchers and government officials on this point, they did so by turning the argument on its head. "The policy of restriction," said Delaney, addressing the 1988 meeting of the Infectious Diseases Society of America, "is itself destroying our ability to conduct clinical research." Delaney explained: "AIDS study centers throughout the nation tell of widescale concurrent use of other treatments; frequent cheating, even bribery, to gain entry to studies; mixing of drugs by patients to share and dilute the risk of being on placebo; and rapid dropping out of patients who learn that they are on placebo. . . . Such practices are a direct result of forcing patients to use clinical studies as the only option for treatment." If these policies continued, Delaney warned, "it will soon be impossible to conduct valid clinical AIDS research in the US." [82]

This was a forceful argument that spoke to researchers' basic interests while playing on their fears. Continuing in his role as the defender of good science, Delaney proposed the solution: "If patients had other means of obtaining treatment, force-fitting them into clinical studies would be unnecessary. Volunteers that remained would be more likely to act as pure research subjects, entering studies not solely out of a desperate effort to save their lives." Their motivations for doing so might be altruism or a desire to obtain other tangible rewards of clinical trial participation, such as access to free, high-quality medical care.

Over the next few years, treatment activists would pursue a three-pronged agenda, one that Delaney's solution in many ways suggested. First, they would fight with the FDA over what counted as sufficient proof of safety and efficacy in a medical emergency, speeding up the approval of a number of drugs, particularly ones that treated opportunistic infections associated with AIDS. Second, in the case of experimental drugs still being tested, they would press for institutionalized mechanisms of "expanded access" outside of the framework of clinical trials. And third, they would seek to transform the clinical trials themselves, to make the trials more relevant, more humane, and more capable of generating trustworthy conclusions. This complex agenda would require a thoroughgoing engagement with the biomedical establishment—an encounter that would have important implications for the practice of medical research, the dynamics of the movement, and the establishment of certainty or uncertainty about specific experimental treatments.

LEARNING NEW LANGUAGES

The shift in attention from the FDA to NIAID raised important questions about the capacity of laypeople to intervene in science. Put bluntly, how did these activists know what they were talking about? What was the source of their expertise? It was one thing to educate oneself about one's own illness and thereby shift the dynamics of power in the relationship between doctor and patient. It was quite another to suggest that one had a role in the actual conduct of scientific research.

Part of the explanation lies in issues of organization, resources, and community. Patients with heart disease who want to share information or organize a critique of medicine have to seek out like-minded individuals and find points of commonality with them. People with AIDS—particularly in gay communities—already knew how to find one another, and they benefited from a history of political and social organization.[83] By 1988 there was an entire infrastructure encompassing treatment publications and buyers clubs, advocacy groups and grassroots activists—a firm foundation that could then support the widespread dissemination of medical knowledge. And by this point, these organizations' knowledge about AIDS often exceeded that of the average practicing physician. "When we first started out, there were maybe three physicians in the metropolitan New York area who would even give us a simple nod of the head," said the director of a New York City buyers club in 1988: "Now, every day, the phone rings ten times, and there's a physician on the other end wanting advice. [From] me! I'm trained as an opera singer!"[84]

This was the base on which the treatment activists could build as they turned their attention to clinical trial design. To be sure, not every AIDS treatment activist started without scientific training. Iris Long, for instance, had worked for twenty years as a pharmaceutical chemist before she decided to join ACT UP/New York; she quickly made herself indispensable as a teacher of raw recruits.[85] Andy Zysman, who would become a key activist addressing issues of cancers associated with AIDS, was an emergency physician at Kaiser Hospital; he joked that his professional background caused him to be "viewed as a reactionary Republican" when he joined ACT UP/San Francisco.[86] More typically, however, the stars of the treatment activist movement were science novices, but ones who were unusually articulate, self-confident, and well educated—"displaced intellectuals from other fields," according to Jim Eigo, a New York City treatment activist with a background in the arts.[87] Often these activists were able to parlay other social and personal advantages into a new type of credibility—to convert their "capital" from one form to another, as Bourdieu would put it.[88]

The trajectory of Mark Harrington, a de facto leader of ACT UP/ New York's Treatment & Data Committee, exemplified one pathway to expertise among the key treatment activists. Harrington studied German critical theory in college at Harvard and had worked as a coffeehouse waiter and a freelance writer. When he discovered ACT UP, Harrington was writing scripts for a film company.[89] "The only science background that might have proved relevant was [what I had] when I was growing up: my dad had always subscribed to *Scientific American*, and I had read it, so I didn't feel that sense of intimidation from science that I think a lot of people feel," Harrington recalled.[90] Taking quick stock of his ignorance about science and the federal bureaucracy, Harrington stayed up one night and made a list of all the words he needed to understand. That list evolved into a fifty-page glossary that was distributed to ACT UP members.[91] Harrington's frequent collaborator on the Treatment & Data Committee, Jim Eigo, authored poetic critiques of scientific practice that were peppered with references to Shakespeare. These were intellectuals, to be sure, but they represented the "humanistic" wing of the intelligentsia, a fact that shaped the contours of their engagement with the other, "technical" wing.[92] They learned their science, but their engagement with it rested on moral principles and an ethic of commitment, which they juxtaposed with images of the clinical detachment of the scientists and the bureaucrats. "I have a face in my mind for every AIDS-related condition I can describe to you," said Eigo, ". . . every one the face of a friend."[93] Science and bureaucracy, by contrast, were cold and passionless—epitomized, in activists' eyes, by the FDA's Ellen Cooper, whom some labeled the "Ice Queen."

Steven Shapin has noted, in an analysis of the historical constitution of the expert/lay divide, that the question of who possesses "cultural competence" in science is "one of the most obvious means by which we, and people in the past, discriminate between 'science' and 'the public. . . .'"[94] The most crucial avenue pursued by treatment activists in the construction of their scientific credibility has been precisely the acquisition of such competence—that is, learning the languages and cultures of medical science. Through a wide variety of methods—including attending scientific conferences, scrutinizing research protocols, and learning from sympathetic professionals both inside and out-side the movement—the key treatment activists have gained a working knowledge of the medical vocabulary. While activists have also insisted on the need to bring "nonscientific" language and judgments into their encounters with researchers, they have nonetheless assumed that the capacity to speak the language of the journal article and the conference hall is a sine qua non of their effective participation. In a learning approach that one activist, G'dali Braverman, has frankly characterized as "ass-backwards," activists often began with the examination of a specific research protocol in which patients had been asked to enroll and, from there, went on to educate themselves about the mechanism of drug action, the relevant "basic science" knowledge base (such as considerations of the viral replication cycle of HIV or the immunopathogenesis of AIDS), and the inner workings of "the system" of drug testing and regulation, including the roles of the pharmaceutical companies and the relevant government advisory committees.[95]

Other activists have explicitly used the metaphors "foreign language" and "foreign culture" to describe their initiation into treatment activism. Brenda Lein, a San Francisco activist, described the first time she went to a local meeting of the Treatment Issues Committee of ACT UP: "And so I walked in the door and it was completely overwhelming, I mean acronyms flying, I didn't know *what* they were talking about. I thought, 'Oh, they're speaking Greek and I'm never going to understand this language.' ... Hank [Wilson] came in and he handed me a stack about a foot high [about granulocyte macrophage colony–stimulating factor] and said, 'Here, read this.' And I looked at it and I brought it home and I kept going through it in my room and ..., I have to say, I didn't understand a word." But after reading it "about ten times," Lein concluded: "Oh, this is like a subculture thing; you know, it's either surfing or it's medicine and you just have to understand the lingo, but it's not that complicated if you sit through it. So once I started understanding the language, it all became far less intimidating."[96]

And indeed, the remarkable fact is that once they acquired a certain basic familiarity with the *language* of biomedicine, activists found they could also get in the doors of the *institutions* of biomedicine. Once they could converse comfortably about Kaplan-Meier curves and cytokine regulation and resistance-conferring mutations, activists increasingly discovered that researchers felt compelled, by their own norms of discourse and behavior, to consider activist arguments on their merits. Not that activists were always welcome at the table—to quote Lein again: "I mean, I walk in with . . . seven earrings in one ear and a Mohawk and my ratty old jacket on, and people are like, 'Oh great, one of these street activists who don't know anything. . . .'" But once she opened her mouth and demonstrated that she could contribute to the conversation intelligently, Lein found that researchers were often inclined, however reluctantly, to address her concerns with some seriousness.

THE "IMPURITIES" OF ACTIVISM

Few social movements are inclined to mix "moral crusades" with "practical crusades."[97] Treatment activism in the late 1980s was distinctive for the powerful fusion of these two forms. A case in point was the presentation made by activists in early 1989 before a special governmental committee charged with reviewing procedures that concerned cancer and AIDS drugs—generally called the "Lasagna committee" after its chair, Dr. Louis Lasagna of Tufts University, in Massachusetts, an authority on clinical trials and FDA approval policies. What particularly caught Lasagna's attention was the extraordinary contrast between the AIDS activists and the spokespersons for other illnesses. On one hand, there was the "very well behaved," "well-dressed" woman dying of breast cancer, who testified before the committee in moderate tones about the need for new cancer therapies. On the other hand, there were the noisy AIDS activists who "came dressed in any old way almost proud of looking bizarre." The activists' "penchant for the dramatic" was well evidenced at the hearings, Lasagna later recalled: "About fifty of them showed up, and took out their watches and dangled them to show that time was ticking away for them." But the activists' message did not rest on theatrics alone. "I'd swear that the ACT UP group from New York must have read everything I ever wrote," said Lasagna. "And quoted whatever served their purpose. It was quite an experience."[98]

Even as activists creatively blended moral and scientific claims-making, they were burrowing progressively deeper into the institutional structures of the federal health bureaucracies. In consequence, activist identities were being reshaped—that was part of what the construction of credibility entailed. As Mark Harrington recalled after contributing to the activists' testimony before the Lasagna committee:

"There was a lot of euphoria, but there was also a wistfulness about crossing over. From then on we were sort of inside/outside, and not just outside; and [we] sort of lost innocence. I knew that we would never be so pure and fervent in our belief that we were right, because we were actually going to be engaged and, therefore, be more responsible for some of the things that actually happened."[99] As treatment activists sought to mobilize supporters and construct their own frames for the problems with AIDS research, they experienced the tensions—endemic to many social movements—between "prefigurative" and "accommodationist" politics. On one hand, they sought to "live their values" and see them inscribed on the inner workings of the institutions of medicine and science. On the other hand, they strove for effectiveness within the system as constituted.[100] The tension between these goals would lead to cleavages and fractures in AIDS activist organizations over the succeeding years.

A broadly similar contradictory impulse could be observed in the educative strategies of the grassroots treatment organizations and in the conceptions of science that they put forward. Project Inform, for example, didn't simply advise people with AIDS or HIV infection what to do or what to think, it also sought to educate them about how to weigh scientific claims, read between the lines of the journal articles and the news reports, and make informed treatment decisions—how, in other words, to *assess credibility* in science. In the October 1987 issue of its publication, *PI Perspectives,* Project Inform set out the dilemma: "What is a reasonable strategy in the absence of hard scientific conclusions? How do I choose something that is likely to help without throwing money away?"[101] It's not "reasonable," the article maintained, to put much faith in unscientific "personal testimonials"; "to avoid being misled by personal enthusiasm or stifled by the turgid pace of science, one must focus as much as possible on objective, measurable indicators." When considering a new treatment, one should first ask what formal research data are available on this treatment. Next, who conducted the research? ("We must look to the reputations of the authors and institutions they are working for.") Where was the research published? ("The best shows up in major journals, such as *New England Journal of Medicine, Lancet, JAMA,* and *Science.*") Do the research data lack "apparent validity"? ("Are there obvious internal inconsistencies or misleading statements"?) What controls were employed in the study? How many people were studied? Is there a plausible theory for the mechanism of antiviral action? How is antiviral activity measured? ("Viral culture methods are notoriously inconsistent.")

In essence, Project Inform was proposing that people with AIDS or HIV infection pursue the same interpretive strategies as do doctors and scientists themselves when they read a scientific journal article: they should weigh the markers of credibility that attest to the validity of scientific claims. Indeed, if anything is surprising about Project Inform's advice, it is the utter *conventionality* of their assumptions about the telltale indicators of good science. There were no suggestions here, for instance, that forces may sometimes conspire to keep articles out of the prominent journals or that new ideas may spring from unlikely sources. Nor, in the reliance on "objective, measurable indicators," was there any truck with relativist notions about truth being in the eye of the beholder.

This strategy for the knowledge-empowerment of the movement represented one face of AIDS treatment activism and, indeed, one face of Project Inform. At times, the movement asserted its faith in science (or a particular, positivist conception of it): it believed that "only by following the rules of investigation will we ever be certain of a treatments' [*sic*] usefulness. We differ with the scientific establishment mostly in regards to the pace of research and the degree of certainty required before a treatment should be made available." [102] At other times, the movement posed fundamental challenges to the conventional scientific wisdom about who produces knowledge and what social practices ensure its validity. This unresolved tension—between reformist and revolutionary critiques of scientific practice—would surface with regularity in the debates over treatment in the years to come.

CHAPTER 7

THE CRITIQUE
OF PURE SCIENCE

AZT and the Politics
of Interpretation (1989–1990)

SIGNS OF RAPPROCHEMENT

By early 1989, it began to appear that AIDS treatment activists had won a partial convert to the cause: Anthony Fauci himself, the head of NIAID and the government's AIDS research program. To a greater extent than his counterparts at the FDA, Fauci had cultivated good relations with treatment activists, opening up channels of communication with people like Martin Delaney of Project Inform and Mark Harrington and Jim Eigo of ACT UP/New York's Treatment & Data Committee. "In the beginning, those people had a blanket disgust with us," Fauci told the *Washington Post* in 1989: "And it was mutual. Scientists said all trials should be restricted, rigid and slow. The gay groups said we were killing people with red tape. When the smoke cleared we realized that much of their criticism was absolutely valid." [1] When activists complained about the FDA's slowness in approving a drug called ganciclovir that appeared to prevent blindness in people with AIDS suffering from a viral infection of the retina called CMV retinitis, Fauci went to bat for them and helped to put pressure on the FDA. [2] In an article in the journal *Academic Medicine* published early in 1989, Fauci defended established scientific methods but also acknowledged some of the points that activists had been making. "Clearly, there is a need for greater access to clinical trials of investigational drugs by a broader spectrum of the infected population," wrote Fauci.[3]

The turning point came at the Fifth International Conference on AIDS, held in Montreal in June. Activists took center stage at the conference—disrupting the opening ceremony, staging protests against pharmaceutical companies that had been identified as profit-hungry, and presenting formal poster sessions with titles like "AIDS Drugs and the Politics of Biomedicine" and "Drug Regulation Gone Wrong: The Saga of Ganciclovir."[4] Behind the scenes, Larry Kramer of ACT UP/ New York met with Fauci—a man he had called "an incompetent idiot" and worse in print—and solidified Fauci's support for "parallel track," a new concept that had been developed by Jim Eigo and other New York activists.[5]

The parallel track program was, in effect, the solution to the sort of dilemma that Martin Delaney had described at the meeting of the Infectious Diseases Society a few months before (a meeting that Fauci had attended): when researchers coerced people into trials by giving them no other means of access to experimental treatments, participants likely wouldn't comply with the study protocols, and as a result the data would be unreliable. To avoid such difficulties, as Fauci told the press in June, a parallel track program "would provide promising drugs to some people with AIDS at the same time as the drugs are undergoing rigorous [Phase II] clinical trials."[6] Patients would be eligible to receive free drugs in the parallel track program "if they were unwilling or unable to participate in the normal clinical trial"—for example, because they failed to qualify for the study or because they lived too far from the study centers.

In essence, Fauci adopted the activist line on this issue, as his comments quoted in the front-page *New York Times* article made evident: "'Previously, there was a great concern that if we did this, then no one would be in the clinical trial,' Dr. Fauci said. But he added that he has changed his mind and now thinks it is unnecessary 'to hold a gun to their heads' to induce people to join clinical trials."[7] Fauci explained that NIAID could pursue parallel track under its own authority without the need for any new, enabling legislation; indeed, he was prepared to start the program soon with the drug ddI, pending support from the manufacturer, Bristol-Myers.[8] Unlike the FDA's more limited compassionate use policies, parallel track promised to provide large numbers of AIDS patients with easy access to drugs that had passed only Phase I trials. "I came out and stuck myself out on a limb . . . and everybody here in Washington fell off their seats and said 'What is he doing?'" Fauci later recalled. But "I thought it was the right thing to do, and I figured the only way we could get it done was to just say that I was in favor of it and apologize later. And as it turned out, I didn't have to apologize, because everybody then jumped on the bandwagon. . . ."[9]

Optimism among activists about their successes in changing federal policies was matched by more upbeat attitudes on the part of researchers and clinicians about therapeutic prospects. With AZT, with prophylaxis against PCP, and with better treatment strategies against other opportunistic infections, AIDS patients were living longer. Other antivirals like ddI and ddC were on the horizon. By combining or alternating the use of these and other drugs (as was often done in cancer treatments and for some bacterial infections), doctors might be able to keep the virus in check while preventing the onset of drug resistance. In Montreal, a new conventional wisdom emerged: HIV infection might soon become a "chronic manageable illness," not fully curable but something that a person might live with.[10]

AZT: "THE TIME HAS COME"

This notion that HIV disease could soon become a chronic manageable illness received a sharp boost in August 1989 with the release of the latest news about AZT. "The drug AZT can delay the onset of AIDS in people who are infected with the virus but have no symptoms," began a front-page *New York Times* article.[11] ACTG 019, as the ACTG-sponsored study of AZT use in asymptomatic HIV-infected patients was dubbed, had just been halted upon the discovery by the Data and Safety Monitoring Board that the participants on placebo had been twice as likely to develop AIDS-related symptoms as those taking AZT. Just a few weeks earlier, ACTG 016 had also been ended, with the conclusion that AZT helped prevent HIV-infected people with mild symptoms from progressing to full AIDS. Out of 713 people in that study, 36 taking a placebo had progressed to AIDS, versus only 14 of those on AZT. Dr. Jerome Groopman had called it "the first clear proof that early intervention makes a difference."[12] Now, with the results from 019, the verdict seemed to be in. "Today we are witnessing a turning point in the battle to change AIDS from a fatal disease to a treatable one," said Dr. Louis Sullivan, the Bush administration's secretary of health and human services.[13] It was indeed a turning point, though 019 would prove to be one of the most-debated studies in the history of AIDS clinical trials.

The 019 study finally made its way into the *New England Journal* the following April, with Paul Volberding of San Francisco listed as the first author.[14] About 1,500 patients at thirty-two trial sites around the country had participated in the study for an average time of fifty-five weeks. Though none of them had AIDS symptoms upon entry, all of them were immune deficient, with T cell counts below five hundred per cubic millimeter of blood. One third had received fifteen hundred milligrams a day of AZT—by the time the study ended, this was generally believed to be an unnecessarily high dose—and 14 patients in that group had developed an AIDS-defining illness. Another third had received five hundred milligrams a day, with 11 developing AIDS. And of the final third, the patients on placebo, 33 had developed AIDS. AZT did not *stop* patients, as an aggregate, from developing AIDS, but it appeared to slow the process down, at least over a fifty-five-week period. Furthermore, the subjects receiving AZT (either high or low doses) showed, on average, statistically significant increases in their T-cell counts as well as decreases in their "p24 antigen levels" (p24 is one of the core proteins that make up HIV, so a measure of p24 is a crude measure of how much virus is present in the bloodstream—also called the "viral load"). These markers provided additional evidence that AZT was boosting immune functioning while curtailing viral replication.

What about the rumors of "cheating" by patients seeking to avoid the placebo? Did this skew the study and make the results untrustworthy? "There were lots of stories circulated in the press about people sharing drugs, analyzing drugs," recalled Volberding. But lab tests to detect the presence of AZT in the blood of the placebo patients suggested that drug sharing in fact "was an incredibly small problem."[15] In any event, noncompliance actually strengthened the results of the study, the authors of the study results argued, since it "would tend to give results that underestimate the true effect of zidovudine" (the generic pharmaceutical name for AZT).[16] Noncompliance effectively blurred the differences between the treatment arm and the placebo arm, so the demonstration of a statistically significant difference became all the more impressive.

Volberding and his coauthors included a series of important disclaimers.[17] Since the trial had been ended early, there was still no definitive evidence about the *long-term* benefits or safety of AZT: "Thus, it is possible that the eventual risks of disease progression in the three treatment groups could become similar after a longer time period." This might prove true particularly if AZT were to lose its effectiveness after extended use, as the virus mutated to resist the drug. (Such "resistance-conferring mutations" had already been observed in the test tube.) Finally, said the authors, "it is possible that even if zidovudine persistently delays the onset of AIDS, it may not have an ultimate effect on survival." On first glance, this was a surprising and paradoxical notion: how could a drug delay the progression to AIDS without extending the patient's life span? Volberding and his coauthors didn't elaborate, but the implication was that once progression did occur, the downhill course might then be rapid. Such cases were not unknown in cancer treatment research, where a drug might shrink the size of a tumor yet not confer any survival benefit upon the patient.[18]

The accompanying editorial, by Dr. Gerald Friedland, acknowledged these various uncertainties and also spoke of the psychological implications of putting asymptomatic people on AZT: "The decision to start therapy . . . converts an apparently healthy person into a patient probably committed to lifelong treatment."[19] The initiation of therapy in effect transformed the infected person's identity; this was not an act to be undertaken lightly.[20] Nor was there any hard evidence from 019 about the best time to take such action: Was it when the patient's T-cell count dropped to seven hundred per cubic millimeter? Five hundred? Three hundred? But despite these words of caution, the overall tone of the editorial was upbeat, and the title conveyed the basic message: "Early Treatment for HIV: The Time Has Come." Friedland wrote: "The results of this study strongly support a recommendation to institute zidovudine therapy at a dose of five hundred mg per day [the lower, less toxic dose used in the study] in persons with asymptomatic HIV infection and CD4 + cell counts [T-cell counts] below five hundred per cubic millimeter."[21]

Treatment recommendations in an editorial in the *New England Journal* carry considerable authority, but in a certain sense these were moot. Everyone had known about the study for eight months. Moreover, in early 1990 the FDA's new Antiviral Advisory Committee (one of more than forty standing committees of experts charged with giving independent scientific advice to the agency) had already recommended changing the labeling for AZT to include all HIV-positive patients with T-cell counts below five hundred. Despite concerns about the development of drug resistance, the vote this time was unanimous.

The FDA's Ellen Cooper had reservations about the recommendation—after all, the vast majority of people in each arm of the study had done *well* over the course of fifty-five weeks; the percentage of "events" (progression to AIDS) was small. Did it really make sense to begin mass administration of AZT to hundreds of thousands of relatively healthy people in order to prevent a small fraction of them from progressing to AIDS each year? As Cooper would later acknowledge, this was ultimately less a scientific question than "a matter of judgement and generalization." [22] In the end, the FDA adopted the advisory committee's recommendations on March 2, and the NIH issued new guidelines for physicians concerning when to prescribe AZT.[23] Burroughs Wellcome's potential market thereby increased by a factor of more than ten: In the United States alone, there were fifty thousand reported living AIDS patients, but an estimated six hundred thousand HIV-infected people with no AIDS-defining illnesses and with T-cell counts below five hundred.[24] In England, the stock value of parent company Wellcome PLC increased by 1.4 billion pounds.[25]

In practice, the findings of the 019 study, announced only in preliminary form to the media by NIAID, had provided the basis for regulatory policy making before the full results had even appeared in a peer-reviewed journal, where they could be scrutinized by other experts. Project Inform praised NIAID for its "efforts to release important news without waiting the extra 6 months or more needed for acceptance and printing of a completed journal article." [26] For some time, activist groups had been insisting on the rights of people with AIDS to have access to medical data, and they had criticized the tendencies of some medical journals to monopolize control of information by threatening not to publish studies that had been disclosed to the press.[27] But others, both within the AIDS movement and the scientific establishment, would condemn the practice of "science by press release." [28] As far as Fauci was concerned, however, he really didn't have much of a choice, given the widespread interest in the 019 trial and the extensive monitoring of science by the AIDS movement: "Very, very quickly, everyone would have known the study was terminated. . . . It would have been unacceptable to everyone to make them guess why." [29]

POISON? OR JUST MEDIOCRE?

In fact, neither NIAID's press conference, nor the FDA's approval, nor even the article in the *New England Journal* and the accompanying editorial succeeded in bringing closure to debates about AZT. This was true both within the AIDS movement and among the scientific establishment. In gay communities, controversy about AZT had been bubbling away ever since the original licensing of the drug in early 1987 for use by people with full-blown AIDS. The *New York Native,* the gay newspaper most closely associated with the promotion of heretical views, had been calling AZT a "poison." Its administration "was an act of genocide on the scale of the kinds of 'medical experiments' conducted in Nazi Germany," the newspaper argued.[30] "AZT's alleged benefits are not backed up by hard data, and are not sufficient to compensate for the drug's known toxicities. . . . Do not take, prescribe, or recommend AZT," read the *Native*'s cover in June 1987; an article by John Lauritsen, the HIV dissenter and ally of Peter Duesberg's, accompanied it.[31]

Since Lauritsen did not believe that HIV caused AIDS (see part one), it followed that he would not support the use of an anti-HIV agent as a treatment for the syndrome—especially one that was a DNA chain terminator with potentially serious effects on healthy body cells. But Lauritsen, like Sonnabend, Callen, and other HIV dissenters, also argued that the Phase II AZT study had been methodologically flawed in ways that cast doubt on its substantive conclusions. "In practice, the study became unblinded almost immediately," wrote Lauritsen, recapitulating the various rumors about problems in conducting that study. Though, as with 019, it could be maintained that any noncompliance by participants actually strengthened the results, Lauritsen turned the argument around by proposing that the failure to maintain perfect double-blind conditions had pernicious effects on the research process. Since the research staff knew from lab test results which patients were receiving AZT and which were taking the placebo, he argued, they may have provided better overall care to the AZT patients, whether "unconsciously or deliberately"; this difference in care, rather than the administration of AZT, might explain the difference in progression to AIDS.[32]

Lauritsen's was a textbook case of how to deconstruct a scientific study. "Scientists constantly face uncertainty," Susan Leigh Star has emphasized. "Their experimental materials are recalcitrant; their organizational politics precarious; they may not know whether a given technique was correctly applied or interpreted; they must often rely on observations made in haste or by unskilled assistants."[33] Yet precisely because contingency, confusion, misgivings, and indecision tend to be "written out" of scientists' published work as part of their normal persuasive practice, nonscientists often have mistaken notions about the degree of certainty behind the knowledge that science generates. As Harry Collins has concluded, "There is a relationship between the extent to which science is seen as a producer of certainty and distance from the research front."[34] Thus one strategy for undercutting the credibility of scientific claims is to bring the audience in for a closer look, so as to recapture the contingency and messiness: "Irrespective of whether the critic describes 'truly disqualifying' acts of clumsiness or incompetence, or irrelevant details, the mere act of describing an experiment as a piece of ordinary life reduces its power to convince."[35]

Although dissenters in the AIDS causation controversy universally rejected AZT, criticisms of the drug were not limited to this group. Particularly in New York City—which Martin Delaney characterized as "almost unique in the nation in its anti-AZT hysteria"[36]—there were numerous pockets of suspicion of AZT. Throughout the epidemic, the New York gay community had been—depending on one's perspective—either more radical in its skepticism toward authority or more possessed of a debilitating paranoia than its counterparts in San Francisco and elsewhere around the country. From early on, New Yorkers had seemed to show more interest in conspiratorial theories about the origins of AIDS. With the advent of the HIV antibody test in 1985, even the more mainstream organizations like the Gay Men's Health Crisis had advised against taking the test, on the grounds that those testing positive might be rounded up and quarantined or at least discriminated against; by contrast, San Francisco organizations like the AIDS Foundation had taken a more neutral approach, while Project Inform had advocated in favor of testing as the necessary first step in a program of early intervention. Randy Shilts has suggested that such political and attitudinal differences reflected the relative degrees of comfort of the two gay communities as they evolved in the years before the epidemic, with New Yorkers more "closeted" and concerned about threats to their social privilege and San Franciscans more out-of-the-closet, secure, and influential vis-à-vis their city government.[37]

Whatever the structural or psychosocial roots of these dispositions, they surfaced as well in debates over AZT. Though the "AZT is poison" argument was always a minority view among treatment activists and the communities at large, it was less of a fringe perspective on the East Coast than it was on the West Coast.[38] Indeed, a 1989 gay health conference at Columbia University in New York erupted into a debate between Delaney and Sonnabend over AZT. Interestingly, Delaney agreed that there were "some problems" with the original AZT study but also "[took] some responsibility for those problems": "We as a community screamed and hollered to move that drug through the system and study it as fast as humanly possible." Counseling pragmatism over a methodological purism, Delaney told the audience that to obsess about any deficiencies in that study "is a little like having study groups on the Council of Trent." [39]

In its treatment newsletter, *PI Perspectives,* Project Inform expanded on the view that it was willing to accept a certain degree of uncertainty about drugs as a trade-off for more rapid approval: "Patients and their advocates, including Project Inform, pushed the regulatory and research system hard to make AZT available as soon as possible. We should not be surprised that the drug came into common use while our understanding of it was still very crude." [40] The irony is that, when it was first approved, "there was widespread belief that AZT would be quickly replaced by other drugs with similar benefits and fewer side-effects." That hope had proven to be misplaced, so now patients and advocacy groups found themselves having to make the best of a not so great situation, forced to depend on a mediocre drug. But in response to this predicament, Project Inform advocated judicious risk taking over what it saw as denial and defeatism.

Having committed itself to an interventionist therapeutic strategy, Project Inform in a sense depended on AZT, the only approved anti-HIV drug and the only such drug with widespread public credibility. AZT was, at the moment, an "obligatory passage point": Project Inform needed the drug to advance the group's mission. [41] With the news about ACTG 019, Project Inform pushed its critique of the AZT dissidents: "This latest information should (but won't) sound the death knell for the views of those who have bitterly opposed AZT for the last 3 years." [42] The only real question now, Project Inform's newsletter proposed, was whether every HIV-positive person shouldn't begin immediate AZT use, even if his or her T-cell count was higher than five hundred per cubic millimeter. "At the very least, it is one rationally supportable course of action, perhaps more so than the opposite view."

TWO COMMITTEES, TWO CONCLUSIONS

Critiques by the AZT dissidents would continue after the results of the 019 study were announced. But perhaps more noteworthy (though in practice little noted at the time outside of the scientific press) was the lack of consensus in *mainstream science* about the merits of early intervention with the drug. All mainstream authorities agreed that AZT should be prescribed to patients with AIDS. But should it be recommended for use by every HIV-infected person with fewer than five hundred T cells (let alone those with more than five hundred T cells)? Here the gap in perception was not between the two coasts of the United States, but rather between the opposite shores of the Atlantic Ocean. While the *New England Journal of Medicine* had promoted the message that the "time had come" for early intervention, *Lancet,* the most important British medical journal, suggested that "clinicians should change their prescribing habits with caution."[43] The 019 study, according to *Lancet,* had simply shown that AZT could prevent a small number of people from progressing to AIDS over a short time period. Could these results be extrapolated to the majority of patients, who would progress more slowly in any case? Did the drug really halve the progression rate, or did it simply delay progression for a period of months until the onset of drug resistance?

According to Anthony Pinching, a British immunologist and AIDS clinical trials investigator, the difference in judgment "was exacerbated by the 8-month delay between the announcement of some preliminary results and publication [of the study]"—a delay that Europeans, including the British, had found irritating. During this time, while the rest of the world was waiting to see the data, the NIH and the FDA had effectively given their blessing to AZT use in asymptomatics. In the United States, hopes had coalesced into certainty; elsewhere, scientists and patients were in limbo. At root, said Pinching in an editorial about "knowledge and uncertainty" in AZT use, the problem was that U.S. authorities had "extrapolated" beyond the limits of the actual data—even if one considered the full data from the published study. They had been led beyond the limits of legitimate scientific deduction by "the widespread desire to see progress achieved and the wish to be seen to have made such progress." To illustrate his point about extrapolation, Pinching listed fifteen questions about AZT use in asymptomatics that still remained to be answered, even after the conclusion of 019.[44]

The issue of what remained to be answered was very much on the minds of researchers throughout Europe, for some of them were smack in the middle of their own study when the media began trumpeting the news about the termination of 019. A consortium of researchers in Britain, Ireland, and France was conducting a trial dubbed "Concorde" that was substantially similar to 019. As in the United States, the European researchers had dealt with the ethics of placebo-controlled trials; as in the United States, the Europeans had had to justify to community groups why such trials were necessary in studying AZT use in asymptomatics.[45] But now—even after the results from 019 had been reported—the Concorde researchers were intent on continuing the study. As far as they were concerned, a state of equipoise still held: "The results we have seen," said Jean-Pierre Aboulker, the head of the study on the French side, "do not allow us to give a strict recommendation to give AZT."[46] In deference to those who trusted the results of 019, they would modify the protocol to allow participants to begin "open-label" use of AZT, if they chose not to run the risk of being given the placebo. This change would introduce methodological complications into the interpretation of the data. But it would satisfy ethical objections while allowing Concorde to continue.

"Two committees looking at one set of data have come to radically different conclusions about the anti-AIDS drug AZT," was how a reporter for *Science* characterized the transatlantic dispute.[47] In practice, everyone agreed on which questions they would like to have answered—questions about long-term risks and benefits, about the development of resistance, about whether early use would squander the limited efficacy of the drug against the virus. The different actions taken had to do with different judgments about the *implications* of what was known and what wasn't. How and when should a particular balance of certainty and uncertainty about a drug inform clinical practice? And what is the *feasibility* of continuing a placebo-controlled trial, once a specific (but not conclusive) benefit had been shown?

"I think there is generally a greater skepticism in the U.K. about the value of treatments than in the U.S.," commented biostatistician Susan Ellenberg, reflecting a widespread perception in the U.S. biomedical community. "I think there is much more reluctance [in Britain] to treat unless it is absolutely necessary."[48] Such cultural differences were compounded by differences in the sheer magnitude of the epidemic in the two countries, not to mention the more vociferous character of AIDS treatment activism in the United States. Continuing the 019 trial "was not a conceivable possibility when the data were first seen . . . by those of us who were on the executive committee of the ACTG," researcher Martin Hirsch later recalled. "There was no choice but to stop the study given what the results were. . . . If we had withheld that kind of information we would have been strung up on trees. And if we had given out the information and said we were going to continue the placebo control trial anyway, we would have been strung up even quicker."[49] Similarly, the principal investigator for Concorde in Britain, Dr. Ian Weller, suggested to *Science* that the large numbers of AIDS patients in the United States had generated greater pressures there for the immediate translation of research into results.[50] And once the formal guidelines had been issued, all the remaining uncertainties, though never denied, had in a practical sense been bracketed, largely to be ignored by the media, most practicing physicians, and most patients. Concorde, by contrast, chose to put uncertainty in the foreground. With the goal of obtaining definitive answers about early intervention with AZT, the Concorde trial would keep running all the way to 1993. Ironically, the results of Concorde, when finally available, would provoke more controversy than any AIDS antiviral study ever.

Activism and the Manufacture of Knowledge (1989–1991)

METHODOLOGY TO THE RESCUE

As treatments activists followed, or contributed to, the debates surrounding AZT, they also devoted increasing attention to new drugs, such as ddI and ddC, that appeared likely to be the next additions to the therapeutic armamentarium of HIV antivirals. Since these drugs were chemically related to AZT, few thought that any of them would be an ideal therapy; but nothing else was anywhere near approval, and ddI and ddC at least showed promise. Perhaps they could provide alternatives for those who couldn't tolerate AZT's toxicity or for those who, over time, had stopped benefiting from AZT. Or perhaps some combination of these nucleoside analogues would prove more effective than AZT alone. Throughout 1989 and 1990, as AIDS treatment activists pursued the approval of these drugs as well as others that treated opportunistic infections, they became ever more enmeshed in the minutiae of clinical trial design—a set of topics that, increasingly, they would debate face-to-face with researchers and officials from the NIH and the FDA. This direct engagement with the terms of clinical research would both establish the scientific credibility of the activists (or certain of their representatives) and ultimately alter the pathways by which specific treatments came to seem credible in different quarters.

As with the parallel track initiative, a turning point came with the Montreal conference in the summer of 1989. ACT UP/New York had distributed an *AIDS Treatment Research Agenda* blasting the ACTG program and detailing the activists' demands: more compounds in clinical trials, an end to placebo-controlled trials that required "body counts" to prove efficacy, greater access to clinical trials by all social groups affected by the epidemic, and more flexible protocols with broader entry requirements. Susan Ellenberg, the chief bio-statistician assigned to the ACTG trials at NIAID, recalled seeking out the ACT UP/New York document in Montreal in response to her own curiosity: "I walked down to the courtyard and there was this group of guys, and they were wearing muscle shirts, with earrings and funny hair. I was almost afraid. I was really hesitant even to approach them. . . ." But after picking up the document, Ellenberg quickly found her-self "scribbling madly in the margins." Though most of her marginal notes reflected dismay at activists' failure to understand, "there were many places where I found it was very sensible—where I found myself saying, 'You mean, we're not doing this?' or 'We're not doing it this way?'"[51]

Ellenberg brought the ACT UP report back to Bethesda and shared it with her colleagues in a working group of statisticians who had been meeting to discuss challenges posed by the AIDS epidemic. "I've never been to such a meeting in my life," said Ellenberg. According to David Byar, the chief of the biometry branch of the Division of Cancer Prevention and Control at NCI: "I think anybody looking at that meeting through a window who could not hear what we were saying would not have believed that it was a group of statisticians discussing how trials ought to be done. There was enormous excitement and wide divergence of opinion."[52] Soon afterward, with Fauci's consent, Ellenberg expanded her Statistical Working Group by inviting representatives from ACT UP and other community-based organizations to participate.

In a sense, the agenda of these meetings of the Statistical Working Group was to find methodological common ground that would satisfy competing ethical concerns. In more public arenas, activists were effective in seizing the moral high ground, and researchers were easily put on the defensive. Activist theater—like serving "Kool-AID" at public speeches by ACTG researchers to compare them to Jim Jones orchestrating mass suicide in Jonestown, Guyana—acted on researchers' sensitivities but risked alienating them as well.[53] In more private negotiations, by contrast, there was at least tacit acknowledgment of ethical claims on both sides.

On one hand, activists often criticized trials in terms of the rights of research subjects; on the other, researchers defended the trials with utilitarian arguments about the benefit to society. But as Rebecca Smith of ACT UP/New York and AmFAR, who became close to several of the biostatisticians, explained in a letter published in *Science,* the solution was precisely to find points of convergence between "the immediate short-term needs of people with AIDS" and the "long-term goals of medical research."[54] To the extent that methodological solutions could be engineered that would make all parties comfortable, people with AIDS and HIV infection would willingly participate in the trials and conform to the protocols, and scientific knowledge would be advanced.

Still, AIDS researchers often found this agenda threatening. At a 1990 community forum on clinical trials held in San Francisco, Donald Abrams commented: "My concern is we may never be able to study *anything* again to see if it works." But ACT UP/San Francisco member Michelle Roland argued at the same conference that perhaps the problem had less to do with any inherent limitations of science than with the ways in which doctors are socialized to imagine that clinical trials ought to be conducted. "We need to design realistic clinical trials that do a better job of meeting people's needs," said Roland, calling for a "revolution in clinical trial design." She acknowledged that such trials were "going to be more difficult to analyze. But we've got to do it."[55]

The biostatisticians at NIH proved to be an important ally in this struggle: they did not always agree with activists, but some of them also had their criticisms of biomedical researchers. In the view of these biostatisticians, the reliance of principal investigators on "overly narrow and unimaginative" rules for conducting clinical trials betrayed their failure to entirely comprehend the underlying statistical principles.[56] "Statisticians had been trying to say a lot of these things for years," Rebecca Smith recalled. "And we came along, and from a somewhat different perspective said a lot of them."[57] Or as Ellenberg put it: "What the activists wanted pretty much was what we wanted too, and what we had every confidence that we were eventually going to be able to persuade the investigators of. . . ."[58]

At a panel discussion at the 1990 Annual Meeting of the Society for Clinical Trials to which Ellenberg invited activists, Jim Eigo explained the kinds of obstacles that stood in the way of carrying out effective AIDS research. "Investigators have traditionally had to deal with people who are sick in a *single* way"; they therefore had been able to study the effect of a single drug on a single condition. But in the case of AIDS, where patients might be taking a range of drugs to treat their opportunistic infections, this was an "unreasonable preference" and one that had "made a shambles of the efforts to enroll AIDS clinical trials." Investigators routinely eliminated people who were on various medications and then found they could not fill their trials, explained Eigo, giving an example of recent trials for the antiviral drug ddI: at one New York site researchers had screened 150 people with AIDS and found only 3 who were "eligible" to participate in the study.[59]

The point was that activists had insights about "accrual" of subjects into studies and "compliance" with the conditions of studies, two of the most vexing issues for clinical investigators: What trials would patients sign up for? Under what conditions could patients be relied on to follow the study protocols? It wasn't that researchers couldn't speculate about the answers to these questions; as one prominent researcher, Douglas Richman, insisted: "It's not like we're completely out to lunch. We sit and we talk to the patients. We've got some incredibly good nurses at the study center who spend all their time with the patients and think about the inefficiencies and the problems with the protocols and why patients are not happy with some protocols and happy with others."[60] In practice, however, many researchers had tended to view accrual as essentially a technical problem and compliance as a management issue. From the investigators' standpoint, noncompliant subjects were "bad" subjects; from the activists' perspective, "noncompliance can be taken as a surrogate marker of the extent to which [doctors] have been able to explain things to patients." In fact, "if people don't comply," said Rebecca Smith, "that means they're not buying in, on some level."[61]

Activists, as the research subjects' representatives or as subjects themselves, possessed grounded knowledge that many researchers found valuable in the design of trials—"an extraordinary instinct . . . about what would work in the community," as Anthony Fauci summarized it, and "probably a better feel for what a workable trial was than the investigators [had]."[62] This was the expertise that researchers began to find attractive, and that made it worthwhile for activists to be invited onto the local community advisory boards and institutional review boards that oversaw protocols for clinical trials at hospitals and research centers. Furthermore, activists could work as intermediaries, helping to explain to people with AIDS and HIV exactly what a clinical trial was and how one might decide whether to participate. Rebecca Smith considered one of her most important activist projects to be the production of a booklet called "Deciding to Enter an AIDS/ HIV Drug Trial."[63] Published by the AIDS Treatment Registry in New York, this booklet was designed precisely to give people with HIV the capacity to make an informed decision about whether to participate in clinical research. It offered an overview of the drug approval process, a glossary of terms, and a long checklist of questions that the potential research subject should consider.[64]

THE QUESTIONS OF REAL IMPORTANCE

Of course, activists also had quite a bit of learning to do about clinical trials, and biostatisticians played an important role in that education process. Both Susan Ellenberg of NIAID and Mark Harrington of ACT UP/New York pointed to David Byar (who died of AIDS himself in August 1991) as the key "charismatic" figure who helped bridge the gap between worlds. Byar suffered no fools— whether statisticians, activists, or researchers—but was happy to expound on the inner logic of the controlled clinical trial until his audience grasped the issues.[65] Inevitably, the greater exposure to the science of clinical trials caused activist opinions to begin to shift.

An interesting example concerned the debate over the ethics of placebos. The idea that placebo-controlled trials were inherently unjust in life-threatening illnesses had endowed treatment activists with a moral claim, and it had made for some catchy slogans. But ironically, the same argument that had helped mobilize the AIDS movement to pay attention to clinical trial design had little currency once activists sat down at the table with the wizards of statistics. Simply by accepting the terms of the debate—that properly conducted, controlled trials should guide the selection of therapies—treatment activists became bound, at least to some extent, by the inner logic of these evaluative methods. And that logic, as David Byar insisted, at times favored the use of placebos as the shortest route to a meaningful answer: placebos were "sometimes . . . in the patients' best interest, whether they realize it or not, and no matter how many signs they paint and march around New York City with. . . ."[66]

As D. Bruce Burlington of the FDA explained, the FDA did not necessarily insist on placebo controls as the only mechanism for conducting a controlled study that could lead to a drug's approval. For

example, "the agency can, and frequently does, accept . . . the historically controlled trial," where patients receiving an experimental treatment are compared with a matched group of untreated patients who
were followed at some point in the past. But drug sponsors relying on
historical controls "bear the burden of establishing the natural history
of the disease," that is, proving that the progression of illness within
the untreated cohort was representative of the disease in question. The
problem, according to Burlington, was that AIDS had no single, constant natural history, given "the dramatic changes in demographics
and the marked improvement in diagnosis and management of [HIV-
infected] patients."[67] The natural history of AIDS was in flux; so what
would the treatment group be compared against?

Some activists, like Jim Eigo, rethought their assumptions: at another panel discussion in 1991, he acknowledged that although he
originally had seen no need for placebos ever, he now recognized the
virtues of using them in certain situations, where a short trial could
rapidly answer an important question.[68] More generally, activists
maintained that the point was not so much placebos versus no placebos, but whether a trial asked a meaningful, real-world question that
the patient community wanted answered. As Eigo put it in 1989 at a
symposium entitled "Methodological Issues in AIDS Clinical Trials,"
sponsored by NIAID and the FDA: "If every arm of every trial asked
a question of real importance to people with acquired immune suppression, enough of those people would find every arm of every trial a
viable treatment option and, therefore, if they knew about the trial,
could be accrued for that trial."[69] This, in a sense, was a new definition of "equipoise" reframed from the vantage point of the community of patients rather than the community of scientists. If a trial compared different treatment options (including one option that was the
control), if patients didn't know which option was best, if patients
wanted to know which option was best, and if every option provided
patients with quality medical care in all other respects, then patients
would sign up for the study, regardless of the type of controls used.
The prescription, therefore, was for better and more profound communication between researchers and the subject population (or their
activist representatives) before studies got off the ground—indeed, before they were even proposed. "When we talk about methodology,"
Mark Harrington told the participants at the "Methodological Issues"
conference, "we usually talk about how we are going to answer the
questions that we set out to ask." This begs the prior question of "how

. . . we decide what are the important questions. As patients become more involved in the design and execution of clinical trials," said Harrington, "it is crucial to recognize that patients' questions are very important and deserve to be answered."[70]

The questions that regulators or researchers wanted answered were often too academic, too removed from the day-to-day realities of patient care; and the resulting trials didn't provide participants with attractive options. Only an active engagement and negotiation between researchers, doctors, and the AIDS movement could ensure that the most important therapeutic questions were being studied; only such an engagement could rescue researchers from the not infrequent difficulties in recruiting patients to participate in their trials. As Paul Volberding acknowledged in his presentation at the same conference, "examples abound of clinical trials that are elegant in their design but fail because of limited accrual of subjects."[71]

CREDIBILITY AND REPRESENTATION

Even if researchers were dubious about the patient community's ability to gauge what research was most important, they certainly recognized the practical virtues of cooperation and negotiation in order to ensure accrual. In this sense, a basic "credibility achievement" of treatment activists has been their capacity to present themselves as the legitimate, organized voice of people with AIDS or HIV infection (or, more specifically, the current or potential clinical trial subject population). This point is easily missed, but important, since the three groups—activists, people with AIDS or HIV, and clinical trial participants—overlap but are not isomorphic, and it is a complicated question whether in fact activists *do* meaningfully represent the diverse groups in the United States that are affected by HIV. Even within gay communities, the question of representation can be complex, in part because the activists are often politically more radical than the gay mainstream on whose behalf they speak, and in part because gay researchers and health professionals may also make plausible claims to representation. "What right do these people have to think that they are representing the gay community, when I'm also here and just on the other side of the fence?" Donald Abrams complained.[72]

Looking back at her experience with treatment activism, Michelle Roland reflected with some candor, "I *never* represented 'people with AIDS.' I represented *activists*. And those are different people, you know. They are a subset of people with AIDS." [73] Yet the extraordinary success of treatment activists (who have always been a relatively small group and whose ranks have been further depleted by burnout, illness, and death over the years) stemmed in large part from their capacity to convince the biomedical establishment not only that they spoke for the larger body of patients but also that they could mobilize hundreds or thousands of angry demonstrators to give muscle to their specific requests. And once activists monopolized the capacity to say "what patients wanted," researchers could be forced to deal with them in order to ensure that research subjects would both enroll in their trials in sufficient numbers and comply with the study protocols. On the basis of their credibility, activists constructed themselves as an "obligatory passage point" standing between the researchers and the trials they sought to conduct. [74] Of course, by the same token, the activists *wanted* to see the trials conducted, so the point, really, is that the relationship became a powerfully symbiotic one.

ACCESS, HETEROGENEITY, AND PRAGMATISM

One area in which activists succeeded in placing considerable and effective pressure on the biomedical establishment was the question of opportunity to participate in clinical trials. In part this concern grew out of the earliest debates about the true purpose of trials: were they scientific experiments or a means of access to unapproved treatments? The activists engaged in debating clinical trial design had no desire to pose the question in either/or terms, and certainly they were in favor of conducting experiments. On the other hand, they objected to the exclusion of individuals from trials on grounds that seemed to them arbitrary. Typically, the protocols specified various lab test levels as cutoffs for entrance into a study; a person with results outside the normal or expected range on these lab tests was excluded, ostensibly in order to avoid the introduction of extraneous variables into the study. In some cases, such rules actually threatened to derail the study. At the "Methodological Issues" conference, Harrington gave an example of a worthwhile study that was enrolling at a "snail's pace" because the protocol required that potential participants test positive for the p24 antigen, a marker of active viral replication, but one that in practice is hard to detect. [75]

Principal investigators insisted on the virtues of "clean data." But in the name of this lofty goal, people who were currently taking other medications, or had taken them in the past, found themselves excluded by study protocols, while sometimes those enrolled in studies who took so much as an aspirin without explicit permission were threatened with expulsion. Terry Sutton, a San Francisco activist who was going blind from CMV retinitis but who was denied entry to a test of a drug to treat that condition because he had already used another (unsuccessful) drug, summed up his frustration: "The idea of clean data terrifies me, because it punishes people for trying to treat early. My roommate . . . has made the decision not to treat early because of the pure subject rule. What he says is 'I want to be a pure subject so that I can get access to the best protocol once it starts to move.' You only get to be a pure subject once." [76]

Rebecca Smith described a similar, but more hopeful story that pointed to the virtues of activist intervention. A patient who believed that his AIDS-related dementia was being kept in check by AZT also wanted to take an experimental drug to prevent blindness from CMV infection of his eyes. But in order to enroll in the trial for the CMV drug, he was told by his doctor that he would have to go off AZT. The patient "told me that . . . he was being asked to choose between his vision and his sanity," Smith recalled. But with Smith's support, the patient persisted, asking his doctor if there was any medical reason that one couldn't take both drugs, and whether anyone had ever studied the conjoined effects of the drugs. The end result of these discussions was the enrollment of the patient in a new study that alternated regimens of the two therapies. [77]

In the skirmishes over these poignant dilemmas, activists found an ally in some of the biostatisticians. David Byar, for example, argued that as long as a study had been properly randomized from the outset, research subjects could simultaneously receive other medications, such as PCP prophylaxis, without threatening the statistical interpretation of the study results. [78] Similarly, Byar insisted there was no statistical barrier to the simultaneous participation of patients in multiple trials, and he argued against excluding potential research subjects simply because they had abnormal results on lab tests. "Sometimes rigid entry criteria are defended because the investigators desire to study homogeneous groups, but this reasoning is usually difficult to justify," said Byar. "It is important to study patients with abnormal baseline values, because such patients will receive treatments shown to be effective, and we need to know in advance whether or not they can tolerate them." [79]

Byar's argument pointed to a larger debate between two competing understandings of the very purpose of clinical trials—a debate with a history independent of AIDS or AIDS activism. In a 1983 article in the *Annals of Internal Medicine,* Dr. Alvan Feinstein, a professor at the Yale University School of Medicine and an authority on clinical trials, had distinguished between two warring conceptions of such trials, which he called the "pragmatic" and "fastidious" perspectives. Proponents of the first perspective look to trials "to answer pragmatic questions in clinical management." The trial design, in their view, should "incorporate the heterogeneity, occasional or frequent ambiguity, and other 'messy' aspects of ordinary clinical practice." Those who approach clinical trials with the perspective that Feinstein called fastidious "fear that [the pragmatic] strategy will yield a 'messy' answer. They prefer a 'clean' arrangement, using homogeneous groups, reducing or eliminating ambiguity, and avoiding the spectre of biased results" in order to produce rapid and secure findings.[80] This theoretical dichotomy was linked to an even older power struggle that Harry Marks has characterized as intrinsic to the history of the use of controlled trials in medicine—between academic researchers who would like to impose scientific judgment on clinical practice and primary-care physicians who struggle to preserve autonomy over clinical decision making.[81]

Feinstein's distinction between fastidious and pragmatic clinical trials was described by Dr. Robert Levine, a professor of medicine and ethicist at Yale University, in his 1986 book, *Ethics and Regulation of Clinical Research;* from there, the distinction made its way into the pages of *AIDS Treatment News.*[82] The pragmatic perspective made sense to activists, as it did to community physicians with whom they were often allied. Clinical trials are experiments, to be sure, but they are real-world experiments with real-world implications. They should be designed not to answer ivory-tower theoretical questions but to inform day-to-day clinical practice and help patients and doctors make meaningful decisions when confronted with treatment dilemmas. If, for example, patients in the real world take different pills simultaneously, why not study the combined effects of the drugs? By contrast, many FDA regulators, academic researchers, and researchers for drug companies were more inclined, by training and institutional logic, to adhere to the dictates of fastidiousness. But by the late 1980s, many parties to the controversy could appreciate that there were valid arguments on each side. Indeed, Paul Volberding, in his talk at the

"Methodological Issues" conference, presented the case of entry restrictions as a simple trade-off: strict entry criteria promised an efficient trial, but one that might lack generalizability; broad criteria meant that findings would be generalizable but that the trial would be less efficient in the short run.[83]

What was "real" and what was "artificial"? Precisely because *every* scientific experiment is by definition a stand-in for reality, *any* experimental method is, in principle, open to being taken apart by those who claim reality is not adequately represented.[84] In this case, where there was an ongoing dispute between experts about which method was truer to "nature," activist pressure stood a good chance of tipping the balance. Because activists were able to enroll allies from fields such as biostatistics and bioethics, they succeeded in endowing the pragmatic perspective with additional credibility. "Once statisticians and activists started to talk, [this] was one of the things that there was immediate agreement on, from different points of view," recalled Ellenberg. "The activists were screaming that people couldn't get into trials. . . . The statisticians [were concerned] that the results of the trials weren't going to apply to anybody. . . ."[85] Working together, activists and biostatisticians successfully called for a number of modifications in trial design, many of which were already in common use in trials for other illnesses such as cancer. These included the use of broader entry criteria, more diverse subject populations, and concomitant medication.[86]

THE POLITICS OF PURITY

Taking on a more profound challenge, one suggested by Terry Sutton's poignant comment, activists interrogated the presuppositions of scientific "cleanliness." Did "clean" data come only from "pure" subjects? Was "messy," "impure" science necessarily bad science? The debate between fastidious and pragmatic approaches to clinical trials already pointed to these questions; AIDS treatment activists pressed them even further. People with AIDS were not in awe of that "strange and abstract god, clean data," Jim Eigo told a Senate health subcommittee.[87] Similarly, John James argued that "Good Science, like God, patriotism, and the flag, are rhetorical devices designed to be impossible to argue against—devices often used in the absence of a good case on the merits."[88] Academic researchers could be counted on to come up with "elegant" research designs, but were these the ones that would most effectively answer the burning questions?[89]

The metaphors varied, but the implication, in each case, was similar: the defense of science put forward by mainstream researchers was an *ideology* designed to promote *the kind of science they happened to do* as the only kind that could be called science.[90] Purity and cleanliness, in this sense, were not intrinsic to the scientific project; they were legitimating metaphors that imbued modern scientific institutions with an appearance of the sacred.[91]

Building on concepts like Feinstein's notion of "pragmatic" trials, activists hinted at (though never fully described) what they saw as a preferable kind of science, which would be more accurate, more useful, and more responsible. This science would be less preoccupied with the formal rules that prevent "contamination" and more open to the varying of experimental design in recognition of practical barriers, ethical demands, and other "real-world" exigencies. "The truth is that [clinical trial] research is muddy, and people need to start acknowledging that," San Francisco activist Michelle Roland explained. "You can't get good clean answers, the world does not work that way. Patients tend to not work that way unless you totally manipulate them. And this is not a population that is going to be easily manipulated. So you either have muddy research that you *know* is muddy, and you can at least say, 'This is where it's muddy,' or you have muddy research and you don't even know how muddy it is."[92]

The championing of "real-world messiness" was also the strategy of Martin Delaney of Project Inform when he decided, in 1989, to conduct research on "Compound Q" (tricosanthin), a drug obtained from a Chinese cucumber that had been shown to kill HIV-infected macrophages in the test tube. Believing that the official study of Compound Q was too small and that it was using inadequate dosages, Project Inform initiated its own study with the cooperation of a number of doctors and laboratories and forty-two participants in three cities. No placebo controls were used.[93] The following year, Delaney reported his cautiously optimistic findings at the main panel on clinical trials at the Sixth International Conference on AIDS, in San Francisco. Delaney acknowledged that Project Inform had "stretched the rules" by including research participants who were simultaneously taking other medications. But rather than accept that such procedures contaminated the study, Delaney argued that the "real-world conditions" of his study were precisely its virtues and the warrants of its validity. "This is the real-world laboratory," Delaney proclaimed. "This is not the artificial world of clinical trials."[94]

Needless to say, the Compound Q trial sparked considerable controversy, and it prompted an FDA investigation, though in the end Project Inform was allowed to proceed. At an earlier juncture in the study, when two participants went into comas, Delaney was blasted by Paul Volberding, who was directing the official study of the drug at the University of California at San Francisco. "It doesn't take a genius to hand out drugs," said Volberding, "but it takes a certain amount of discipline to ask questions in a rigorous way."[95] And at the AIDS Conference, Delaney was attacked by co-panelist Arnold Relman, editor of the *New England Journal of Medicine*, who defended the "proven methods of science." "Let's not go back to the days of black magic," Relman exhorted.[96] For his part, Delaney continued to defend his "real-world laboratory," but the experience of designing and conducting a study also made an impact on him. "The truth is, it does take a lot longer to come up with answers than I thought before," he admitted at a community forum in 1990.[97]

HETEROGENEITY AND SOCIAL DIFFERENCE

Having campaigned against narrow inclusion criteria, activists pushed the question of access to trials even further: they opened up the issue of the social demographics of clinical trial participants. In public, the research establishment was on weak ground in this debate: since AIDS activists had successfully promoted the notion that access to trials was potentially beneficial, ordinary notions of equality and justice suggested that this social good should be distributed widely and fairly. Just the opposite was in fact the case, at least in the trials funded through NIAID's ACTG program.

As a 1989 front-page *Los Angeles Times* exposé by Robert Steinbrook had revealed, "blacks, Latinos and intravenous drug users, the groups increasingly afflicted with AIDS virus infections, are significantly under-represented in federally sponsored AIDS clinical trials. . . ."[98] Using documents obtained from NIAID under the Freedom of Information Act, Steinbrook showed that while blacks and Latinos accounted for 42 percent of adult U.S. AIDS patients, they made up only 20 percent of the research subjects in the ACTG trials. Only 11 percent of the ACTG subjects were injection drug users, though this population accounted for 28 percent of AIDS cases. A later study by New York activists that was presented at the Seventh International Conference on AIDS in 1991 showed that women comprised only 6.7

percent of ACTG trial participants. While women accounted for only 9.8 percent of overall AIDS cases according to the CDC's statistics, activists argued that many actual cases of women with AIDS were not captured by the CDC's surveillance definition.[99]

In fact, most trials were populated largely by adult, white gay men who had contracted HIV through sexual transmission. Other demographics groups, such as men of color and women and children of all races, were underrepresented; so were those who had contracted HIV through drug use or contaminated blood products. The reasons for these exclusions were multiple. Certainly it didn't help that there were no AIDS Clinical Trials Units in five of the thirteen cities that contributed the greatest numbers to the CDC's statistics for U.S. AIDS cases— Houston, Philadelphia, Atlanta, Dallas, and San Juan, Puerto Rico. Injection drug users were rarely targeted for recruitment because they were considered to be "bad" research subjects. "They are alienated, disorganized and distrustful," one doctor told the *New York Times* in 1988. "They don't keep appointments; you can speculate about why, but they just don't do it."[100] (In response, other doctors maintained that those drug users who were participating in drug treatment programs made perfectly good research subjects.)[101] Some observers also cited "real-life barriers" to the participation of working-class and poor people in trials, including the cost of transportation and the lack of child care.

In the case of minority groups, particularly African-Americans, it also could not be assumed that people were *anxious* to volunteer for trials. Whites may have been banging on the doors demanding to be put to use as "guinea pigs," but many blacks had vivid historical memories of precisely what such use entailed. As one Dallas health educator testified before the National Commission on AIDS, "So many African American people that I work with do not trust hospitals or any of the other community health care service providers because of that Tuskegee Experiment."[102] The fact that many researchers had targeted Africa as the site of origin of AIDS aroused further distrust in African-American communities. In one survey of black church members, 35 percent of the respondents expressed agreement with the claim that AIDS might actually be a form of genocide perpetrated by the U.S. government on minority communities.[103] Given such sentiment, it was unlikely that the AIDS Clinical Trials Units would draw many African-Americans simply by posting an announcement and waiting for the phone to ring. At a minimum, serious recruitment would have required a concerted outreach effort that presupposed gaining the trust of community leaders.

Finally, the very same reforms in the protection of human subjects that incidents such as the Tuskegee study had engendered also created pressures to exclude various groups from clinical research. According to this logic, experimentation was something that vulnerable populations were to be *protected from*. Children, for example, were generally not to be the subjects of clinical trials until after a drug had been proven safe and effective in adults. (Partly as a result, AZT was not widely distributed to children with AIDS in the United States until October 1989, more than three years after adults had gained broad access to the drug.[104])

The situation with women was even more restrictive. Until 1986, women "of childbearing age"—regardless of whether they were pregnant or had any intention of becoming so—were barred from trials as a matter of course out of fear of causing damage to fetuses (or out of fear of resulting lawsuits). Though the NIH formally changed its rules in response to protests, research protocols (for AIDS and other illnesses) often continued to exclude women, and the FDA continued to ban women from early research on new drugs. Some women with AIDS charged that even after they had offered to undergo sterilization, they were still told they would be unable to join the clinical trials for drugs that the women considered to be promising.[105]

In practice, such policies meant not only that women lacked access to experimental therapies that might help them but also that doctors lacked certainty about the effects of drugs in women's bodies. "American women have been put at risk," said Representative Pat Schroeder, citing a study begun in 1981 that sought to investigate the role of aspirin use in preventing heart attacks, which had enrolled twenty-two thousand male doctors. "[NIH] officials told us women were not included in this study because to do so would have increased the cost," commented a congressional investigator. "However, we now have the dilemma of not knowing whether this preventive strategy would help women, harm them, or have no effect."[106] Another female member of Congress, Olympia Snowe, described a federally funded study on the relation between obesity and cancer of the breast and uterus; the pilot study had used only men. "Somehow I find it hard to imagine that the male-dominated medical community would tolerate a study of prostate cancer that used only women as research subjects," Snowe commented.[107]

Men's and women's bodies are manifestly different, and it seemed not unreasonable to suggest that drugs might have different effects in the different genders. Some experts claimed that the same was true for members of different racial groups; Asians, for example, were said to metabolize an antidepressant drug called desipramine more slowly.[108] As to whether such differences might reveal themselves with AIDS therapies, researchers remained uncertain. Anthony Fauci would comment in 1994 that such a basic question as "whether the drug has an antiviral effect" is something "you could determine . . . by giving it to people who live on . . . Park Avenue and 69th Street in New York City and not worry about the rest of the world. . . ." But that's different, Fauci went on to say, from the question of precisely how best to use particular drugs in particular populations—an issue to be determined by administering drugs to a heterogeneous collection of patients.[109]

Whether or not there truly are significant variations in how drugs affect different social groups, the fact remains that the existence of such variations is widely considered plausible by a society that increasingly tends to understand social difference as something rooted in biology.[110] The body of a gay white man, therefore, was seen as an inappropriate location for generating predictions about the effects of a drug on a straight white man, or a gay Latino man, or a gay white woman. The complexities involved in such debates became evident in 1991, when yet another AZT study, conducted in Veterans Administration hospitals by the Department of Veterans Affairs, purported to find a difference in response to AZT between white and minority patients. "AIDS Study Suggests Drug May Have Racial Limits," declared a *Washington Post* headline.[111] Dr. Wayne Greaves, an infectious disease specialist at Howard University in Washington, D.C., told the *New York Times* that he would "counsel black and Hispanic patients that in light of the new data they had to decide for themselves whether to take the drug."[112] But as scientists and activists scrutinized the data, they discovered that the Veterans Administration researchers had in fact made their claims about a racial category they called "minority." Lacking sufficient numbers of Latinos and African-Americans to draw statistically significant conclusions, the investigators had simply decided to lump the two groups together. Ron Johnson of New York City's Minority Task Force on AIDS blasted the "sloppy" methodology: "Until they do a credible study, they're just playing with us, throwing out confusing and conflicting bits of information."[113] Underlying this response, however, was the prior reification of racial categories: "black" and "Hispanic" were considered to be "real" markers of biological difference (and thus potential predictors of differences in response to treatment), in a way that the hybrid category "minority" was not.

The issue was indeed one of credibility, as Johnson indicated, and in U.S. society at the time, a drug would simply not be perceived as credible across the board if it had not been tested in a diverse range of social groups. As Vivian Pinn-Wiggins, a pathologist at Howard University and the president of the National Medical Association (an organization mainly of African-American physicians) put it in 1990, "some of our physicians are a little leery" of certain medications because "we can't be certain whether minorities have been participants" in the clinical trials.[114] Of course, as Ellen Cooper pointed out at the "Methodological Issues" conference, there are many kinds of heterogeneity, and there are no a priori grounds for singling out particular instances, such as racial and gender differences, and assuming that these are the ones that will manifest differences in response to treatments.[115] These categories are simply the ones with greater *social* and *political* salience.

Two sets of issues came together in the debate over homogeneity and heterogeneity in a study population: the need for a morally credible policy promoting fair access to experimental drugs and the need for a scientifically credible policy for acquiring generalizable data. Between these two sets of issues, AIDS treatment activists had plenty of room to play. Defenders of the notion that a "clean" trial required a homogeneous research population, by contrast, found themselves increasingly on the defensive. The activist critique demonstrated the back-and-forth movement between ethical and epistemological claims-making that AIDS treatment activism had perfected: heterogeneous trials were not only fairer, they were also better science. Though it would not always prove so easy, in this case, the goals of "access" and "answers" could be made to coincide.

OLD DOGS AND NEW TRICKS

Two astonishing, back-to-back "Sounding Board" articles in the *New England Journal of Medicine* in October 1990 attested to the activist success in shifting biomedical norms governing the acquisition of knowledge through AIDS clinical trials. One article, by David Byar and many prominent biostatisticians, argued for restructuring the "phases" of the FDA approval process, dismissed the requirement of homogeneity in a clinical trial population, and called for more flexible entry criteria. The authors concluded with a call for "patients and their organizations to participate in the planning of clinical trials. Such participation is likely to ensure greater agreement with the objectives and design of the trial and to make people with AIDS more aware of the opportunities to enter trials."[116]

The other article, by Thomas Merigan, an ACTG researcher from Stanford, was called "You *Can* Teach an Old Dog New Tricks: How AIDS Trials Are Pioneering New Strategies." Praising the "new level of rapport" and the "partnership of patients, their advocates, and clinical investigators," Merigan argued that "all limbs [of a trial] should offer an equal potential advantage to patients, as good as the best available clinical care"; that no one in a trial should be denied treatment for opportunistic infections; that trials should not be "relentlessly pursued as originally designed" when "data appeared outside the trial suggesting that patients would do better with a different type of management"; and that "the entry criteria for trials should be as broad as scientifically possible to make their results useful in clinical practice."[117]

Medical ethicists had also come on board; they wrote elsewhere of "the beginnings of a new consensus . . . on basic principles and policies that ought to guide HIV/AIDS clinical research."[118] Such principles emphasized the "routine use of community consultation," but also called specifically for such practices as broad entry criteria for trials. One ethicist, Robert Levine, argued against "boilerplate exclusions" that ruled out whole groups of potential research subjects on the basis of abnormal lab test values—and acknowledged that the issue "didn't occur to me until I had it explained to me by Mark Harrington."[119]

Few of these "reforms" were actually new, and many were standard practice in cancer research. As Byar commented, the reaction to his paper in the *New England Journal* was "Well, that's not terribly exciting, I mean we knew that stuff already." But, Byar continued, "there was plenty of evidence that if they *knew* it, they weren't *using* it."[120] What the two articles marked was not the birth of new ideas but the successful passage of those ideas into commonsense understandings about how AIDS trials should be done. Moreover, these were the ideas that had been pushed by the activists, and their ascension was widely understood as a testament to the activists' forceful argumentation and successful mastery of the *arcana*.

On one hand, activists had "denaturalized" the randomized clinical trial—taken it off its pedestal and subjected its presuppositions to scrutiny. Clinical trials "are a product of recent history," argued Jim Eigo in a presentation at the conference of the American Academy for the Advancement of Science: they are not an "unassailable gold standard." On the other hand, activists had presented themselves as the collective voice of reason that could restore order to the scientific method. Theirs was "not a call for the abolition of clinical trials," Eigo assured his listeners at the same conference, but "rather a call for their revision and augmentation." [121]

In retrospect, this was a high point—though few activists marked it at the time, being preoccupied with keeping themselves, their friends, and their lovers alive. Activists had reframed how clinical research should be conceived, and they had established the proposition that the desires of the patient community must be factored into the design of clinical trials. They had situated themselves as an "obligatory passage point" on questions of trial methodology, and they had enrolled at least a number of statisticians, ethicists, researchers, and government officials behind their program. For the moment, it appeared that activists could be the voice of principled morality for their communities *and* the voice of principled science in the inner circles of biomedicine—without undue strain arising out of conflict between these roles. The challenges of the early 1990s would pose complications to this impressive agenda.

CHAPTER 8

DILEMMAS
AND DIVISIONS IN
SCIENCE AND POLITICS

Combination Therapy and the
"Surrogate Markers" Debate (1989–1992)

THE ORIGINS OF A BANDWAGON

By the late 1980s, the guiding assumption was that "combination therapy" was the most fruitful avenue of therapeutic investigation in treating HIV infection. AZT, the only approved antiviral, seemed to benefit patients for a while, until the virus mutated to resist the drug's action. Combining drugs would in theory delay the development of resistance while, perhaps, permitting lower doses of each drug to be used, thus reducing the exposure of the patient to toxic side effects. This was the model in fighting tuberculosis and other diseases; it was generally extrapolated to HIV infection.[1] Researchers and activists alike were anxious to proceed with the testing of combinations of nucleoside analogues (drugs like AZT) as well as drugs with other mechanisms of action. But activists, researchers, government officials, and pharmaceutical companies would have to negotiate the crucial details of the testing process: What evidence was required to demonstrate the safety and efficacy of combination therapies? How quickly could these drugs be released?

At the Sixth International Conference on AIDS, held in San

Francisco in June 1990, researchers presented the preliminary results of a clinical trial called ACTG 106, a small-scale study of the combined use of AZT and ddC. One of the first in vivo studies to test a combination therapy, ACTG 106 was carried out in two sites, under the direction of Margaret Fischl at the University of Miami and Douglas Richman at the University of California at San Diego. As a preliminary study, the main purpose of the trial was *not* to determine efficacy but simply to monitor for toxicity and determine an appropriate dose for use in subsequent, larger studies. There were only fifty-six patients, and they were randomly assigned to six different "dosing regimens" of the combination therapy of AZT plus ddC and followed for an average of forty weeks. Because the study was not meant to measure efficacy, there was no control group.[2]

The study succeeded in its explicit goal of determining an optimal dose and assuring that the side effects of the two drugs, while certainly unpleasant and potentially quite serious, were still manageable. (With AZT the main concern was liver damage; with ddC, peripheral neuropathy, or nerve damage in the hands and feet.) But this was not what attracted attention. "To everyone's surprise," according to John James, the editor of *AIDS Treatment News,* "not only did the combination seem safe, it also appeared to work much better than any other anti-HIV treatment known."[3] Though the participants were severely immune suppressed, with fewer than 100 T cells per cubic millimeter upon entry, they experienced sharp increases in their T-cell counts—a mean increase of about 120 cells per cubic millimeter in the patients receiving higher doses. "Although these results must be interpreted with caution," the authors noted in the published report of the study, which finally appeared in early 1992, "the response rates of CD4 lymphocytes [helper T cells] seen in our patients differ sufficiently from those reported in previous studies to merit comment."[4]

Activists were less restrained in expressing the widespread enthusiasm. "There was *nothing* at that point in time that was comparable to that sort of jump, particularly at late stage of disease. And at late stage of disease, everybody had run out of their options," recalled G'dali Braverman, an activist with ACT UP in San Francisco.[5] The problem was that the study was small, lacking a control, and too short in duration to determine if the therapy prolonged life. Confirmation of the efficacy of AZT/ddC combination therapy would have to wait several years for the completion of ACTG 155, a much larger, Phase II study that was already under way. That study had randomly assigned patients, in blind fashion, to one of three treatments: AZT alone, ddC alone, and the two drugs in combination. Meanwhile, according to John James, "long before the scientific paper was published, the results of [ACTG 106] had established a de facto standard of care among many of the best-informed patients and physicians." As James expressed it in the pages of *AIDS Treatment News,* researchers and people with AIDS simply "drew different practical conclusions" from ACTG 106. "Scientists who run clinical trials are interested in maintaining scientific standards, in doing studies correctly so that they get solid, trustworthy results. People with life-threatening illnesses, on the other hand, are interested in using whatever knowledge is available to make the best treatment decisions they can."[6]

Belief in the efficacy of the ddC/AZT combination regimen swept through the AIDS movement with the force of a juggernaut. Of course, no doctor could prescribe ddC to his or her patients at this point. Some people with AIDS were able to obtain free ddC from the manufacturer, Hoffman-LaRoche, under the new parallel track program (also called "expanded access") that provided experimental drugs to people not in clinical trials. But one particular fact about ddC really fueled the bandwagon: unlike other nucleoside analogues, such as AZT and ddI, ddC could be manufactured cheaply and easily from common chemical ingredients.

Soon ddC was being pumped out of basement laboratories and passed on to the buyers clubs and, from there, distributed to people with AIDS and HIV around the country. And the FDA, for the most part, was turning a blind eye. If the estimate put forward by Derek Hodel, then director of the PWA Health Group, a New York City buyers club, can be trusted, as many as ten thousand people nationwide may have been receiving bootleg ddC by late 1991.[7] Hoffman-LaRoche representatives were, not surprisingly, upset about the infringement on the company's patent, and they voiced concerns about quality control in the underground manufacturing process. Experts on clinical trials complained that the access to ddC threatened to undermine ongoing trials of the drug. After all, if you are in a ddC trial and become convinced that ddC works but don't know for sure whether you are receiving ddC or are in the control group, *and* if you can get ddC at bargain-basement prices around the corner, are you going to bother staying in the trial? Thomas Chalmers of Harvard University, a medical researcher and expert on clinical trials, told the *New York Times* that the buyers clubs were "terrible," "the most serious step backward I've seen in a long time."[8]

One of the most noteworthy aspects of the controversy, however,

was the fact that a considerable number of practicing physicians tolerated, and even encouraged, the bootleg use. One San Francisco doctor
well known for his involvement in AIDS care, Marcus Conant, acknowledged that as many as three hundred of his patients were taking
bootleg ddC.[9] "If I were in their shoes I would be doing the same
thing," Conant told a reporter for *Nature*.[10] A manufacturer of the
bootleg drug told the gay newsmagazine the *Advocate:* "Doctors from
around the country are calling us and their local buyers clubs to get
ddC for their patients."[11]

Some of these doctors may simply have been acknowledging the
inevitable: given the existence of the buyers clubs, they no longer stood
as the "gatekeepers" between their patients and the medication that
might help them. At the same time, both doctors and patients recognized the practical virtues of cooperation: these were serious drugs,
and it behooved patients to find doctors willing to monitor the use of
their ddC in case of toxicity or adverse reactions. Other doctors may
have found it easier to hand out the buyers club phone number than
try to navigate Hoffman-LaRoche's restrictive parallel track program,
which required complicated paperwork certifying that the patient had
already tried both AZT and ddI and had failed on both drugs.[12] Finally, many doctors quite simply believed that the AZT/ddC combination was state-of-the-art medicine and preferable to ddI, given the results from existing studies. "I'm not going to wait for my patients to
lose any more T cells before advising them to get ddC on the underground," said one Washington, D.C., physician, delivering a personal
manifesto. "For me and a lot of other doctors, we're out and we're
not going back."[13]

These community physicians had precisely the overlapping affiliations that the term suggests: they aligned themselves, in complicated
ways, both with their communities and with their professions. Or to
put it another way: by the early 1990s, AIDS treatment activism had
become a movement that cut across professions, not just one that pitted
professionals against laypeople. These physicians, moreover, were
quick to insist on the evidence of their own eyes. Clinical trials or no
clinical trials, *their* patients benefited from the combination therapy.
Such attitudes, of course, have a long history, as practitioners have resisted the encroachment on their professional authority that the scientization of medicine represents. Medicine, in this view, is an "art," not a
"science." "While science may be considered a symbol of legitimacy
and source of power for the medical profession," Deborah Gordon has

noted, "physicians' clinical expertise may be regarded as their personal power and private magic."[14] The tacit knowledge and skills of everyday practice, not the results of randomized clinical trials, were the basis of these doctors' claims to professional autonomy. They were the ones on the front lines of patient care; they saw themselves as best suited to make clinical judgments about what was best for their patients.

By late 1991, the credibility of the combination therapy—or at a minimum, widespread belief in its *potential* efficacy—had been established in the United States, less through the formal claims of infectious-disease researchers than through the interventions of less authoritative actors, including AIDS activists and community-based physicians. The FDA, meanwhile, though mandated to assure the safety and efficacy of drugs, was taking a backseat. In an intriguing analysis published sometime afterward, John James defended this peculiar, de facto endorsement of an underground drug as perhaps "the best possible solution to a deeper structural problem, a confusion about what we as a society use FDA approval for." Was the purpose of the FDA sanction to *permit* access to a drug, or to *recommend* a drug as the standard of care? "In theory the FDA does not regulate the practice of medicine"; in practice, doctors relied on FDA approvals to decide what to prescribe, while insurers often declined to reimburse the cost of a drug used outside of its indicated labeling. Given this basic confusion, what could the FDA do? "With only one small study available, it would have been difficult to say, 'Here, take this' to tens of thousands of people. Yet it would also be unacceptable to say, 'You can't have this' to those who had studied the matter and made an informed choice," James concluded.[15] Much as a rumor on Wall Street can circulate uncontrollably and inflate the value of a stock, any positive signal from the FDA would have had widespread repercussions, augmenting the credibility of the drug. Since the FDA had no mechanism for permitting access to a drug without appearing also to recommend it, turning a blind eye to the buyers clubs was a convenient, and perhaps necessary, holding action.

SURROGATE MARKERS TO THE RESCUE

But how to get ddC, along with ddI and other new drugs, formally approved by the FDA? *That* was the true goal, in the eyes of most AIDS activists—not relying on compounds cooked up in somebody's kitchen. No one thought these drugs were magic bullets.

As Mark Harrington wrote in his column in the gay and lesbian magazine *Outweek,* "At best, [ddI] will be a less toxic alternative to AZT
[and] at worst, it will be an alternative with less antiviral activity and
unpleasant side effects."[16] Nonetheless, the issue was "vitally important," wrote John James, "because there are tens of thousands of
people unable to use AZT, or no longer able to benefit from it."[17]

The obstacle, in James's view, lay "not with any one agency, company, or other institution, but with a professional consensus which
crosses organizational boundaries"; this consensus, if not disrupted,
would effectively prevent "any decisive treatment advance from being
available for years."[18] The entire research enterprise was geared toward what James called "dinosaur trials"—huge, costly, multicenter
trials that would take years to complete. Why did the trials take so
long and require so many subjects? As James explained in *AIDS Treatment News,* the chief impediment was that "the FDA has insisted on
the slowest measure of clinical improvement," namely death or opportunistic infections in the control group. "This means that the drug
being tested is not measured by improvements in the patients who
receive it, but [opportunistic infections] or deaths in those who
do not."[19]

The alternative measure of drug efficacy that activists proposed was
one with a long history in biomedicine but none whatsoever in AIDS:
the use of "surrogate markers" to demonstrate the efficacy of a treatment. A drug shown to reduce serum cholesterol or blood pressure,
for example, may be approved to treat heart disease on the assumption
that such improvements correlate in the long run with an overall clinical benefit. Similarly, the amount of reduction in tumor size is sometimes used as a surrogate marker for the effectiveness of a cancer drug.
Approving a drug on the basis of a surrogate marker necessarily implied greater uncertainty about the actual effects of the drug against
the disease for which the marker is a stand-in. But it was a more or
less accepted course of action for life-threatening diseases, since it
could speed up the decision-making process considerably.

The difficulty, however, was that no marker had yet been proven to
function as a surrogate for the effectiveness of an antiviral AIDS drug.
A good marker would be one with "face validity" and "biological
relevance"; it would also be easily measurable in some objective and
reliable fashion.[20] But a high-profile workshop called "Surrogate Endpoints in Evaluating the Effectiveness of Drugs against HIV Infection
and AIDS," sponsored by the Institute of Medicine of the National

Academy of Sciences and held in September 1989, had failed to arrive at a consensus on such a marker or markers.[21] Anthony Fauci, the director of NIAID and the government's point man on AIDS research, backed the most obvious and oft-discussed marker: CD4 counts (the technical name for T-cell counts). Another logical choice was the level of p24 antigen, the core viral protein, but it was found only inconsistently in the blood. Debate also focused on other indicators of disease progression in the blood of HIV-infected people, such as a rising "β_2 microglobulin" count or "neopterin" count. But these latter measures were nonspecific, Fauci argued, since they are common in many illnesses. "Nobody dies from elevated levels of β_2-microglobulin or neopterin," said Fauci, "but nobody can make it without CD4 cells."[22]

T-cell depletion was the very hallmark of AIDS; to an immunologist like Fauci, AIDS could almost be *defined* in terms of HIV's direct and indirect effects on T cells. Any drug that staved off T-cell decline had to have some value. To Fauci, and certainly to many activists, this made such intuitive good sense that any opposition seemed almost frivolous.[23] The biostatisticians and the FDA regulators had their doubts, nonetheless. As a measure, CD4 counts were notoriously labile, fluctuating depending on the time of day the blood was drawn, how much sleep the patient had the night before, what the patient ate for breakfast, or which laboratory was doing the analysis.[24] More fundamentally, as NIAID biostatistician Susan Ellenberg pointed out, the problem was that something might be a good prognostic marker of the future course of illness in the natural history of a disease (and no one doubted that CD4 counts filled this role in AIDS), but that didn't *prove* it could function as the endpoint of a clinical drug trial. That is, researchers can predict the future of an HIV-infected person (speaking in probabilistic terms) if they know his or her CD4 counts, but that doesn't necessarily mean they can predict the effect of a *treatment* on the person's prognosis simply by knowing the effect of the *treatment* on his or her CD4 counts.[25] Such an association remained to be demonstrated.

Some of the New York activists, like Mark Harrington, promoted the use of surrogates but also argued that surrogate markers were only part of the answer. He called for careful attention both to quality-of-life indicators and the pathogenetic mechanisms of HIV infection that presumably underlay the surrogate markers.[26] But others, particularly in San Francisco, saw surrogate markers as *the* critical issue. Martin Delaney, the director of Project Inform, for whom the virtue of CD4 as a surrogate marker was "intuitively correct," blasted what he saw as the head-in-the-sand insistence on definitive proof. "Such a view may be valid from a scientifically conservative, purist perspective," Project Inform's newsletter contended, "but it is hardly a progressive position in the context of a raging epidemic. . . . How much does one have to know about the scientific nature of combustion when the house is burning down?"[27] Yet researchers and regulators presented examples from other diseases to argue that their concerns were more than mere pedantry. James Bilstad, an FDA official, described to a *JAMA* reporter in 1991 the recent "very disturbing" finding that certain cardiac arrhythmia drugs improved the commonly accepted surrogate markers for heart disease but tripled the risk of mortality from sudden cardiac arrest.[28]

Books about AIDS drug development have tended to portray the struggle over surrogate markers as one in which stodgy defenders of the status quo were eventually won over by well-informed activists who were in possession of what was indisputably the "right" answer.[29] No doubt this is partly because these books were published before 1993, when the use of CD4 as a surrogate marker was seriously challenged. However, from the start the issue of surrogate markers in AIDS clinical trials had scientific arguments on both sides that were passionately defended. (Indeed, activists themselves were not insensitive to the arguments against surrogate markers, particularly the sole reliance on CD4. James, for instance, was more impressed by a technique called quantitative PCR [polymerase chain reaction] that measured plasma viremia; he and others advocated combining laboratory markers with markers of apparent health, such as a doctor's ranking of the patient's overall state of being.)[30] Here, once again, an activist victory depended on the capacity of activists to intervene in a complex scientific controversy by adding their moral authority—and political muscle—to one particular side in a methodological and epistemological controversy. The existence of competing expert interpretations of how knowledge was to be constituted gave AIDS activists an opening from which to conduct their campaign.

Activist pressure on the surrogate marker issue was destined, in turn, to hold profound consequences for the public negotiation of belief about the efficacy of drugs like ddI and ddC. The debates over whether ddI and ddC "worked" would proceed hand in hand with a debate over the very mechanisms by which efficacy might be established in an AIDS antiviral trial. Given these circumstances, controversy about the licensing and use of these drugs was almost inevitable.

In general, for a clinical trial to "work," its results must be taken to "stand for" [31] the effects of a drug were the drug to be administered widely to patients outside the artificial, experimental setting. A trial resting on surrogate markers, therefore, derives its credibility from a two-stage process of representation: it must first be agreed that the short-term effect of the drug on the marker represents the long-term effect of the drug in reducing mortality—and *then* the trial results must be understood to reflect what would happen in the everyday world of patients who consumed the drug. When articulation of the linkage between "experiment" and "real world" becomes so complex—and when the stakes are nothing short of life and death—not only is there more space for argument about the meaning of trial results, but the capacity of "outsiders" to intervene and assert claims becomes all the more potent.

THE "FUTURE THAT WE ALL ENVISIONED"

By 1991, the uncertainty about surrogate markers was on a collision course with the widely felt need to license ddI and ddC. Everyone knew these drugs had a certain value, activists contended; the issue was simply one of finding the appropriate mechanism for making them available. Expanded access, the San Francisco activists had decided, was a step in that direction but simply not good enough: It "only works when there is a public-spirited and well-financed drug company, willing to spend money to save lives when sales of the drug may be years away," wrote John James.[32]

The Phase II trials—those vast, costly, and inefficient endeavors—were ultimately of little relevance, activists argued, because they were designed "to produce a single bit of information, one yes-or-no answer," namely, the question of statistical significance: in the event that these drugs were useless, was the chance of falsely concluding that they had benefit less than five percent? This, in James's view, was simply the wrong question to be asking. Doctors and patients needed pragmatic advice about the best ways in which to use these drugs. In that sense, "the real issue with ddI is not whether it works. A growing working consensus holds that it probably does. . . . The most important questions now are long-term toxicity, and when and how to use ddI most effectively in various groups of patients."[33]

Particularly for San Francisco activists, two solutions to the "dinosaur trials" dilemma became effectively joined: the FDA could speed up approval by relying on a surrogate marker such as CD4 counts, and it could make that approval *conditional* upon evidence to be obtained from subsequent studies. A proposal for a new FDA policy of "conditional approval" therefore emerged as a strategy for managing the greater uncertainty that the reliance on surrogates would entail.[34] Such a policy, as activists imagined it, would put the burden on the drug companies to fund and conduct "postmarketing studies" to provide additional evidence of drug safety and efficacy. If evidence was not forthcoming, the FDA would revoke the license for the drug and it would be taken off the market. However, as soon as a drug was conditionally approved, the manufacturer could begin selling it and insurers would reimburse for it. The advantage over expanded access was that the latter program had provided only weak incentives for drug company cooperation. At most, as David Feigal of the FDA suggested, participation in expanded access enhanced a drug's credibility as an effective treatment: "It cements [the perception] that this is an up-and-coming drug, one valuable enough that it's being made available early."[35] Conditional approval, by contrast, was designed with the explicit goal of enlisting the pharmaceutical companies by giving them a chance to do what they liked best: earn profits. The idea of conditional approval was quickly endorsed by the deregulation lobby and by the Quayle Competitiveness Council, the vice president's commission dedicated to the elimination of regulatory barriers for U.S. industries.[36]

New York activists, who had pushed through the expanded access mechanism, were less enthusiastic about the idea. David Barr commented: "We have never said we are not interested in collecting good data. I have concern that if conditional approval is not done the right way we will lose our ability to collect data."[37] Members of Congress who promoted consumer protection, such as Ted Weiss and Henry Waxman, were even more dubious. In April 1991, Waxman wrote to David Kessler, Bush's newly appointed head of the FDA and an advocate of change at the agency, expressing his concern that conditional approval, unlike the expanded access program, "could allow promotion and sale of drugs that did not meet previous standards for safety and efficacy."[38] Soon afterward, Martin Delaney sent off a blistering letter to Waxman defending the policy and demanding that he cease and desist. Conditional approval "is not about lowered standards or opening the floodgates to harmful or worthless drugs," Delaney told Waxman. "It would be a very limited program accessible only in life-threatening situations and for drugs which show safety and clear

promise on the basis of surrogate markers." Insisting that Project Inform was not the "dupe" of the Republican party or the pharmaceutical industry, Delaney demanded that Waxman "put a muzzle" on one
of his aides who had been speaking against the policy.[39]

Meanwhile, as the various parties debated the merits and dangers
of conditional approval, the question of surrogate markers also moved
to the fore. By late 1990, Ellen Cooper, director of the Antiviral Drug
Division, was describing herself as "encouraged" about the use of
CD4 counts as a surrogate marker for AIDS antivirals, but she told
JAMA that "we are not there yet" regarding reaching agreement in
the research community.[40] Delaney's analysis was that the FDA preferred to share the decision-making risk by forging a consensus with
other federal agencies rather than go out on a limb.[41] Cooper herself,
however, seemed resistant to joining any consensus she did not genuinely support or to approving drugs based on standards she felt were
inadequate. That, at least, was the general conclusion drawn when she
suddenly resigned her position on December 19.[42]

To consider the role of surrogate markers in approving antiviral
AIDS drugs, the FDA convened a special meeting of the Antiviral Advisory Committee in February 1991. Among various scientific presentations was one by Anastasios ("Butch") Tsiatis, a statistician from
Harvard, who had gone back over the data from the original Phase II
AZT study. Tsiatis found that those patients whose T-cell counts went
up after receiving AZT did better overall than those patients who did
not experience a rise. In other words, by looking at the effect of AZT
on CD4 counts, one could predict who would benefit most from
AZT. On the other hand, it also appeared that the people who received
AZT in the study experienced *more* of a benefit from the drug than
the rise in CD4 alone could explain. But to Delaney, the issue wasn't
whether CD4 told us *everything* as long it accurately predicted some
significant portion of a drug's potential benefit.[43]

"I think the reality is that we are not going to have this future that
we all envisioned here," warned Martin Delaney in his testimony at
the meeting, explaining that "body count" trials with survival as an
endpoint simply were no longer *feasible,* regardless of whether they
were desirable. "Survival . . . studies with each passing day of this
epidemic become less and less possible. As more data accumulate on
each of these drugs, as we take more time to compare one to the next,
fewer and fewer patients are willing to sit still in studies that take two
to three years. Fewer will stay on those studies as newer and better

compounds come along. . . ."[44] Delaney was certainly right in insisting that regulators not conceive of AIDS antiviral trials as abstract laboratory experiments whose purity could be protected from external influences. These were concretely situated and inevitably messy enterprises, enormously dependent on the behavior and attitudes of the research subjects and carried out within a certain historical field of possibilities, with each trial having ramifications on concurrent and subsequent ones. Where Delaney was being more than slightly disingenuous was in his failure to acknowledge the extent to which organizations such as his own accelerated the kinetics (or the psychodynamics) of this system. Project Inform, for example, held regular "Town Meetings" and published reports in its newsletter detailing the latest thinking about the experimental AIDS drugs, in effect encouraging patients to believe or disbelieve, to comply with protocols or switch to other studies.

At the end of the day, the Antiviral Advisory Committee unanimously endorsed the use of CD4 counts as a surrogate marker for demonstrating the efficacy of nucleoside analogues in the treatment of AIDS. The way was paved for Bristol-Myers Squibb, the sponsor of ddI, and Hoffman-LaRoche, the maker of ddC, to file their applications with the FDA. Existing data on toxicity and efficacy, combined with CD4 data, would be enough to warrant licensing these drugs, Jim Eigo predicted. "Maybe a year down the road we'll find we made a mistake," David Barr told *JAMA*. "But the choice on the other side is no treatment."[45] Ellen Cooper, who had sat out the meeting as a spectator, came up to Delaney toward the end. "You have to be careful with this, or you could do yourself more harm than good," she told him.[46]

BETWEEN "SCIENCE" AND "POLICY"

A long and divisive two-day meeting of the Antiviral Advisory Committee in July 1991 resulted in the recommended licensing of ddI, though not by unanimous vote. The clincher came on the second day, when the committee considered data that had been obtained, on special FDA consent, from a peek at the ongoing Phase II trial. In the study, patients who had already been on AZT for twelve months or more were randomly assigned either to continue AZT or to receive ddI. The results so far showed a T-cell decline in those who stayed on AZT, compared with a modest rise in those who had been switched to ddI. After what Project Inform referred to as "endless hand-wringing by some committee members," the committee voted in favor of approving ddI for adult and pediatric AIDS patients no longer responsive to AZT; the vote was five to two.[47] As it almost always does, the FDA endorsed the recommendations of its advisory panel sometime afterward.

Project Inform's newsletter, commenting on the approval, called it "in many ways the single most important victory in 6 years of AIDS activism" and described the FDA as "courageous."[48] Kessler himself characterized the vote as "a milestone in drug review." "We're in the midst of a medical emergency," Donald Abrams, one of those who voted for approval, told a reporter for *JAMA*. "One person dies of AIDS in the United States every 8 minutes," Abrams added, repeating what was in fact a common ACT UP slogan.[49] Later, when asked about his vote, Abrams described his role in essentially political terms, as one of "representing" doctors and patients from San Francisco, groups that wanted ddI to be approved.[50]

Normally, as Sheila Jasanoff describes it in a study of regulatory science, the use of independent scientific advisory bodies allows agencies such as the FDA to "harness the authority of science in support of its own policy preferences." The experts on these panels "seem at times painfully aware that what they are doing is not 'science' in any ordinary sense, but a hybrid activity that combines elements of scientific evidence and reasoning with large doses of social and political judgment."[51] Nonetheless, the experts normally speak in the language of science, and this has the important effect of legitimating the policies that are ratified. In the case of ddI, however, the scientific basis was so contested and the political pressures so extreme that panelists sought to disentangle their separate roles as scientists and policymakers—to make clear that as far as *they* were concerned, their vote was a scientific endorsement of neither ddI nor the use of CD4 counts as a surrogate marker, but rather a pragmatic policy decision. The panelists were going to allow patients to assume the risks that patients themselves, their activist representatives, and their physicians were demanding that they be allowed to assume.

Some refused to take this step, however. Deborah Cotton, a Harvard Medical School professor who was one of the "no" votes, expressed concern that the approval had set a bad precedent that "creates incentives" for other drug companies to press for approval with inadequate data. She worried, moreover, that it would be "a real challenge to explain to participants in the controlled trials why it is so important for the trials to continue and for them to remain in them."[52] Now, more than ever, it was necessary to complete the trials and make sure that the effect of ddI on a surrogate marker would translate into a genuine clinical benefit and decreased mortality. But once the FDA had given its blessing to the drug, based on data that seemed to show that ddI was *better than* AZT for those who had been on AZT for some time, why would anyone stay in the trial, at the risk of being in the AZT arm? Why not just drop out of the study and have one's doctor prescribe ddI? Belief had now hardened into relative certainty; in such an environment, was a clinical trial possible?

Paul Meier, a statistician from the University of Chicago who said he voted for approval reluctantly, noted that the committee would have preferred to make the approval conditional upon future studies, "yet had to take full approval because there is no such option." [53] He commented to the *New York Times:* "I really genuinely worry that we are ratcheting down what has been a good standard for the F.D.A." Some New York activists, while supporting the decision, were also concerned about the inconclusive nature of the data. "This whole situation makes all of us very nervous," David Barr told the *New York Times.* [54]

THE GENIE IN THE BOTTLE

It was in the wake of these decisions that the FDA's Antiviral Advisory Committee sat down in April 1992 to consider the approval of ddC. First the committee turned back to ddI, looking at the data that had since been accumulated from the first of the Phase II trials to be completed. With a collective sigh of relief, the panel concluded that faith in ddI had apparently been borne out: its impact on CD4 counts had indeed predicted its clinical benefit. Nor had the approval of ddI impeded the successful completion of the trial, as committee members like Cotton had feared. "We took a risk in approving DDI and today I think that on balance we did it right," said Kessler, expressing the philosophy of what some were calling the "new FDA." "We cannot wait for all the evidence to come in when people are suffering and dying from these devastating diseases." [55]

With renewed confidence in the use of CD4 counts as a surrogate marker, the committee then turned to ddC. A week before the meeting, Kessler had made official the new option of what would now be called not "conditional" but "accelerated" approval, along the lines originally proposed by activists. [56] According to David Feigal, who would replace Ellen Cooper as head of the Antiviral Drug Division, Kessler emphasized that such approvals should indeed be thought of as "conditional." But Kessler couldn't call the policy by that name for fear that third-party payers might decline to reimburse patients for their purchases of such drugs. Here again, the FDA was forced to be acutely sensitive to the vast financial and human consequences of the signals the agency sent out—despite the fact that, officially, "our approvals are not intended to be the basis for reimbursement decisions." [57]

Hoffman-LaRoche asked that ddC be conditionally approved as a monotherapy (that is, for use by itself) for patients who were intolerant to AZT; but there was no evidence to support such a labeling, and the committee quickly nixed the idea. Instead, the committee turned to the evidence from ACTG 106 and other small studies that showed positive effects of ddC/AZT combination therapy on CD4 counts. Ironically, as Michael Botkin, an activist and writer on AIDS treatment issues for a San Francisco gay newspaper, described it, Burroughs Wellcome "[pulled] their rival's chestnuts out of the fire." [58] In past years, Burroughs Wellcome had been decidedly uncooperative about research involving the use of AZT and the products of other companies. But with the growing interest in combination therapy, and with the widespread recognition that AZT alone was no solution to AIDS, the company stood to gain from an official endorsement of the ddC/AZT combination. They presented data from a study the company had commissioned that corroborated the results of ACTG 106 by showing the drug combination's effect on T-cell counts. By an eight to three margin, the committee voted in favor of conditional approval of ddC when used in conjunction with AZT. (Final approval would depend on the outcome of other studies, particularly ACTG 155.) [59] As Botkin commented, that put Burroughs Wellcome in the "delightful position of proving that their rival's treatment is effective—but only when taken with their own product!" [60]

The FDA ratified the advisory committee's recommendation on June 22, in what Health and Human Services Secretary Louis W. Sullivan described as "another step forward for patients with AIDS." [61] Many treatment activists, like Delaney and James, were pleased by the outcome. Others were decidedly cynical. "For once, politics played in our favor," said G'dali Braverman of ACT UP/Golden Gate, adding that the Antiviral Advisory Committee meeting had a "scripted" feel, with dissenters being "strong-armed" by Kessler. [62] In Botkin's analysis, Kessler had been seeking support from all sides, playing to the AIDS activists and the deregulation advocates by adopting accelerated approval, while placating consumer protectionists with simultaneous, well-publicized campaigns to beef up vitamin and food labeling.

Meanwhile, the underground ddC was a threat and a growing embarrassment. "The only answer, from Kessler's perspective, was to co-opt the buyers clubs by quickly approving ddC, thus demonstrating that the government is moving fast enough to introduce new AIDS treatments and that independent efforts aren't needed." [63]

Comments by some committee members supported these activists' perceptions that the results had been foreordained. Deborah Cotton, who voted against approving ddC just as she had voted against ddI earlier, told *Science* that in her view, the committee had been asked to "pound [the data] into a scientific conclusion." [64] FDA Commissioner Kessler "clearly wanted it," Cotton afterwards recalled. "David spent the entire two days at the table, which is usually how you tell that he's invested in an issue. . . ." [65] From Cotton's standpoint, the ready reliance on surrogate markers was a mistake, because it threatened to *delay* the process of obtaining solid data about treatments. "We really have to ask whether relying on surrogate markers will hasten a cure or hinder it," Cotton told the reporter from *Science:* "We're getting into a situation of such complexity that we may have a large number of agents being used and no way of distinguishing among them." She added: "It's sad that we may have nothing to offer people in 1992. . . . It's sadder that in 2000 we may have nothing, too. In 2000 we'll look back and say, 'If only we'd done this in a more rational way.'" [66]

Kessler assured the worriers that accelerated approval demanded careful postmarketing studies. If the surrogate marker evidence didn't hold up, the FDA would then "[put] the genie back in the bottle." [67] Yet as Kessler's own phrasing perhaps inadvertently suggested, removing an approved drug from circulation might be easier said than done. Short of a truly catastrophic result in the postmarketing study, was it really likely that the political environment would permit the withdrawal of one of only three antiviral drugs approved against HIV? Or had the construction of belief passed the point of no return?

Inside and Outside the System

NEW ANTIVIRAL RESEARCH AND THE "RECEDING" BOTTLENECK

One irony in the push to license ddI and ddC is that, long before the drugs were approved, the hopes of researchers, doctors, and activists had moved well beyond the infertile terrain of the nucleoside analogues. Officially, the research establishment continued to tout the potential virtues of combination therapy with the nucleosides and to promote the goal of turning AIDS into a "chronic manageable illness," though increasingly it appeared that the announcement in Montreal of its advent had been more than a little premature. Activists were less sanguine about the pace of progress. By the time of the San Francisco conference in 1990, ACT UP/New York had concluded: "This year, the hopes of many in the AIDS communities have reached a low ebb. It is clear to all that anti-HIV agents such as AZT, ddC and ddI will not, in any conceivable combination, stop the progression of HIV infection—at most, for those who are lucky, they will significantly slow it."[68]

Writing in *Outweek* in 1990, New York activist Larry Kramer put the position in his own inimitably vituperative style. He accused researchers like Margaret Fischl and Paul Volberding of having "pumped AZT down the throats of AIDS patients like they were Strasbourg geese being fattened up for the kill." Kramer averred: "AIDS is not a manageable disease, and there is nothing at present that makes me think that it is going to be a manageable disease in my lifetime or the lifetime of the other 20 million HIV infected. ANYONE WHO TELLS YOU OTHERWISE IS A LIAR."[69]

ACT UP/New York's Treatment & Data Committee analyzed the predicament in the 1990 update of its *AIDS Treatment Research Agenda,* distributed at the San Francisco conference. The ACTG was concentrating its resources on "massive Phase II trials of stop-gap first generation nucleoside analogues," to the exclusion of just about everything else. Hardly any compounds were in Phase I trials, even though dozens were known to act against HIV in vitro (the report listed sixty of them, along with many immune therapies, anti-infectives, and other drugs that awaited testing). Given the backlog, and given the ACTG's apparent priorities, the emergence of a new generation of antiviral treatments was necessarily years away. In that sense, the problem was no longer the FDA, the Treatment & Data Committee concluded. "As activists make increasing headway with regulators, the bottleneck in AIDS drug development seems to recede towards the beginning of the process, when compounds are taken from test tube and animal studies and administered to humans for the first time."[70] Mixed metaphor though it may have been, this notion of the "receding bottleneck" served to orient treatment activists in the years to come.

For patients, the pace of AIDS antiviral research was measured in relation to their own life expectancy; but researchers, whose point of reference was the rate of scientific progress for other diseases, found the advance of knowledge both swift and encouraging. "We have learned more about the AIDS virus than any other virus that affects humans," Dr. William Haseltine told *New York Times* reporter Gina Kolata in late 1990, reciting what had become almost a mantra in AIDS research circles. "Molecular biologists and drug development experts have climbed rapidly from a valley of despair to a peak of expectation in their struggle to combat the AIDS virus," wrote Kolata, focusing on a recent publication in *Science* by NCI scientists Hiroaki, Yarchoan, and Broder that identified "13 major chinks in [the virus's] armor, each one of which may in time yield to therapeutic attack." "There really is a large and growing menu" of ways to interrupt the cycle of viral replication, Broder told Kolata: "I think it's a very important time." [71]

John James agreed there was room for "cautious" optimism, especially with regard to three promising sets of "designer drugs" that were farthest along in development. [72] First, there were new drugs that acted at the same point in the virus's replication cycle (reverse transcription) as AZT, ddC, and ddI but didn't belong to the dideoxynucleoside family. These so-called non-nucleoside reverse-transcriptase inhibitors included the "L drugs" made by Merck (formally labeled "L-697,661" and "L-697,639") and a drug called nevirapine developed by Boehringer Ingelheim Pharmaceuticals.

Second, Hoffman-LaRoche had been developing a "tat inhibitor," which was designed to block the protein produced by the viral gene called *tat*. This protein, required for the replication of HIV, acted "downstream" of reverse transcriptase in the replication cycle; it was responsible for "transactivation," a speeding-up of the manufacture of the new viral particle. In vitro, the tat inhibitor was synergistic with AZT, meaning that the drugs might conceivably be given in combination to deliver a one-two punch against the virus. Unlike the reverse transcriptase inhibitors, a tat inhibitor would, in theory, work against chronically infected cells such as macrophages; such cells behave abnormally but are not killed by the virus. In addition, some believed that a tat drug also showed promise against Kaposi's sarcoma. Finally, Hoffman-LaRoche's drug seemed particularly promising because it was chemically related to diazepam (Valium), a well-known drug that had already been used extensively in humans. [73]

The third exciting set of compounds, still under development, were called protease (or proteinase) inhibitors. These drugs would block the action of a different enzyme, protease, that plays a role at yet a later stage in the viral life cycle. After being assembled, the newly produced virus that buds from the infected cell is in an immature state; the protease enzyme then processes the genetic material to complete the virus's development. Only at that point does the new virus become infectious. In the presence of a protease inhibitor, therefore, the new virus released into the bloodstream would be harmless, incapable of infecting other cells. At least, that was the theory being pursued by a number of pharmaceutical companies, including Hoffman-LaRoche.

These were the practical applications of the intense scrutiny of HIV by molecular biologists; one problem, however, was that scientific knowledge about the virus far outstripped an understanding of the immunopathogenesis of AIDS in the human body—that is, how the virus directly or indirectly contributed to the eventual collapse of immune functioning. As David Baltimore and Mark Feinberg wrote in an editorial in the *New England Journal of Medicine* toward the end of 1989: "Humans are genetically heterogeneous, lead idiosyncratic lives, and become infected through a number of routes, and important practical and ethical considerations constrain clinical experimentation. As a result, we are rapidly learning about the role of each of HIV's approximately 10,000 nucleotides, but remain largely ignorant of rudimentary aspects of the processes underlying the development of AIDS in humans."[74] It was believed at the time, on the basis of blood work done with cohort studies, that there were three stages to "HIV disease." First, soon after infection with the virus, there was an initial stage of acute infection marked by a high viral load in the blood, a strong antibody response, and in many cases, symptoms such as a low-grade fever and swollen lymph glands. Then a long, middle stage of "latency" would set in, during which the viral load measurable in the blood was relatively low but the T-cell count gradually declined. In most cases this was succeeded—eventually—by a final stage of crisis, coincident with the onset of opportunistic infections (and, usually, a T-cell count below two hundred per cubic millimeter), in which the viral load once again became high. Increasingly it was also becoming apparent that "latency" was a misnomer, because although the infected person was outwardly healthy, and although the virus might indeed be dormant in some infected cells, the process of viral replication continued throughout the middle stage.

The implication of this clinical picture was that the infected person's immune system initially succeeded in controlling the infection and keeping the virus in check, but over time lost that ability quite dramatically—for reasons that were not at all well understood, though hypotheses certainly abounded. Some, like Luc Montagnier, argued that simultaneous infection with other agents ("cofactors") speeded up the process of immune breakdown. Others pointed to syncytia formation (the clumping together of infected T cells) or to abnormalities with cytokines (the proteins released by immune system cells that signal other immune cells) or to autoimmune mechanisms. These competing hypotheses sometimes led to contradictory implications for treatment strategies. For example, researchers such as Jonas Salk were working on a "therapeutic vaccine" designed to bolster the immune response in people already infected with HIV; but those who believed that HIV progression was a result of "overactivation" of the immune system feared that such a therapy might actually make the infection progress faster.[75] Clearly, in the absence of a good working knowledge of pathogenesis, it was difficult to elaborate a coherent therapeutic approach that aimed at preventing the development of AIDS and not just the replication of the virus.

A SEAT AT THE TABLE

Treatment activists in the early 1990s followed the reports of novel therapies with intense interest. How could these drugs get into development faster? How could researchers be induced to focus on them and on the promising anti-infectives for treatment of opportunistic infections, rather than devote federal funds to what activists saw as increasingly arcane trials of different regimens of the nucleoside analogues? To have influence over such questions, activists needed a seat at the table—specifically, places on the committees of the ACTG, where decisions were made about the research priorities that determined how federal funds would be distributed. As activists saw it, the big names in AIDS antiviral research—Paul Volberding, Douglas Richman, Thomas Merigan, Margaret Fischl, Martin Hirsch—dominated the committees that voted, predictably, to fund the kinds of studies that these researchers did. Treatment activists wanted to situate themselves as a counterpower to assert their own priorities.

That they might achieve such a lofty goal was plausible only because the activists already were winning their credibility in the methodology wars—the debates over such matters as inclusion criteria, concomitant medication, and surrogate markers in clinical trial design. At the same time, activists hadn't simply studied science and "played nice." Throughout 1990, ACT UP put the same kind of direct pressure on NIAID that the FDA had been made to endure a few years earlier. One thousand demonstrators from around the United States made a show of force at NIH headquarters in Bethesda, Maryland, on May 21, occupying the office of Daniel Hoth, Fauci's assistant and head of the ACTG program. Activists held banners and shouted slogans: "Ten years, one billion dollars, one drug, big deal." Eighty-two of them were arrested.[76]

Demonstrations had an important function in building the movement and drawing in new activists. Yet it was difficult for treatment activists to frame their critique of NIAID and the ACTG effectively, in a way that would mobilize the masses and capture the media spotlight. In that sense, as John James noted, the change in the rallying site from Rockville in 1988 to Bethesda in 1990 represented "much more than just a different subway stop." "The public does not understand the NIH issues (by contrast to the FDA, which it can easily picture as the 'heavy' keeping promising treatments away from patients). NIH issues center [on] scientific judgments and priorities; it is hard for the public to judge whether or not criticisms have merit."[77] In a word, any critique of NIAID and the ACTG demanded *expertise*. Even educating the AIDS movement base, let alone the general public, about the problems with the ACTG was a daunting task, though Harrington did his best in passionate screeds published in *Outweek* and the *Village Voice*. "The U.S. has poured over a quarter of a billion dollars into the AIDS Clinical Trials Group . . . , making it the most generously endowed clinical research network in history," wrote Harrington. "Yet the ACTG has managed only to test old drugs inefficiently and new drugs not at all. . . ."[78]

One of Harrington's recurrent themes was that the ACTG operated like a secret society, and he took it upon himself to air the dirty laundry. The ACTG was not some neutral advisory body; its meetings were a political field, and the principal investigators who comprised its advisory committees all had vested interests. "Card-carrying virologists" dominated the all-powerful executive committee that made final decisions behind closed doors about which studies to fund. The executive committee ensured that the bulk of the resources went to the giant, high-profile trials of the antivirals, while researchers studying anti-infectives were starved for funds. The only solution, the activists insisted, was to throw open the doors of the ACTG and put community representatives on every last committee, from the executive committee on down.

To Fauci and others in NIAID, ACT UP members like Harrington and Eigo, and certainly more mainstream figures such as Delaney, were known quantities. These activists had in some respects been incorporated into the AIDS establishment; by the time of the Sixth International Conference on AIDS in 1990, they spoke from the podium, rather than shouting from the back of the room.[79] "When it comes to clinical trials, some of them are better informed than many scientists can imagine," Fauci himself insisted in a speech at the conference, adding that researchers "do not have a lock on correctness."[80] For Fauci, there was no great threat in granting the activists' demand to attend ACTG meetings.

Indeed, Fauci may have deemed it both strategic and useful to incorporate activists into the process: as he later commented, his assumption was that "on a practical level, it would be helpful in some of our programs because we needed to get a feel for what would play in Peoria, as it were."[81] But many of the principal investigators sitting on the ACTG committees were leery of opening the door to the activists. In 1989, according to the account by Bruce Nussbaum, Fauci had told Hoth to get the researchers "used to the idea"—"to tell them that Eigo and Harrington were 'good guys,' smart enough to understand the science. . . ." But the researchers balked. Nussbaum quotes "one key member of the ACTG" as having told Hoth: "What are you going to do if you want to have a serious scientific discussion about a promising agent and you've got someone from the Provincetown PWA Coalition who thinks that [the drug] Peptide T is the greatest thing since sliced bread . . . ?"[82]

After members of ACT UP/New York's Treatment & Data Committee crashed a meeting in late 1989, an initial compromise position was offered: a Community Constituency Group (CCG) would be formed, a demographically diverse advisory body of representatives from all communities affected by AIDS that would meet with the ACTG at its quarterly meetings. But by this point activists refused to accept token participation; they sought to open up the closed-door meetings of the key committees—and even to obtain voting rights for the activists, just as the principal investigators enjoyed.[83] After a yearlong campaign that included the demonstration at the NIH campus, Fauci gave the activists what they wanted and forced the researchers to play along. All ACTG meetings would be opened up, and each of the twenty-two representatives of the CCG would have a regular seat on one of the ACTG committees, including the executive committee. In exchange, according to Arno and Feiden's account, "Fauci wanted the rhetoric toned down." These authors quote Fauci as saying: "If [activists] are trying to get into the system, they may have to modify some of their activist modes, but that doesn't mean they have to become Uncle Toms." [84]

THE RECONSTITUTION OF IDENTITY

Victory or co-optation? Such a stark opposition is inadequate to capture the nuances and micropolitics of activist engagement with the ACTG. Activists certainly were aware of the risks; for some time, they had been elaborating a complex strategy of intervention as both "insiders" and "outsiders." The NIH demonstration was a case in point. Fauci told the *New York Times* that he "knew the leaders of the protest well and was surprised to hear 'irrational' language on the street from people he had worked with in meetings." [85] But activists, and surely Fauci as well, knew that the language of the street and the language of the meeting room served different purposes and had different intended audiences. Activists, for their part, had been concerned about not jeopardizing the existing working relationships with NIH personnel, as Harrington later recalled: "When we did the NIH demo, Peter [Staley of ACT UP/New York] said, 'Oh, let's call Tony [Fauci] and go and have dinner with Tony and tell him about this demo. . . . In a way, we'll give him an advance heads-up. But we'll also be saying: "Look, even though we're doing this demo, we still want you to understand that we have a relationship where we can discuss and debate our issues. . . ."'" [86]

Such maneuvering was a tricky business. Yet the politics of simultaneous insider and outsider activism might well have continued smoothly had it not been for two crosscutting sets of pressures. First, AIDS treatment activism was becoming increasingly *diverse,* and the establishment of the CCG would make it more so. But different constituencies had different priorities, goals, and degrees of access to federal officials—and, therefore, different opinions about the purposes and the relative merits of insider and outsider strategies. Second, AIDS treatment activism was becoming increasingly more *complex* (as John James had suggested in comparing NIH issues to FDA issues). The established treatment activists knew about much more than clinical trial methodology and design—by this point they could speak fluently about a host of technical issues that were surfacing in research on AIDS treatments. These activists had become experts of a sort, and they could engage with researchers, government health officials, and pharmaceutical companies in a way that their fellow activists could not. The practical consequence was that it became harder for individual activists to locate themselves simultaneously on the inside and the outside. Activism tended toward a de facto division of labor—some people working on the inside, others on the outside—thus relocating the expert/lay divide to a position within the movement itself.

THE DIVERSIFICATION
OF TREATMENT ACTIVISM

Treatment activism began in gay communities for the same reason that AIDS activism in general began in gay communities—because gays asserted "ownership" of the social problem and had the material and symbolic resources with which to organize themselves and confront adversaries.[87] But even within the predominantly gay male social movement organizations like ACT UP, various constituencies had asserted their priorities. In New York City, for example, the Women's Caucus of ACT UP had been pursuing treatment issues since 1988 at some distance from the work of the Treatment & Data Committee (the home of Harrington, Barr, Eigo, and others), made up mostly, though not entirely, of men.

Activists in the Women's Caucus, and their counterparts around the country, confronted a complexly interwoven set of obstacles in bringing attention to the health needs of women with HIV and AIDS. In a book on women and AIDS, Gena Corea has described the "crazy-making politics of knowledge" that seemed to bar women from scientific consideration and medical treatment: the Centers for Disease Control's definition of AIDS, created largely with reference to the opportunistic infection contracted by gay men, systematically "exclude[d] the symptoms appearing exclusively in women," such as pelvic inflammatory disease. In very practical terms, this meant that women were not receiving the health and disability benefits that accrued from an AIDS diagnosis. ("Women don't get AIDS, they just die from it," to quote the ACT UP slogan.) However, the definition couldn't be changed to include women's symptoms, the CDC maintained, because of the absence of data proving a causal link between those symptoms and HIV infection. But the necessary data *couldn't be generated,* because "women of childbearing potential" had largely been excluded from clinical trials (putatively out of concern for their potential fetuses), and when they were included, no pelvic exams were performed. This meant not only that we failed to learn about the effects of HIV in women, but also that women were denied access to experimental treatments that might have helped keep them alive.[88]

Women activists linked their critique of these practices to an analysis of the history of the medical profession's treatment of women: women had long been considered medically "other." In the case of AIDS, activists charged, biomedicine ignored women except to consider them as "vectors" or "vessels"—as transmission routes to men or to babies, or as carriers of precious fetuses that required protection.[89] Eventually, women activists pressed successfully for a change in the CDC case definition. They also pressured Daniel Hoth and Anthony Fauci to hold a National Conference on Women and HIV Infection in December 1990. According to Maxine Wolfe of the Women's Caucus: "Although men in ACT UP had, by now, been routinely meeting with NIAID officials, in order for women AIDS activists to get *just a meeting* with them we had to stage a sit-in at the offices of Dr. Daniel Hoth . . . , make constant phone calls, send him several letters threatening a repeat sit-in, and 'zap' him in front of 5,000 of his colleagues at the Sixth International AIDS Conference. . . ."[90]

Gay men and lesbians of color also formed caucuses within ACT UP chapters around the country, and some of them, too, became concerned with treatment issues. But, as Cathy Cohen notes in her study, activists of color in ACT UP found themselves "in the precarious position of not being trusted by many in communities of color because of their ties to ACT UP and at the same time not being fully supported by influential members inside of ACT UP."[91] And as Moisés Agosto, who became involved in AIDS activism after moving from Puerto Rico to New York City, discovered, it was often hard to convince members of racial minority communities of the *need* for activism on treatment issues, given the wide range of concerns confronting them. To the extent that these communities became open to AIDS activism, it was on issues of prevention and care. Treatment activism, Agosto found, was generally perceived as "an upper-middle class, white gay-boy thing to do"—though Agosto tried to demonstrate the importance of the work by translating treatment information into Spanish.[92]

Finally, by the early 1990s, some hemophilia activists had also moved into the arena of treatment activism. Despite the very high incidence of HIV infection among people with hemophilia, this community had been slow to mobilize. Eventually people with hemophilia would organize forcefully around the question of the culpability of the blood-banking industry in the infection of people with hemophilia through contaminated blood products, and they would pursue legal remedies. But "it's a very geographically dispersed community, there's not a lot of us, [and] we're dying at the rate of one a day, which is a lot considering that there were only probably eight or ten thousand of us infected to begin with," explained Jonathan Wadleigh, a founder of the key hemophilia activist group, the Committee of Ten Thousand. Gay men organizing an activist response didn't need to search far and wide to find others affected by AIDS. By contrast, "with an incidence of one in ten thousand [in the] population, normally you're lucky if you meet one person in a lifetime who has hemophilia."[93]

When Wadleigh decided to begin attending meetings of ACT UP/ Boston in the late 1980s, he was "often the only straight person" in the room as well as "the only person with hemophilia." But given the inaction he perceived on the part of the New England Hemophilia Foundation, Wadleigh "began to quickly associate [himself] more with the gay community and . . . to relate to the brand of activism that was going on there." Recognizing that the level of information about treatments in the hemophilia community was very low, Wadleigh started up a treatment newsletter, summarizing articles from the established grassroots publications such as *AIDS Treatment News,* the San Francisco AIDS Foundation's *BETA,* and Project Inform's *PI Perspectives.* He also became involved in methodological debates about the inclusion criteria for AIDS trials. Boilerplate language in trial protocols routinely excluded anyone with elevated liver enzymes—but people with hemophilia (along with injection drug users) quite often show signs of liver disease and hence have elevated enzyme levels. Wadleigh's fight to liberalize the entry criteria so that more people with hemophilia could participate in clinical trials was, in his view, one of his most significant contributions in the domain of treatment activism.[94]

THE POLITICS OF CLEAVAGE

In agreeing to establish a Community Constituency Group that would attend ACTG meetings, Hoth and Fauci proposed that the group include representatives of a wide range of constituencies—gays, racial minorities, women, injection drug users, people with hemophilia, and children. Whether NIAID officials deliberately sought to dilute the impact of gay male treatment activism, or simply considered it good politics to broaden the community representation, the significance of the CCG was that it became the first place where activists from all these various communities came together to talk about AIDS treatments. Particularly for activists representing communities of color, this was a long-awaited opportunity to present their views before government officials and scientists, and their agenda was broad. The established treatment activists, however, saw it as inappropriate to use the CCG as a forum for issues beyond the purview of the ACTG. They wanted to talk about the science of clinical trials, and they urged the newcomers to "get up to speed." Almost immediately, tensions rose sharply.

At an AIDS Treatment Activist Conference held just prior to a CCG meeting, some called the ACT UP/New York Treatment & Data Committee's agenda a "white male" approach to health care, focused solely on drug development to the exclusion of issues like health care financing, which were of primary interest to women, minorities, and poor people.[95] One ACTG committee meeting ended in chaos, when members of ACT UP/New York's Women's Caucus, most of them white, blasted a planned clinical trial of pregnant women with HIV as "bad science" and "unethical." (The study, ACTG 076, was designed to test the use of AZT in interrupting transmission of HIV from mother to fetus. The activists objected to, among others things, the apparent prioritizing of fetuses over adult women in clinical research.) In response, several African-American women who were involved in running the study denounced the activists, leading a number of black and Latino members of the CCG to cry that ACT UP was "racist." [96]

On the local level, similar pressures fractured individual ACT UP chapters. Flush from its triumphs at the Sixth International Conference, where it had mobilized hundreds of people into the streets around the conference center for a weeklong series of demonstrations, ACT UP/San Francisco swelled with new members in the latter part of 1990 and then rapidly exploded. Ostensibly, the debate concerned whether the group should continue to operate according to the consensus process, allowing a single voice of dissent to paralyze decision making. At a deeper level, most commentators agreed, the split was between those (mostly gay white men who were HIV positive) who supported the basic goal of "drugs into bodies" and those (including many of the women and people of color in the group) who sought a more thoroughgoing engagement with the class-based inequities of the

U.S. health care system and with the racist, sexist, and homophobic dimensions of biomedicine and, indeed, of U.S. society as a whole.[97] From the standpoint of the latter group, the privileged white men were insensitive to any issues but their own; from the vantage point of the former, the forces of political correctness were engaged in utopian phrase-mongering while *they* were busy saving lives. The former group seceded from ACT UP/San Francisco to constitute a new chapter, ACT UP/Golden Gate.

Similar splits soon occurred in ACT UP/Chicago and ACT UP/Portland. Meanwhile, women in the Women's Caucus of ACT UP/New York became increasingly disturbed by the incorporation of "the boys" into the ACTG system. Though the Women's Caucus members had succeeded in pressuring Fauci to hold the National Conference on Women and HIV Infection in December 1990, they had never enjoyed easy access to NIAID officials, and the conference itself proved to be a tense and acrimonious event. "So imagine our fury," wrote Risa Dennenberg, describing the occasion in *Outweek,* "when, like ships in the night, three of [us] collided in the lobby of the Sheraton at the close of the conference, with members of the Treatment and Data Committee of ACT UP/NY, who were, unbeknownst to us, heading to a social event with these same dreaded government bureaucrats."[98]

Members of the Women's Action Committee proposed a six-month moratorium on face-to-face meetings with government officials—to the utter bewilderment and consternation of the Treatment & Data Committee. "As soon as we got the seat at the table, which we had fought for, and which had been a part of our rhetoric for years, there was a faction in ACT UP that didn't want us to claim it," Harrington recalled with disbelief, several years later.[99] Soon afterward, the core of the Treatment & Data Committee split off to form a new, more exclusive organization, which they called the Treatment Action Group, or TAG. "In New York, we were running a participatory democracy with nine hundred people in the room," commented David Barr, recalling how painful it was to contemplate leaving ACT UP: "You know, you can only do it for so long. . . ."[100]

Gender and racial divisions, as well as debates over internal participatory mechanisms, insider/outsider strategies, and overall priorities and goals, are the kinds of issues that can tear apart any social movement. What particularly complicated the internal battles of the AIDS movement was the additional overlay of the politics of expertise. It was not simply that some people were working on the inside while others were outside—just as important, those who were on the inside were increasingly mastering specialized forms of knowledge with which their fellow activists on the outside did not come into contact. There resulted what Gilbert Elbaz, in an analysis of ACT UP/New York, has nicely described as a gap between the "lay expert" activists and the "lay lay" activists.[101] Stratification by gender, race, class, and education helped to structure access to the "lay expert" identity. "[It's] interesting how similar they are to the people that they're fighting," reflected Michelle Roland, a San Francisco Bay Area treatment activist. "I mean, it's science. And who is raised in this culture to believe that they could be scientists? Smart white men. And who are the treatment activists? Smart white men. All with an education. . . . And then you have . . . the occasional woman who says, 'I can do it too!'"[102]

The CCG should have been a place where possession of knowledge became equalized. In practice, people who not only came from very different backgrounds and had sharply differing priorities but also had widely varying degrees of exposure to biomedical science were thrown together and expected suddenly to perform. The CCG "was a great experiment," reflected David Barr, "but there were people at all different points within the learning curve." Barr explained: "You'd have somebody . . . who had AIDS, who knew a lot about AIDS, [but who] didn't know *anything* about AIDS research—you know, nothing. And never had seen a clinical trial, didn't live in a city where they did clinical trials, on the one end—and then Mark Harrington and Martin Delaney on the other."[103] The solidification of knowledge-based hierarchies was furthered by the difficulties experienced by the first wave of autodidacts in developing a coherent educational strategy that would bring larger numbers of activists into the arena of knowledge-assessment. One activist who remained with ACT UP after others left to form TAG painted a picture of a Treatment & Data meeting circa 1990: the core group of activists "feverishly [tossing] acronyms at each other," complaining that they were overworked and in need of help; the "mostly silent majority of 20 or 30," sitting in the back of the room, "waiting for a revelation."[104]

Another tendency accentuated by the organizational splits and the professionalization of treatment activism was the increasing emphasis on Western medicine and reliance on the pharmaceutical industry, to the relative exclusion of alternative treatments and non-Western conceptions of healing. The main ACT UP chapters had always had committees on alternative treatments, while Project Inform had promoted

Compound Q, derived from the root of a Chinese cucumber, and *AIDS Treatment News* had regularly and consistently promoted a range of nonpharmaceutical products. With the splits in the prominent ACT UP chapters, advocates of alternative and mainstream treatments often ended up in different camps. ACT UP/Golden Gate focused on the ACTG and the pharmaceutical companies, while interest in natural and alternative treatments was pursued mainly by ACT UP/San Francisco and other groups. Similarly, in New York, TAG focused on mainstream science, while alternative treatment activists found ACT UP to be a more congenial environment.[105]

At a national level, too, there was often little room for discussing alternative treatments. Jason Heyman, a San Francisco activist who tried to address the issue at a CCG meeting, recalls being "told to leave the room" by a prominent East Coast treatment activist.[106] In this case as in others, the dominant treatment activists had acquired the power to perform the "boundary work" that distinguished legitimate treatment issues from illegitimate ones.[107] "They were a wall . . . between us and the establishment. They were keeping us out." Heyman had no objection, in principle, to the fact that activists had moved to the inside. But once they had done so, "they changed . . . and they looked at us differently. They were offended by us." And the irony was that "we were doing what they had done. We were just being rude and . . . coming in there and saying, 'Look, this is what we want'— which is just what they had done."[108]

By 1992, the links connecting treatment activist experts with their grassroots base had become increasingly attenuated. Knowledge still flowed "downward" in the form of articles by the treatment activists that appeared in the gay press and the treatment newsletters. But there was less accountability to the broader movement. Perhaps predictably, perhaps inevitably, pressures to democratize science conflicted with pressures to establish new hierarchies of expertise. The tugs toward these different poles coincided with yet another tension, that which existed between "prefigurative" and "accommodationist" politics— between the appeal of a radical critique of medicine and the felt need to save lives now. By the early 1990s, it seemed that the voices of pragmatism had become dominant. Core groups of activists had established themselves as important contributors to the development of knowledge about AIDS treatments—but at the price of increasing distance from what was, in any case, a rapidly splintering movement.

CHAPTER 9

CLINICAL TRIALS
AND TRIBULATIONS

The Search for New Directions (1992–1993)

"OUTSMARTING SCIENCE"

The ever fragile optimism of treatment activists strained to the breaking point in late 1991. The second generation of antiviral AIDS drugs—the non-nucleoside reverse-transcriptase inhibitors that had been engineered specifically to fight HIV and that had looked so promising in vitro—performed poorly in clinical trials. Merck's "L" drugs, nevirapine, and another drug called TIBO were all shown to have little individual efficacy against the virus because the viral gene that produced reverse transcriptase proved capable of mutating in a matter of days or weeks to resist these compounds. For some time now, the avowed goal had been to use the little-loved nucleoside analogues, AZT, ddC, and ddI, to keep people alive just long enough to get better drugs into circulation. Now people would have to depend on the first-generation drugs for much longer—while those who ceased benefiting from them would have no obvious therapeutic recourse standing between them and complete immune collapse.

The news about the non-nucleoside reverse-transcriptase inhibitors "was nothing short of shattering," said Theo Smart of ACT UP/New York. "So many hopes had been pinned to [these drugs'] effectiveness."[1] "Researchers openly wondered, 'What are we going to do next?'" reported Jesse Dobson of ACT UP/Golden Gate and the Community Constituency Group, describing an ACTG meeting in late

1991.[2] "Activists Despondent and the Movement Is Splintering" was
the headline of one of a series of articles in the *San Francisco Examiner*
by reporter Jayne Garrison, describing the state of affairs. Garrison
quoted Peter Staley, a prominent New York activist: "As far as I'm
concerned I'm going to die, Magic Johnson is going to die and the
million Americans who are presently infected will die."[3] Concluded
Garrison: "So far, the virus is outsmarting science."[4]

Martin Delaney, projecting the generally upbeat message of Project
Inform, rejected the "gloom and doom" and stressed instead the continued importance of combination therapy with nucleoside analogues,
the apparently large numbers of "long-term survivors" who had been
living with HIV for a decade or more, and the promised protease inhibitors and tat inhibitors then on the horizon.[5] Unfortunately, the
ongoing saga of Hoffman-LaRoche's tat inhibitor—the only such drug
in development—was hardly reassuring. For reasons that were inexplicable to the Johns Hopkins researchers who had been contracted to
conduct the study, the company summarily postponed its Phase I trial
in May 1991. Activists had generally found this company less cooperative than most; now they could only speculate that Hoffman-
LaRoche wished to avoid subsidizing another parallel track program,
having given out free ddC to more than three thousand AIDS patients.[6]

At first the company announced that it would sell its tat inhibitor
to the highest bidder; then, half a year later, Hoffman-LaRoche
changed its mind, saying it would develop the drug after all. "Apparently the company decided that this drug was too good to sell—especially in view of the disappointing results with the competing class
of non-nucleoside reverse-transcriptase inhibitors," suggested John
James in *AIDS Treatment News*.[7] But throughout 1992, Hoffman-
LaRoche sat tight. In early 1993 activists declared open warfare on the
company with the mass resignation of the members of the Community
Advisory Board that the company had established. "There can be no
more polite dialogue with your company," said TAG and ACT UP/
New York in a letter sent to Hoffman-LaRoche in late January threatening a boycott of its products, laboratories, and home care services.[8]
In his column in the *Advocate*, Delaney proposed that the government
seize the drug "in the national interest": "Eminent domain is frequently used to seize private property for such national emergencies
as highway construction. Is AIDS less important?"[9]

As John James observed, the lesson of the tat inhibitor extended well beyond the cupidity or irresponsibility of a single company. Here was a type of drug that "leading AIDS scientists" considered to be "perhaps the single most promising approach to developing better AIDS treatments"; furthermore, potential tat inhibitors could easily be discovered through known screening methods. There was no reason, in theory, why there couldn't be fifty tat inhibitors in development; "instead, the whole pharmaceutical industry (or rather, that small part of it which has any interest in AIDS) seems to be waiting to see what happens with the only tat inhibitor drug now in human testing. . . ." It was a maddening picture: "In the middle of a major worldwide epidemic, the most promising approach to treatment development has been abandoned to a single project with a single drug in a single company." The problem was not just Hoffman-LaRoche; the problem was the whole notion that the "invisible hand" of the free market would somehow function in the service of the public good and not just private gain—a notion that the NIH was unwilling or unable to challenge. And, separate from the issue of political economy, there remained the additional, nagging question: Why did Hoffman-LaRoche seem to have "so little interest in its own drug"? "What might it know that we don't?" asked James.[10]

A "NEW PARADIGM" FOR TREATMENT ACTIVISM

In keeping with the grim news from the treatment front, the Eighth International Conference on AIDS, held in Amsterdam in June 1992, was "somber" in atmosphere. One striking expression of official pessimism came from the editor of *JAMA*, Dr. George Lundberg, who predicted that AIDS would remain a common disease a century from now. Lawrence Altman, covering the conference for the *New York Times,* noted some of the effects of discouragement: "Even demonstrators who have disrupted previous conferences and attacked health officials and scientists for their slow, step-by-step approach conceded that there was an urgent need to return to basic science," he wrote.[11]

These were the sentiments that motivated the lengthy report "AIDS Research at the NIH: A Critical Review," prepared by Gregg Gonsalves and Mark Harrington and presented by the Treatment Action Group at the 1992 conference.[12] The two authors had sat down and read every NIH grant that had funded AIDS research through each of the NIH institutes, and they had tried to envision a logical, cohesive approach to organizing that research effort.[13] "Since 1987," wrote Gonsalves and Harrington, "the activist critique of AIDS research has worked its way back: from drug approval at the regulatory level of the US Food + Drug Administration . . . , to expanded access for drugs still under study (Parallel Track), to the design and conduct of the controlled clinical trials themselves by the National Institutes of Health . . . , pharmaceutical companies, and community-based clinical trial centers." Now activists had come to realize that in order for their efforts to succeed, they would have to focus their attention on an even earlier phase of the research process: "If the reforms won by activists are not to become mere stratagems for craven pharmaceutical companies swiftly to develop and market a whole series of additional nucleoside analogues (d4T, FLT, 3TC, etc.), activists must become more involved in the basic research process itself, forcing academic and industrial researchers to turn their attention to novel treatment approaches to HIV-induced immune suppression. . . ." This was a tall order, one that "[required] that activists become as familiar with the $800 million AIDS program of the NIH as they have with its major clinical component," the ACTG. The ACTG "is but one eighth of the NIH AIDS program. A cure will never be tested by the ACTG unless it's discovered somewhere else first." Clinical trials were the late stage in the game—to get drugs *into* development, activists had to influence the course of basic AIDS research at the NIH, within NIAID as well as the various other agencies, like the National Cancer Institute, the National Institute of Child Health and Human Development, and the National Institute of Neurological Disorders and Stroke. "This is a new paradigm for AIDS activists," the TAG authors made clear: "We have to familiarize ourselves with a wide range of disciplines."[14]

It was a significant shift, but a risky one, for the course of action that now seemed most crucial also appeared to be one in which activists were by no means guaranteed to succeed. Gonsalves and Harrington grasped the point clearly: "Activists' claim to expertise in clinical trials came out of lived experience. Most of us cannot claim the same for basic biomedical research." At best, activists could "hope to serve as catalysts for better and more coordinated work within the research realm, and as agitators with Congress and the Administration for enhanced resources in the public realm."[15] Indeed, it was in the realm of public policy that the report itself had the most impact. Upon the election of President Bill Clinton, who had promised to prioritize

AIDS research, Senator Ted Kennedy made the TAG report the basis for an amendment tacked onto the NIH authorization bill. Following the blueprint laid out in the report, Kennedy called for a strengthened Office of AIDS Research within the NIH, which would have jurisdiction over all AIDS-related research in each of the NIH institutes.[16]

THE SCIENCE OF "CONCORDOLOGY"

As treatment activists focused on such drugs as the non-nucleosides, the tat and protease inhibitors, and still more experimental approaches, controversy continued to swirl around AZT. This made sense: AZT was still, by far, the most commonly prescribed AIDS antiviral, and it was considered the best drug with which to begin antiretroviral therapy. The drug had a high profile, in part because Burroughs Wellcome's marketing of the drug was sophisticated and relentless: the company's efforts included promotional videos mailed to doctors, a toll-free "AIDS information" hot line designed to peddle the company's product, and mass media and billboard ad campaigns preaching the benefits of knowing one's antibody status and initiating antiretroviral treatment early. Yet questions about the drug's use had never fully been answered to the satisfaction of many.

Longtime opponents of AZT, including HIV dissenters such as John Lauritsen and Chuck Ortleb, attacked those who had climbed aboard the AZT bandwagon. Lauritsen labeled Project Inform and the Gay Men's Health Crisis as "gay quisling groups" for their endorsement of nucleoside analogues, while the *Native* referred to John James as an "AZT pimp."[17] Such attacks became more vehement after some of the treatment activist groups began accepting donations from Burroughs Wellcome. In 1992 Project Inform received a $150,000 grant from the company to upgrade its computer equipment. TAG and ACT UP/ Golden Gate received small donations, but TAG also brokered a $1 million grant from the company to AmFAR in support of community-based research.[18] "If I have to take money from the devil to save my life and the lives of my friends, I'll do it," said Peter Staley of TAG.[19] Yet even if the donations came without strings attached, the acceptance of such funds left treatment groups vulnerable to attack by opponents of AZT. One leaflet that made the rounds in San Francisco in 1992 and purported to come from a group called "ACT UP/Underground" described Burroughs Wellcome's "blood payment" to Project

Inform. In a memorable phrase, the leaflet accused the organization of having "promised to deliver its own community to nucleoside slavery, bound in the chains of corporate greed!"[20]

At a different volume level, mainstream authorities continued to debate the merits of early intervention with AZT in people who were asymptomatic. "After 5 Years of Use, Doubt Still Clouds Leading AIDS Drug" was the *New York Times* headline of a 1992 article by Gina Kolata that charted the undercurrents of uncertainty.[21] No study had yet demonstrated that AZT actually prolonged life in people who started taking the drug when they had fewer than 500 T cells, although the Veterans Administration study, once completed, indicated that AZT did prolong the length of the disease-free state.[22] (Concerns about racial differences in response to AZT based on a preliminary report from the study were generally allayed by retrospective analyses of earlier studies that showed no treatment differences based on race.)[23] This study was considered too small to provide a definitive answer to questions of survival; instead, researchers now looked to the completion of the Concorde study in Europe.

Meanwhile, doctors and patients grappled with uncertainties: Was it better to start treatment early, before the immune system had deteriorated and while the patient could more easily tolerate a serious drug, in the hope of delaying the onset of symptoms, thus keeping the patient healthy until more effective drugs arrived on the scene? Or was it better to wait, sparing outwardly healthy patients a toxic drug that could cause anemia or liver damage and avoiding the development of resistance, so that the drug would be effective later in the course of illness at the point when there was clearer evidence that it actually provided a benefit? As a 1992 survey of 448 physicians reveals, the vast majority simply followed the NIH guidelines and the FDA labeling, prescribing AZT for anyone with fewer than five hundred T cells per cubic millimeter.[24] But doctors and patients who tracked the science of AIDS more closely were often less certain about the best course of action.

Still, nobody seemed quite ready for the news when the Concorde researchers released their preliminary report on April 1, 1993, in a brief letter to the editor in *Lancet*.[25] Eight hundred seventy-seven patients, asymptomatic upon entry into the study, had been randomized into the "immediate treatment" arm of the study and had received one thousand milligrams of AZT daily; 872 had been placed in the "deferred treatment" arm, receiving a placebo unless they became symptomatic, at which point they were put on AZT. In total, the study provided 5,328 person-years of data, making it the largest and longest study of its kind. The researchers reported that the patients in the "immediate treatment" arm experienced more a CD4-count boost, on average, than those in the "deferred treatment" arm. However, "by contrast with the differences in CD4 count, there was no significant difference in clinical outcome between the two therapeutic strategies." The three-year survival rate was 92 percent for those who had begun taking AZT early and 93 percent for those who were put on the drug later. And similarly, there was no significant difference between the two groups in terms of disease progression and the development of opportunistic infections.

In the eyes of the Concorde investigators, Ian Weller in Britain and Jean-Pierre Aboulker in France, the study did not so much contradict 019 and the other studies of AZT use in asymptomatic patients as *subsume* them by proceeding for a longer period of time. The investigators had found an initial trend suggesting benefit in the early use of AZT, similar to that found by Paul Volberding in ACTG 019. But since the trend wasn't statistically significant, the trial was kept going, and as time passed the benefit simply disappeared. The bottom line, according to the *Lancet* report, was this: starting AZT early, as opposed to starting it later, did not extend survival or even the disease-free state. And CD4, the "surrogate marker" that had been employed in the licensing of ddI and ddC in the United States, could not be considered predictive of long-term treatment differences.

It was a painful moment that left many people dazed—or defensive, or angry, or jubilant, depending on their previous commitments in the AZT controversies. "Rarely have a mere eight paragraphs sparked such fury, hysteria and hyperbole," said an article in a San Francisco lesbian and gay newspaper.[26] Not long afterward, one researcher with the World Health Organization would suggest that "a whole tropical rain forest has disappeared as a result of this study," which ushered in a brand new domain of scientific inquiry he dubbed "Concordology."[27] And in the space of a few days following the report in *Lancet,* the stock value of Wellcome PLC dropped by more than $500 million.[28]

Billed as the "definitive" study of AZT use in asymptomatic HIV infection, Concorde initially appeared to settle nothing; it seemed almost infinitely malleable in the interpretations it could generate. "You can interpret [Concorde] as your bias dictates," said the director of inpatient services at San Francisco General Hospital.[29] Weller, the British principal investigator, who described himself as having *already* been "very conservative in the use of zidovudine [AZT] monotherapy in asymptomatic patients," now said: "Those physicians like myself who tended to wait until symptoms appeared are going to be more sure they were doing the right thing."[30] Douglas Richman, one of the principal investigators in the AZT studies in the United States, commented: "This is a chronic active persistent infection. It's inconceivable to me that not treating it is the way to go."[31] One "knowledgeable and compassionate AIDS doctor told [GMHC's publication, *Treatment Issues*] privately that he would continue to prescribe AZT for his asymptomatic patients even if it did not work. He said there was nothing else for him to do."[32]

Those who wanted to score political points had plenty of opportunity. Larry Kramer, for instance, used the study to highlight the overall failure of the research effort in an overwrought editorial he penned for the *Advocate,* entitled "AZT Is Shit."[33] Other responses followed predictable patterns. "Advocates of the AZT-is-poison school have had a field day," wrote Tim Kingston, a reporter for the *San Francisco Bay Times.* "Not only do they assert that early AZT intervention is ineffective, but also that *all* AZT treatment and *all* HIV antiretroviral therapies are ineffective."[34] One example was the comment of HIV dissenter and AIDS activist Michael Callen, quoted in the *Los Angeles Times:* "Taking AZT is like aiming a thermonuclear warhead at a mosquito."[35] A San Francisco gay newspaper whose AIDS writer had been opposed to AZT ran a cover graphic of a hand tipping a gigantic bottle of Retrovir (the brand name of AZT), with capsules spilling onto tombstones in a graveyard.[36]

A Los Angeles–based group of AZT dissidents, called Project AIDS, International, sought to spread the word to AZT "victims": "You need to know your rights. Ask yourself the following questions: Were you misled by the U.S. studies or information that was given you through the FDA or CDC? Were you pressured into taking AZT . . . by your doctors or an AIDS organization? . . . If you have answered yes . . . , you have a right to compensation. . . ."[37] In London, newspapers reported that the widow of a person with AIDS was suing Wellcome PLC, claiming that her husband had died from the effects of AZT.[38] And a London group calling itself Gays Against Genocide picketed an AIDS organization and a hospital where a clinical trial of AZT in children was in progress, accusing their targets of "murder" and "baby-killing," respectively.[39] Meanwhile, opponents of these views argued that if Concorde did anything it *disproved*, once and for all, the notion that AZT is poison: after all, a large number of people had taken a high dose of AZT for four years and only a small percentage experienced adverse reactions to the drug.[40]

European AIDS authorities, by and large, tended to accept the study conclusions as given. But U.S. authorities rushed to explain that nothing really had changed. Until more data were available, "no physician or patient should change the approach they're using based on this study," Daniel Hoth of NIAID told *USA Today*.[41] David Kessler, the FDA commissioner, told the *New York Times* that the results of Concorde were not a surprise, since experts "have known that AZT has real but limited benefit"; this of course sidestepped the issue of the FDA's labeling of AZT for use in any HIV-infected person with fewer than five hundred T cells.[42]

East Coast AIDS groups, less well-disposed overall to the nucleoside analogues, criticized the official "spin control." GMHC's publication, *Treatment Issues*, commented: "The blizzard of press releases responding to Concorde reveals the extent of the personal and professional investment many U.S. researchers have in AZT's efficacy. While one should expect a profit-driven corporation like Burroughs Wellcome to interpret the data favorably, U.S. government agencies should be held to a different standard."[43] But West Coast groups like Project Inform and publications like *AIDS Treatment News* that were more committed to early intervention reacted quickly to the study, and they rushed out their methodological heavy artillery. Fighting against the "black-boxing" of Concorde, they strove to highlight as much contingency, messiness, and uncertainty as they possibly could.

First, patients in the study had received an unusually high dose of AZT—twice the dose that had become standard by the time of the study's termination. From the "pragmatic" perspective on clinical trials, this meant that the study had questionable relevance to the real-world treatment decisions of 1993. A larger concern was the modification of the study protocol in midcourse, after the results of ACTG 019 had come out. To satisfy ethical requirements, the Concorde investigators had allowed patients with fewer than five hundred T cells to choose at any point to begin open use of AZT rather than remain in the double-blinded trial. In all, 282 of the 872 patients in the deferred treatment arm had switched from placebo to AZT. The accepted statistical practice, however (called the "intent-to-treat" rule), was to analyze patients *as if they remained in the original groups to which they had been randomly assigned.* That is, the 282 patients who began taking AZT prior to progression to illness were analyzed as if they had been on placebo all along.[44]

The purpose of the intent-to-treat rule in biostatistics is to put the burden of proof on the drug whose efficacy is under investigation.[45] For example, if some subjects in the placebo arm of a trial accidentally receive the study drug, researchers continue to count them in the placebo group. Then, if a difference in outcome is still found between the two arms of the study despite the blurring of regimens that occurred, the researcher can be especially confident about the results. The problem, however, is that if *no* difference is found, the researcher might reasonably wonder: is the drug really useless or did the contamination of the original study design prevent a true difference from manifesting itself? No one representing the Concorde study was suggesting that the change in the study protocol might account for the negative outcome—that if no placebo patients had switched to open-label AZT, the "deferred treatment" arm would have done worse relative to the "immediate treatment" arm. But to many U.S. researchers (and certainly to Burroughs Wellcome) this seemed eminently plausible.[46] In effect, they argued, two *roughly similar* groups were being compared, so it was no surprise when the outcomes were similar.

John James also raised questions about the surrogate markers issue, which, as he noted, was so vital to the program of accelerated approval of new drugs. The *Lancet* letter had reported only that the *median* CD4 counts over time failed to predict the outcomes of the two arms of the study. Most U.S. researchers, wrote James, thought it was insufficient to look just at the median counts: "This question must be addressed by case-by-case analysis of whether individual patients whose T-helper counts rose after starting the drug seemed to show improved prognosis as a result."[47] Meanwhile, treatment activists around the country worried that the initial reports from Concorde would fuel a backlash against the changes that had been instituted at the FDA to approve drugs more rapidly. "The spin, I predict, will be 'This is all the activists' fault,'" wrote Larry Kramer. "*New York Times* chameleon Dr. Lawrence Altman said as much in his ineptly reported article. . . ."[48]

Altman had written a follow-up to his initial news article on Concorde, a commentary entitled "AIDS Study Casts Doubt on Value of Hastened Drug Approval in U.S."[49] The article explained how Concorde researchers had "persisted" against the prevailing construction of belief about AZT, continuing their study even after ACTG 019 had ended. That persistence had paid off in a finding that overturned the conventional wisdom. Furthermore, "in challenging the reliability of the CD-4 count in evaluating AZT, the Concorde study rekindled a long simmering dispute between many European and American researchers over the validity of surrogate markers in H.I.V. and AIDS," wrote Altman, noting that the British government had refused to license ddI on the basis of surrogate markers. Altman quoted Ian Weller, the British principal investigator, about the "lesson" in the Concorde study: "Don't stop trials too early.... Whatever the pressures are, keep going as long as possible."

Some reacted defensively to such charges, while others were despondent. Yet all the responses seemed to reflect the same underlying disquiet. It wasn't just the study; it was the whole state of the science, and Concorde was merely the last straw. An editorial in GMHC's *Treatment Issues* did a good job of capturing the sentiments that seemed to feed many of the reactions to the study: "Concorde underscores the uncertainty many AIDS researchers and clinicians feel. A few years ago, many physicians believed that the nucleoside analogs ... would transform AIDS into a so-called 'chronic manageable' condition. There is now a deep and growing sense among many that some of the basic assumptions underlying AIDS drug development need to be reexamined." [50]

BERLIN

These were the clouds hanging overhead as thirteen thousand people from 166 countries assembled in Berlin's vast and labyrinthine conference center in June for the Ninth International Conference on AIDS. A cover story by *Science* reporter Jon Cohen had set the stage for the scientific proceedings. "The more we learn, the less certain we are" was the message Cohen had gleaned from a survey he conducted of 150 leading AIDS researchers: "After more than a decade of struggling in frustration as the epidemic gallops on, researchers are being forced to reexamine assumptions they once held without question." Even as "politicians and AIDS activists [were] demanding results immediately," researchers confronted a series of "collapsing certainties," including the virtues of antiretroviral therapy in asymptomatics, the trustworthiness of surrogate markers in evaluating treatments, and the reliability of certain key vaccine experiments. In addition, "many researchers who once believed almost all the damage caused by HIV could be explained by the virus's direct killing of cells now think indirect mechanisms must also be at work."[51]

Progress certainly was being made in the understanding of pathogenesis, as conference presentations by top scientists such as Fauci and Jay Levy made clear.[52] On one hand, better laboratory techniques such as PCR had revealed higher concentrations of infected cells throughout the body (and not just in the bloodstream); this lent credence to claims that direct cell-killing could play an important role in AIDS, while arguing against those, such as Duesberg, who had been maintaining that HIV could not be the true cause of AIDS if so few cells were infected (see chapters 3 and 4). On the other hand, few now thought that direct cell-killing was the only factor at work. Levy's recent, one hundred–page journal article on pathogenesis had listed more than a dozen factors he believed were involved in HIV-induced immune deficiency.[53] HIV and its constituent proteins appeared to have a range of effects on both infected and uninfected cells, as well as on their associated cytokines; aberrant signaling by the cytokines then caused cascading effects throughout the immune system.

Better understanding could be gleaned, perhaps, from the study of so-called "long-term survivors" or "long-term nonprogressors"—this was a direction that activists had been promoting and that was increasingly emphasized in Berlin. "There's a growing sense that there is no magic bullet for AIDS, so we should shift research to see why some people do well . . . ," said ACT UP/New York's Aldyn McKean.[54] But as Robin Weiss had pointed out in an article on pathogenesis in *Science*, there might be nothing "special" about long-term survivors: since "the rates of progression . . . are also consistent with a stochastic, random occurrence of AIDS after HIV infection . . . , 'long-term' survival could be pure luck."[55]

Gallo, in his address, offered a dazzling array of future, high-tech treatment possibilities. Gene therapy and "antisense" therapy might be used to prevent infection of cells. Drugs could be developed that targeted cellular products used by the virus, rather than directly targeting the virus. HIV-infected people could be given a genetically engineered protein of HHV-7 (human herpes virus, number seven), a virus that "competes" with HIV for CD4 receptor sites; the protein would then beat the virus to the CD4 molecules on the T cells and prevent infection.[56]

This was all very nice, but what treatments were available in the short run? What could the assembled physicians (or at least, those from rich countries) go back and tell their patients, symptomatic or asymptomatic, about the options that were open to them? What was the "state of the art"? One crucial set of facts was offered by the Concorde researchers, who presented a range of data that went beyond the limited report in *Lancet*.[57] Overall, the Concorde trial gained in credibility at the conference, though some found ways to bracket or qualify its findings. Martin Delaney claimed there were still data he would like to see, but that it "wasn't worth fighting about." Concorde was "just one of many studies out there" and not a particularly relevant one, at that. Concorde had asked "one question": Does a daily gram of AZT initiated early in the course of disease prevent progression? But since no one routinely took a gram a day of the drug, it wasn't clear "what that means for early intervention in general or even for AZT."[58]

The big story, however, was the result from ACTG 155. This was Margaret Fischl's Phase II study that many had been awaiting in order to see whether the AZT/ddC combination, licensed the previous year, would perform as well in a long-term study as surrogate marker evidence had predicted. At a satellite symposium held in Berlin on the eve of the international conference, Fischl tried to put the best face on the study's outcome. The sad facts were that 42 percent of the subjects receiving AZT, 43 percent of the subjects receiving ddC, and 39 percent of the subjects receiving the combination had progressed to serious illness or death; there was no statistically significant difference between the three treatment arms of ACTG 155. The subjects receiving the combination therapy did get a larger CD4 count boost, just as they had in the promising early study, ACTG 106. But they didn't live any longer in the end.

Nevertheless, Fischl framed the outcome as positive by stressing that the combination therapy did show an advantage in the subset of patients whose CD4 counts at the outset were between 150 and 300 per cubic millimeter.[59] Since these were the subjects with the highest initial CD4 counts in the study, the "spin" that Fischl was pushing was that patients benefited from the combination unless they were already too far along in their illness. NIAID supported this interpretation, issuing a press release with the headline: "Effectiveness of AZT/ddC Combination Depends on Pretreatment Immune Cell Count."[60]

Yet as the distressing word of the study's overall findings spread through the halls of the conference center, reporters witnessed the unusual spectacle of a NIAID representative yanking the press release from the media center and hastily replacing it with a new, more sober one: "The Effectiveness of AZT Alone, ddC Alone or AZT/ddC Combination Is Similar Overall for Patients with Advanced HIV Disease."[61] Fischl, undeterred, repeated her original conclusions at the formal conference session.[62] No sooner had she finished than activists from TAG sprang to the microphone. "The answer to the study you designed is that the study shows *no difference* between combo and monotherapy," insisted a furious David Barr. "You have staked your career on these drugs," yelled Barr. "I have staked my life."[63]

Barr and other activists characterized Fischl's stratification of the subjects by CD4 count as a methodologically unjustifiable violation of the fundamental principles of randomization, indeed, as a post hoc fishing expedition for results that would make the study appear a success. As much as activists had wanted to believe in the combination therapy, they now had no patience for any sugarcoating of the bad news. (Or perhaps, to the extent that they felt disillusioned, Fischl provided a convenient focal point for their anger: it's more satisfying, after all, to direct one's wrath at a researcher who appears to be cheating than at a virus that appears to be winning.) "How much is Roche paying you?" yelled out activists in the audience, referring to Hoffman-LaRoche, the manufacturer of ddC, which had already been the target of an activist protest during the conference's opening ceremonies because of the company's slowness in conducting its own, postmarketing studies of ddC as required by the FDA.

Whether Fischl was casting about to salvage her study or describing a genuinely important auxiliary finding was, in some sense, beside the point. Activist rage had more to do with the predicament the patient community now found itself in. As Mark Harrington noted in a heated challenge to Fischl voiced from the conference floor, the response to Concorde by U.S. experts had been to play it down, to claim that, after all, combination therapy was the *real* standard of care for asymptomatics. "The truth is," said Harrington bitterly, "*we have no standard of care* for asymptomatics." There was no disputing Harrington's point, nor did the conference presentations on non-nucleosides, tat inhibitors, and protease inhibitors suggest that answers lay just around the corner. Insiders already knew the gossip about Hoffman-LaRoche's tat drug: after years of stalling, the company had finally determined that the drug had no efficacy, at least at the dosage tried so far. And the results from the protease inhibitors were preliminary and carried little weight.

DOCTORS, RESEARCHERS, AND "COOKBOOK MEDICINE"

The deep uncertainties about antiviral therapy were aired in Berlin at a "Meet the Experts" session entitled "When to Start Antiretroviral Treatment"—though as Martin Delaney aptly noted, it could just as well have been called "*Whether* to Start Antiretroviral Treatment."[64] The session was an elaborate dance between practicing physicians requesting advice and experts reluctant to commit.[65] Robert Yarchoan of the NCI listed the options as he saw them: You could begin monotherapy early. You could begin combination therapy early. Or you could wait for the development of symptoms or until the CD4 count dipped below 200 and then initiate either monotherapy or combination therapy. In short, no logical option could be ruled out! As Delaney noted, the more we knew about pathogenesis and the extent of covert infection, the more *sense* it made to intervene early; but the more we learned about the therapies that were available, the less confident we became about the current *efficacy* of doing so. The challenge of AIDS, said Delaney, was precisely "to make decisions in the face of uncertainty": "I think maybe 019 gave people the illusion we weren't dealing with uncertainty."

Some doctors in the audience stressed the virtues of case-by-case decision making on the basis of the "art" of clinical judgment—the strategy of "try it and see what happens." "I feel, personally, I learn more about how to treat a patient by treating the patient than by looking at the results of clinical trials," said one physician. Others were anxious for formal guidelines. A member of the audience pressed one of the panelists, the British researcher Anthony Pinching, to say what he would tell a patient who was asymptomatic and had a T-cell count of 300. Pinching explained that he would describe the various studies, analyze the patient's T-cell trend over time, and then present the patient with a choice. "Why do we need all this cookbook medicine?" asked Pinching: "I have yet to meet a patient who is unwilling to make a choice." And if the patient wanted to know *your* opinion? the questioner persisted. Pinching replied that, in his experience, there were "two types of patients": "interveners" and "don't rock the boaters." "If they insist on advice, I try to identify their nature as one or the other."

It was a revealing comment and, by one reading, an enlightened response. Resisting doctors' cries for prescriptive advice, Pinching was emphasizing the patient's autonomy in deciding on a course of treatment. Against reliance on inflexible rules ("Do *this* if your T cells drop below 500, do *that* if they fall below 200"), Pinching was insisting on the uniqueness of the individual patient. And rather than speaking beyond the limits of his knowledge, Pinching was candidly exposing the extent of medical uncertainty. Yet the response was also more than a little disconcerting. Thirteen years into the epidemic, at the key international conference at which leading scientists reviewed the state of the art of antiretroviral treatment, the best advice about early intervention that an eminent AIDS authority could offer to the doctors of the world was a handy bit of folk wisdom about the psychological propensities of patients.

Living with Uncertainty (1993–1995)

AZT: MORE "PIECES OF THE ELEPHANT"

Later that month, the NIH would ratify uncertainty as the new wisdom, dressing it in the language of bureaucratese.[66] After a three-day meeting, an expert advisory panel offered up recommendations: Asymptomatic HIV-infected patients with three hundred to five hundred T cells should begin taking AZT. But not taking AZT, and continuing to monitor the immune system, was "an equally valid option." Patients in stable condition with more than three hundred T cells who were already taking AZT should stay on it, the panel recommended. However, the chair, Dr. Merle Sande of the University of California at San Francisco, told the *New York Times* that "stopping AZT for such people would be a medically sound and logical conclusion from the recommendations." In short, the NIH recommended that patients do X, but if they wanted to do *not-X,* that was "equally valid."

Sande blamed the current predicament on the competing conceptions of the purpose of clinical trials. He complained to Lawrence Altman that the various trials of the nucleoside analogues had been designed with FDA regulatory questions in mind, rather than the clinical questions that doctors wanted answered: "We were in a hurry four to six years ago to get drugs approved, so the studies were designed in that way and not necessarily to answer the clinical medical questions that we face in making decisions today. . . . We are a prisoner of those studies."[67] Altman's article suggested that much of the blame also lay with the activists for having pressed so hard to get drugs approved quickly. In fact, though, it had been activists who had insisted all along that clinical trials were asking the wrong questions—that they should be oriented to the real-life issues confronting patients and doctors rather than the thumbs-up/thumbs-down logic of FDA approval.

To complicate the picture further, barely a month after the new guidelines were issued the *New England Journal* published the results of the European-Australian Collaborative Group study, a three-year, double-blind, placebo-controlled study of AZT use in 993 asymptomatic patients with CD4 counts above four hundred per cubic millimeter upon entry.[68] The study found that early administration of AZT did delay the onset of symptoms, supporting the view "that most patients with HIV infection should be treated," in the words of an accompanying editorial.[69] The study did not address the issue of survival benefit. Merle Sande commented to the *New York Times:* "I think all the studies are showing the same thing: that there is a little benefit from AZT for a short period of time." Douglas Richman stressed the differences in endpoints and follow-up periods compared to those used in Concorde and said: "This study looks at another piece of the elephant. . . . But we can't say if five years from now the two curves of the two different patient groups won't come together. It's part of the complexity of a clinical investigation—but that's life in the big city."[70]

"It's really resulted in incredible frustration," acknowledged Paul Volberding, the UCSF researcher, in 1994: "No one feels they know what to do. No one trusts the guidelines, even though the guidelines have been put together as best as people could do. People want an answer and there isn't one."[71] Volberding's own long-term follow-up study of the participants in ACTG 019 (the study that first had suggested benefit from early use of AZT in asymptomatics) was, in fact, consistent with the results of Concorde. First presented in Berlin and published in *JAMA* in 1994, the follow-up concluded that the benefits of AZT were time-limited and that early administration conferred no additional survival benefit over late administration.[72]

The overall credibility of AZT received a boost in early 1994, when NIAID announced the results of a trial called ACTG 076, which had studied whether administration of the drug to pregnant women could prevent transmission of the virus to their fetuses. The results were striking: more than a quarter of the babies born to women who received a placebo became HIV positive, but only eight percent of the babies whose mothers received AZT became infected with the virus.[73] The study left many questions unanswered: What, for example, were the long-term health risks to the baby when AZT was administered to a woman during pregnancy? Did the benefit outweigh the risks, given that, even without AZT, three-quarters of the babies would emerge seronegative?[74] And the study ignited new controversy about the policy implications: Should all pregnant women now be required to take an HIV antibody test?[75] Such questions notwithstanding, there was room for exultation. For the first time, in one particular context, AZT appeared to mean the difference between life and death.

Unfortunately for Burroughs Wellcome, news about ACTG 076 coincided with formal publication of the Concorde study.[76] Burroughs Wellcome took the occasion to issue a spirited defense of its product: "Several independently sponsored studies have clearly demonstrated the benefits and advantages of early therapy," commented David Barry, the vice president of research, in a press release.[77] There were indications, however, that doctors and patients were drawing different conclusions about the drug. *JAMA* reported that a study in the Canadian province of Ontario showed a 45 percent decline in the number of patients beginning therapy with AZT in the months following the preliminary report on Concorde. Even many patients who were symptomatic were apparently forgoing use of the drug. Burroughs Wellcome acknowledged that sales of the drug were down, particularly in the United States.[78]

THE HOLY GRAIL OF STATISTICS

As dissatisfied as activists were with AZT and its chemical cousins, in practice it was impossible for activists not to invest their energies in staking out positions on the use of antiviral drugs that were most readily available. The problem was that the data concerning combinations of nucleoside analogues such as AZT and ddC did not lend themselves to unambiguous interpretation. ACTG 155, Fischl's study of the AZT/ddC combination, was an important and telling illustration: debates about the significance of ACTG 155 demonstrated the interpretative flexibility that could make AIDS clinical trials a *source* of uncertainty rather than the mechanism by which uncertainty was resolved. "People believe passionately on both sides of the question as to whether [the combination therapy] worked," Deborah Cotton, the dissenter on the Antiviral Advisory Committee, commented more than a year after the Berlin conference. "There are schools of thought. There are the believers and the nonbelievers, and . . . I don't think anything is going to change. I really don't." [79]

The ACTG 155 researchers were quick to insist,[80] and the published study was careful to point out, that the controversial subgroup analysis presented by Fischl in Berlin was not "post-hoc": "The three CD4 cell count subgroups were specified by the study chairpersons in June 1992, which was before any interim review of the primary endpoint data," Fischl and her coauthors argued.[81] But this did not settle the issue, because the subjects were not randomized into treatment arms from the outset according to this particular breakdown in CD4 counts. Biostatisticians are typically cautious about pulling subsets out of clinical trial populations after randomization—or at least, cautious about overinterpreting what they find.[82] Susan Ellenberg, formerly the chief biostatistician for the ACTG trials at NIAID, praised the TAG activists' suspicion of subgroup analyses: "I think that that is the kind of thing that they have learned. They have become very methodologically astute," reflected Ellenberg.[83]

Declaring that "several potential explanations exist for the overall findings in our study," the authors in fact presented a series of arguments for why combination therapy might be advantageous *even though* the trial seemed to suggest otherwise.[84] Because patients had taken AZT before enrolling in the study, it was possible that they were already resistant to that drug. In that sense, what was really being studied was not combination therapy but ddC alone. Or perhaps the best time for combination therapy was simply earlier in the progression of HIV disease, before certain phenotypic changes in the virus associated with late-stage AIDS occurred. Finally, the report pointed to the consequences of "intent-to-treat" analysis. Because of the way the protocol was worded, many patients who experienced strong side effects from either AZT or ddC were taken off all their drugs. But in accordance with the logic of intent-to-treat, these patients were still counted as part of the treatment arm to which they were originally randomized. The effect was potentially to blur the difference between the different arms, creating a higher standard for establishing efficacy. But biostatisticians argued that to remove from analysis the patients who go off a drug can bias trial results, because there is no reason to assume that people who go off medications are typical of those who remain.[85] Some clinical researchers found the logic maddening all the same: How could they study the effects of a drug in patients who weren't even using it? "As a clinician, what I really want to know is, is a drug working while a patient is taking it—not six months after he stopped taking it," commented Martin Hirsch, a virologist and one of the principal investigators on ACTG 155.[86]

The debate over intent-to-treat analysis was a perfect example of the clash in perspective between infectious-disease researchers and biostatisticians. "I don't think that statistics is the holy grail," complained Hirsch, at the same time affirming his strong general support for the methods of the randomized clinical trial. "Many of us clinicians think that an 'as-treated' analysis . . . gives us at least as much information that is useful clinically as does 'intent-to-treat.'"[87] And indeed, the authors of the published report on ACTG 155 undertook "an exploratory analysis to gain insight into the possible association between early treatment cessation and treatment outcome." That is, they performed an "as-treated" analysis, ceasing to count people in the study two months after they stopped their treatment. The results: "combination therapy was associated with a significantly lower rate of disease progression or death than were either [AZT] or [ddC] monotherapy." In other words, from this standpoint, the study was quite simply a success, and combination therapy *worked*. Yet "caution should be used when interpreting this exploratory analysis," the authors quickly added, because "this type of analysis is known to be biased."[88]

For all the careful disclaimers, what was noteworthy about the published report on ACTG 155 was how intent it seemed to be on reaffirming the conclusion from which everyone began—that combination therapy really was better. Douglas Richman insisted that the results from ACTG 155 were "compatible" with those from ACTG 106; he added that ACTG 106 had now been corroborated by the final results from the Burroughs Wellcome study of the AZT/ddC combination.[89] By contrast, Mark Harrington of TAG argued that "the high baseline CD4 group (150–300)—the one with the claimed 'benefit' of combination therapy—was exactly the arm with the fewest clinical events, thus the least [statistical] power." Harrington's bottom line: "Combination therapy with AZT/ddC in the 155 population is 50% more toxic and no more effective than monotherapy with AZT alone."[90]

What were the true "results" of ACTG 155? How, and in what way, can we take data produced by such an experiment and apply them to the real-world dilemmas of patients who demand answers? The point here is that clinical trials do not occur in a vacuum—and when the environment in which trials are conducted and interpreted is so contentious, then these experiments, rather than settling controversies, may instead reflect and propel them. Consider the range of factors and pressures that structured the determination of the "meaning" of ACTG 155 as well as that of its precursor, ACTG 106: the methodological (and jurisdictional) disputes between infectious-disease researchers and biostatisticians; activist demands for access to drugs, plus or versus activist conceptions of "good science"; the social construction of hype; the profound need experienced by patients, and the kinds of pragmatic decisions that patients and research subjects make in response to their immediate perceptions of their interests; the marketing strategies of pharmaceutical corporations and the incentive structures to which these companies respond; the complicated role of practicing physicians in interpreting the data produced by clinical trials; the politics of regulation and deregulation; and the distinctive character of regulatory science as practiced by expert advisory bodies. In such an environment—given these stakes—is it any wonder that the interpretation of key trial results is often up for grabs? AIDS trials are not unique in this regard, as studies of cancer trials make clear.[91] But insofar as the participation of knowledge-empowered activists increases the number of claims-makers and alters the distribution of credibility among them, AIDS trials may be particularly inclined toward conflicting readings.

EAST COAST, WEST COAST

From the perspective of TAG activists, the evidence from trials like ACTG and Concorde was clear enough: neither AZT monotherapy in asymptomatic patients nor combination therapy in patients at any stage of illness had been proven efficacious. And the predictive power of the CD4 surrogate marker, in their estimation, was in grave doubt. In the summer of 1994, as the FDA granted accelerated approval to yet another nucleoside analogue, d4T, and announced an upcoming meeting to review accelerated approval, TAG activists began making noise. In August, the finance magazine *Barron's* ran a cover story called "Rushing to Judgment," which quoted TAG members about the risks of accelerated approval.[92] Similarly, *Time* magazine described the evolution of AIDS activists who in the past "threw smoke bombs at the National Institutes of Health" but now were "changing their minds" about the fast-track drug approval policies they once had promoted.[93] Alarmed, Project Inform circulated a "consensus statement" on the need for accelerated approval and gained the endorsement of AIDS activist organizations around the country.[94]

At the Antiviral Advisory Committee meeting held in September 1994 more than forty activist groups presented their positions, including activists from the Midwest and the South who insisted that neither the East Coast nor the West Coast activists spoke for them on questions of access to drugs.[95] Kessler assured the audience that accelerated approval would continue to be FDA policy, and he promised to issue clearer guidelines for companies to follow in preparing applications for such approval.[96] TAG activists did not call for an end to accelerated approval, but they issued a hard-hitting evaluation of the program to date. Accelerated approval, these activists suggested, might well be creating structural incentives for drug companies to crank out mediocre drugs that resemble the mediocre AZT rather than invest in the development of novel treatments with other mechanisms of action.[97] (Others responded that accelerated approval created *greater* incentives for small companies to move into AIDS research: the alternative, long-term Phase II studies, was too expensive and too much of a risk.) Furthermore, argued TAG members, some of the companies were ducking their responsibility to perform postmarketing studies. "We pay huge amounts of money and we suffer through major toxicities, and we have to take the drug company's word for it that the drugs work. That's supposed to be empowerment?" complained TAG member Spencer Cox in comments to the *New York Times*.[98]

Preserving the policy of accelerated approval, as most players preferred to do, presumed finding a better surrogate marker or markers. By fall 1994, attention had focused on new, high-tech measures of viral load, such as assays that used PCR technology to quantify viral RNA. From the standpoint of Anthony Fauci (the most prominent backer of the use of CD4 counts as a surrogate marker in the early 1990s), viral load was "fundamentally . . . better as a marker. I don't think there's any question about it."[99] Fauci explained: "There's a lot of virus floating around, and when you treat somebody, you can see dramatic decreases in that virus." Here Fauci was referring to an important, recent finding about the pathogenesis of HIV infection: rather than a slow, subdued "latency," it now appeared that HIV disease was characterized by "rapid turnover" of both virus particles and T cells[100]—what the *New York Times* described as "a pitched battle from the very start of infection," with hundreds of millions of virus particles and hundreds of millions of infected cells dying every single day.[101] This new conception of the dynamics of HIV infection implied that viral load was a crucial indicator of disease progression.

Biostatistician Stephen Lagakos, while optimistic about the possible uses of these markers, also pointed to "overstatements" on the part of some of their advocates, and he described stories he had heard reporting "that some of the producers of these [marker tests are] trying to get clinicians to buy gobs of these kits and use them on everybody at $500 a crack."[102] More emphatically, in an article subtitled "When Viral Load Is Crowned King," the Treatment Action Group railed in its newsletter against "frustrated scientists [who] have a new toy and biotechnology companies [who] have a new assay to sell."[103] TAG was calling instead for large-scale trials—so-called "large simple trials" with as many as five thousand subjects—particularly for the upcoming protease inhibitors. The virtue of such trials, these activists argued, was that they could simultaneously tell us "if these new drugs prevent sickness and death" *and* "if the new viral load assays are useful predictors." Hoffman-LaRoche, manufacturer of a protease inhibitor called saquinavir, was in TAG's view "racing" to the FDA with "lukewarm" data, seeking accelerated approval on the basis of a single, twenty-four-week study.[104] TAG proposed instead an expanded access program for saquinavir to accompany the larger, long-term studies.[105]

By this point, the long-simmering dispute in tactics between East Coast groups such as TAG and the San Francisco activists had "become particularly intense and often bitter," as John James explained in *AIDS Treatment News*.[106] In general terms, everyone avowed respect and support for his or her activist compatriots. But from the standpoint of the San Francisco activists, the TAG members had become scientific conservatives seeking to be more rigorous than thou. Said G'dali Braverman of ACT UP/Golden Gate: "There's an interesting evolution in terms of one's personal treatment activism. You reach that point where you start losing your sight of [the idea] 'We really are dealing with patients who need an option now,' and you start trying to think like a scientist." Such a tendency was "a difficult thing to temper," added Braverman.[107] "You know why I really think there's a split?" reflected Brenda Lein of Project Inform. "Because the East Coast folks don't have a constituency of people living with HIV that they work with on a day-to-day basis. I mean, I answer hotline calls from people who want access. They talk to each other." [108]

Needless to say, TAG activists, many of whom were themselves living with AIDS and HIV infection, disputed these characterizations. They insisted they were not necessarily opposed to accelerated approval and certainly not to expanded access: Their motto was "access *and* answers." Nor did they oppose the right of the individual to have access to therapies. But they wanted to counterbalance that right against some conception of the greater good. And they criticized their San Francisco comrades for continuing to promote hype about up-and-coming drugs; they saw themselves as hard-nosed realists who had been burned too many times to ever contribute to the "hype cycle" again. [109] This explained the venom behind TAG's attack on Margaret Fischl in Berlin—the sense on the part of activists that they were led to believe in combination therapy and manipulated into hopping onto a roller-coaster ride of exhilaration followed by despair. Mark Harrington made this point emphatically in his written critique of ACTG 155: "ACTG 155 was riddled with investigator bias and sponsor-disseminated hype from the very beginning. . . . Indeed, as early as August 1990, at a meeting with ACT UP, Roche's Dr. Whaijen Soo told us: 'I'd like to confide a remark of Margaret's. . . . The difference she sees among people on the ddC/AZT combination [in ACTG 106] is a big difference—like the difference between people on AZT versus placebo in the original trial. She can almost tell them apart by looking at their behavior.' Say that around the country for three years and you can create a huge demand for an unproved drug." [110] TAG members were now vigilant against becoming the pawns of the pharmaceutical companies and resistant even to well-intentioned optimism. David Barr commented in 1994: "I've been pulled aside several times in the last couple of months [by people whispering], 'I'm really excited about the protease inhibitors.' . . . I have to say, 'Please, I understand you're saying that to me because you want to help me, but *it doesn't help me.*'" [111]

BACK TO BASICS

In the midst of cleavages on regulatory policies, activists could agree on one point: it was time for brand-new directions in AIDS research—new approaches that could arise only out of discoveries in basic science. Project Inform, for example, had begun assembling leading scientists and activists for periodic "Immune Restoration

Think Tank" meetings to brainstorm research directions in restoring immune system functioning.[112] TAG had endorsed the emphasis on basic research in its report on NIH's AIDS research that it had presented in Amsterdam in 1992. A new report presented at the 1993 Berlin conference was all the more emphatic—and dramatic: "The world of basic research on AIDS is the final frontier for AIDS activists; it is here that we make our last stand," wrote Gregg Gonsalves. "We must forge a partnership with those scientists who have devoted their lives to studying the basic biology of HIV and the immune system and quicken the pace of discovery." [113]

On the assumption that basic research, unlike clinical research, "has not had a powerful constituency to advocate on its behalf," TAG had conducted interviews with thirty-six researchers in the basic sciences—immunologists, virologists, and molecular biologists—most of them at work in academic settings. Above all, said Gonsalves, researchers stressed "the need to take basic AIDS research from the pristine *in vitro* laboratory setting to more difficult, but critical, work with wild-type HIV isolates and clinical samples, often using *in vivo* settings with animal models or humans." This was a restatement of the familiar problem—that scientists knew infinitely more about the structure of HIV than about how HIV causes AIDS. "In vivo veritas" was the slogan that TAG recommended: "Many of the interviewees criticized the relevance of *in vitro* work ('pristine, beautiful, irrelevant systems')." [114]

The long-running activist critique of "purity," "cleanliness," and "elegance" was now applied to a new set of concerns: once again, as with clinical trials, activists were pressing for real-world "messiness" in place of pristine, ivory-tower science. Harrington had made this point in graphic fashion in a presentation the year before at the Amsterdam conference. Using slides of his own lymph tissue as backdrop, Harrington had demanded that scientists attend to "what is going on in our bodies, rather than exclusively in elegant and often artificial laboratory and animal models." [115] With representational strategies such as these, activists could hope to bring the "politics of the body" to bear on the remotest regions of laboratory science.

Needless to say, not all clinical researchers were happy about the new activist agenda. "I think that ... the basic science people now have the activist community in the palms of their hands," complained Donald Abrams in late 1993, "and they're going to run with it for a while. ... I think it's too bad." [116] However, activists were by no means alone in articulating the need for a renewed emphasis on basic research. In May 1994, Gina Kolata wrote in the *New York Times* about a "new consensus ... among many leading scientists that the nation's $1.3 billion AIDS research program is on the wrong track." [117] The article cited an editorial just published in *Nature* by Bernard Fields, chair of the department of microbiology and molecular genetics at Harvard Medical School, entitled "AIDS: Time to Turn to Basic Science." "The focus on drugs and vaccines made sense a decade ago," wrote Fields, "but it is time to acknowledge that our best hunches have not paid off and are not likely to do so." [118] Kolata also quoted Harold Varmus, the new head of the NIH: "Everyone agrees with Bernie's basic precept." And William Paul, the immunologist who recently had replaced Anthony Fauci as director of the newly reorganized Office of AIDS Research, said of the Fields manifesto: "We take that as our marching orders." [119]

At the next International AIDS Conference, held in Yokohama, Japan, in August 1994, Paul made his priorities more explicit. This was the tenth annual conference; since the first such conference held in Atlanta in 1985, the number of cases of AIDS in the United States had climbed from about nine thousand to more than four hundred thousand. The number of AIDS cases around the world was now estimated at four million.[120] "Realism was in the air," according to a commentary on the conference in *Lancet;*[121] and it was in a spirit of realism that Paul announced his intention to cut spending on clinical trials sponsored by the ACTG in order to put more money into the "revitalization and expansion" of basic research.[122] Basic research was the "engine that will drive the entire AIDS research enterprise forward," Paul told the conference participants in his plenary lecture, reiterating the long list of fundamental, unanswered questions about HIV and the pathogenesis of AIDS.[123]

What role could treatment activists play in facilitating the progress of basic science? Arguably, activists had a perspective on clinical trials that made them valuable contributors to the effort to conduct such trials smoothly and adequately. In focusing on basic research, however, it was less clear whether activists possessed a special vantage point from which to augment the production of knowledge. By one reading, the most activists could accomplish in this domain was to call for researchers to get on with it. For Martin Delaney, however, the point of Project Inform's Immune Restoration Think Tanks was not just to urge researchers to conduct basic research but to try to sketch out, in discussion with them, the most fruitful avenues of inquiry. "We feel we have accomplished more and better research in this fashion than we ever could have achieved had we chosen to insist on being the researchers ourselves," said Delaney, suggesting a contrast with such earlier adventures as the "underground" trials of Compound Q.[124]

To get a better feel for the conduct of basic research, TAG members actually began spending time in Anthony Fauci's laboratory at NIAID. "I don't think they make any pretenses that they're immunologists or microbiologists or virologists," said Fauci. "But they want to understand as much of the down-in-the-trenches science as they can." Activists didn't need to comprehend every detail or nuance of the research, Fauci explained, in order "to evaluate the broad strokes of the studies that come out." [125] Activists themselves were forthright about the limitations as well as the possibilities inherent in this new approach. "I can't talk cell lines with the big boys, that's for sure, but who cares?" commented Derek Link of TAG. "That's not my role." [126]

Aiding the activists as they negotiated relationships with the basic scientists was the relative accessibility and openness of these researchers. "Most basic scientists are very different than the star clinical researchers," explained Link. "These are people who labor away in a lab, pretty much in obscurity. They're thrilled to have somebody interested in their work. . . ." Brenda Lein of Project Inform echoed this observation: "If you think about it, it's sort of a lonely profession . . . because it's not like you go to a cocktail party as a scientist and people [say], 'Oh that's so fascinating, and what happened in the cell culture next?' And if you actually have someone who's interested, they're more than anxious to be able to talk about their work. . . . You know, there's not many people who get excited about epitope mapping. . . ." [127]

Activists have cultivated these new relationships to bring the patient's perspective to the foreground in basic research—to force bench scientists to be fully cognizant of the day-to-day realities of sickness and suffering beyond the laboratory walls. In so doing, they have attempted to speed the process by which compounds move from the laboratory to testing in humans. "I probably wouldn't have four drugs in clinical trials without the activists having had some [effect on] me," commented Robert Gallo in 1994.[128] Another way that activists influenced the knowledge-making processes of basic research was by performing a bridging, or "pollination," function, bringing together researchers from different specialty areas who were unfamiliar with one another's work.[129] Gallo, a participant in the Immune Restoration Think Tanks, agreed vigorously that activists have served as a "catalyst" that "forc[ed] people to communicate better" and to see beyond the limits of their individual specialty areas.[130] Derek Link was also emphatic about the utility of this role: "There are numerous, numerous times when I'm talking to researcher X and saying, 'Researcher Y is now [working on such-and-such].' And [they say], 'Well, that's interesting.' And then there's some discussion about that."[131]

"COCKTAILS" AND "SYNERGY"

Basic research had produced one recent finding that held crucial implications for drug development: New techniques for measuring virus in the blood had indicated that HIV disease was characterized not by a long, subdued latency but by what researchers and reporters called a continuous "raging battle." Each day the immune system killed hundreds of millions of viral particles; each day the virus replicated to produce hundreds of millions more, killing T cells in the process. Gradually, the virus gained the upper hand in this high-cost war of attrition.[132] Meanwhile, the more the virus replicated, the more it was likely to mutate. Simple math suggested that over the course of a few years, "every viable mutation at every position in the [viral] genome will occur," noted David Ho in a commentary in the *New England Journal*. The implication was that whatever individual antiviral drug researchers threw at the virus, it wouldn't take long before a mutant had emerged that was resistant to the drug. "Therefore, monotherapy as we know it is doomed to fail," argued Ho. "In the long run, effective treatment must instead force the virus to mutate simultaneously at multiple positions in one viral genome. This is best achieved by using a combination of multiple, potent antiretroviral agents." Ho envisioned a time in the near future when combinations of antivirals would be given to patients as early as possible, ideally just after infection, when the virus was most homogeneous. He argued forcefully that the relative lack of success of combinations of the nucleoside analogues (AZT, ddI, ddC, and d4T) was not an adequate test of the *concept* of early intervention. As soon as we had better antivirals, then it was, as Ho's article declared, "Time to Hit HIV, Early and Hard."[133]

What made Ho optimistic were recent studies of protease inhibitors, as well as one nucleoside analogue combination, AZT plus 3TC. In trials, these drugs not only boosted CD4 counts, they also significantly reduced viral load and did so to a greater extent than the approved therapies. Researchers were beginning to speak in optimistic terms of multidrug "cocktails"—such as AZT plus 3TC plus a protease inhibitor—that might inhibit viral replication for extended periods. "Psychologically we definitely have turned a corner," Robert Schooley, the new chair of the ACTG Executive Committee, told the *Los Angeles Times* in February 1995.[134]

Promising results of two European AZT/3TC trials had been announced toward the end of 1994, and Glaxo, the Canadian drug company that manufactured 3TC, had established an expanded access program.[135] TAG described the combination as "admittedly intriguing," but also warned that the results "are based solely on short-term surrogate marker changes: the same surrogate marker changes that brought us those all-powerful antiretrovirals AZT, ddI, ddC (a real winner) and d4T."[136] Both Glaxo and Burroughs Wellcome were delighted by the apparent synergy of their respective products—especially after the 1995 merger that formed the world's largest pharmaceutical company, Glaxo Wellcome.[137]

Meanwhile, by 1995 three companies—Hoffman-LaRoche, Merck, and Abbott—were conducting large-scale trials of protease inhibitors, and several other companies were following in their footsteps.[138] Patient groups clamored for access to these drugs, but expanded access of the protease inhibitors posed special problems for the drug companies. These compounds were difficult to manufacture, and patients consumed them in much higher quantities than required with other antiviral drugs. In short, there just wasn't enough protease inhibitor to go around—at least, not without jeopardizing supplies for clinical trials.[139] As a result, each of the three companies announced that it would hold a lottery to assign spots in its expanded access program. In summer 1995, 18,500 people competed for about 3,600 slots.[140] Though lotteries seemed the most equitable solution in the short run, many observers expressed concerns about the pressures building for accelerated approval of the protease inhibitors, especially with rumors of the upcoming emergence of "underground" protease drugs.[141]

As antiretroviral research embraced new possibilities, including an even newer class of drugs called integrase inhibitors,[142] the pervasive gloom of 1993 and 1994 seemed to be lifting. And in late 1995, the Antiviral Advisory Committee recommended accelerated approval of two more drugs, based on the drugs' effects in boosting CD4 counts and lowering viral loads: 3TC (to be used in combination with AZT) and saquinavir, the Hoffman-LaRoche protease inhibitor (also for use in combinations). FDA Commissioner Kessler took the opportunity to express his excitement about the protease inhibitors, calling them "the most active agents against HIV we have seen to date." [143] With the agency's rapid endorsement of its advisory committee's recommendations, the number of approved antiviral AIDS drugs had risen from one in 1987 to six at the close of 1995.

Optimism increased in the early months of 1996, as the Antiviral Advisory Committee recommended approval of two other protease inhibitors, Abbott's ritonavir and Merck's indinavir. The FDA, then undergoing close scrutiny by Republican members of Congress concerned with speeding up the drug approval process, acted on the committee's recommendations in a matter of days. Indeed, approval of Merck's drug arrived just forty-two days after the company had first submitted its application to the agency.[144] Abbott's drug, ritonavir, was given full (rather than accelerated) approval after an international study reported that the drug cut the death rate nearly in half in a group of 1,090 AIDS patients: the death rate was 4.8 percent among those who received ritonavir and 8.4 percent among those who received a placebo in place of the protease inhibitor. (Subjects in both groups were also free to take AZT or d4T if they chose.) Still, concerns remained about the long-term efficacy of ritonavir as well as the other protease inhibitors, given the likely development of resistance to the drugs.[145]

None of these drugs was a "magic bullet"—a "penicillin" for AIDS; no expert expected that such a drug could be developed. From the perspective of Daniel Hoth, who came to NIAID originally from the National Cancer Institute, the development of antiretroviral AIDS therapies was—slowly but ineluctably—recapping the progress of cancer therapies. Clinicians started out with single-agent, palliative drugs: "That's cancer in the '50s. Then you go through another generation, you get some better drugs. And you start to get complete remissions, you start to get longer durations of partial remission. . . . And you gradually increase both the depth of the response . . . and the duration of it." This would be the likely pathway in the development of AIDS drugs, Hoth was convinced: "I think we're going to see a formal recapitulation of what happened in . . . cancer." [146]

Whatever the speed of development of therapies, political and economic factors dictated that their distribution would be highly uneven. To the extent that existing antiretroviral therapies had important benefits—for example, in the apparently sharp reduction of transmission of HIV from pregnant women to fetuses—such findings remained, in the mid-1990s, irrelevant to most of the world's population. As *Science*'s AIDS reporter Jon Cohen explained: "Poorer countries can't afford either AZT or the sophisticated clinics used in [ACTG] 076. In addition, 076 calls for repeatedly dosing the mother with AZT during her pregnancy, and many women in developing countries don't visit medical clinics until they are in labor—if then." Nor were the pharmaceutical companies likely to provide the solution. "I doubt very much that it will be Glaxo Wellcome giving away unlimited amounts of AZT," a company spokesperson told Cohen.[147] In countries that spent only a handful of dollars per capita on health care in a year, what, then, was the likelihood that *any* antiretroviral therapy developed in the West would actually see widespread use? Even in the United States, with federally funded health insurance programs such as Medicaid under increasing attack, the ability of people with AIDS and HIV to afford multiple combinations of drugs that were each quite expensive seemed increasingly in doubt.[148]

PROMOTING "GOOD SCIENCE"

The mid-1990s saw the U.S. public engrossed by popular nonfiction like *The Hot Zone* and Hollywood films such as "Outbreak," which presented terrifying images of the sudden and devastating illness caused by the rare Ebola virus.[149] AIDS and the fears it had provoked in the 1980s were often the unspoken subtexts in these representations. Yet ironically the ongoing brutalities of the AIDS epidemic seemed to fade from the public eye—even as the number of cases in the United States passed the half-million mark and U.S. health authorities reported that AIDS had become the leading killer of twenty-five- to forty-four-year-olds.[150] Seen less as a raging plague than as a chronic plight, AIDS, like homelessness and drug use, had merged into the background landscape of late-twentieth-century social life.[151]

Activists struggled to bring AIDS back to center stage. For a while, it had seemed as if a Democratic administration might make a difference, that it might offer a different "political opportunity structure" for movement activism.[152] But whatever President Clinton's sympathies, AIDS was far from the top of his agenda. One apparently promising step was the establishment of an eighteen-member presidential commission, the National Task Force on AIDS Drug Development, designed to bring together representatives of government agencies, the pharmaceutical industry, the research community, and activist groups to recommend ways to streamline the discovery and testing of new AIDS drugs.[153] The panel included Ben Cheng of Project Inform, Peter Staley of TAG, and Moisés Agosto of the National Minority AIDS Council and TAG. Daniel Hoth, who had left NIAID for private industry but was a member of the task force, noted the key difficulty confronting them: "Very few of the problems are amenable to executive proclamation."[154] By early 1996 the group had disbanded, acknowledging that they had been unable to remove the obstacles that stood in the way of faster development of new AIDS drugs, and citing lack of clear support from President Clinton.[155]

In debates over how to improve the drug development system, activists were just one player and held relatively few cards. The pharmaceutical companies, by contrast, could often push research as their interests dictated. Drug companies could collaborate with one another, sharing data when it suited their purposes: fifteen of them had formed an entity called the "Inter-Company Collaboration for AIDS Drug Development" to test combinations of drugs produced by different companies.[156] But drug companies could also go their own ways or exit the arena altogether. Many biotechnology firms, for example, were finding the AIDS arena too risky and were choosing to invest their resources in more promising efforts.[157]

By the mid-1990s, AIDS activism in general was in a period of decline, and the "treatment activist" subset looked considerably different from its incarnation in the late 1980s. The dominant wing of treatment activism—which encompassed groups such as TAG, Project Inform, and subgroups of ACT UP chapters around the country, along with representatives to the CCG and local community advisory boards—was small, committed, relatively expert, and relatively professionalized. As the mainstream treatment activist groups have moved into the mid-1990s, their work has proved to be a vital but less visible, and in many ways less hopeful, political endeavor.

There are many factors that have contributed to the current juncture. While all social movements confront the issue of burnout and renewal, few find that on a regular basis their leaders become ill or die. More generally, much of the difficulty has lain in the vicissitudes of the research process and the sheer intractability of the scientific problem. Garance Franke-Ruta, a TAG activist who was 17 when she first joined ACT UP, recalled the evolution: Activists first gained access to the system at a time of relative optimism, when drugs such as AZT suggested the hope of keeping patients alive until a better drug came along. By the early 1990s, when the much-disliked and marginally effective AZT was still the first-line therapy, activists had come to adopt a longer view.[158] "Most of us are just simply not going to see the answer to this in our lifetime," commented San Francisco activist G'dali Braverman. "And I think there was an excitement in the early days and this feeling that we could change everything—which we *will!*—and that we would live to see it and that the answers were already there, we just hadn't seen them, or hadn't been told them. We know better now."[159]

With this perspective came a further shift in strategic thinking away from the simple strategy of "drugs into bodies" and toward the promotion of "good science." As Moisés Agosto put it, "A lot of treatment activists got involved [in the 1980s] believing that through their activism they were going to be able to save *their* lives." Strategies, therefore, were based significantly on the desire to get something—*anything*—through the pipeline—to get "drugs into bodies" fast enough to matter for the health of the current generation of activists. Agosto continued: "Now, my personal [belief] is, 'No, I'm not going to be able to save my life.'" In the ongoing tension between "access" and "answers," activist strategy had moved toward the opposite pole: "It's about having good science that develops good therapies [so] that we may have a cure or therapy someday."[160]

In this current period of adjustment, groups such as TAG, ACT UP/Golden Gate, Project Inform, and others around the country have accelerated their engagement with the AIDS research effort, but the details of their work have receded from public view. As the issues become ever more complex and technical, they also become more difficult to summarize on a leaflet or in a sound bite. Nor has it proven easy to recruit new activists into a movement with such a high degree of accumulated technical expertise. "The training program is sink or swim," Derek Link commented. "People who are totally intimidated are not going to do well."[161]

To the extent that polarization between "us" and "them" increases the tendency for social movement actors to sacrifice for the cause,[162] the evolution of relatively more cooperative relationships between activists and their interlocutors in research and government may have made it somewhat harder for the movement to stoke the fires of passion. Some activists, such as the novelist Sarah Schulman, who are critical of those in groups like TAG believe that the decline in the use of direct action techniques spelled the end of effective treatment activism.[163] But others reject what they see as a fetishizing of confrontational direct action—trying to "scream a cure out of a test tube"—insisting that tactics should be suited both to the task at hand and to the stage in the evolution of the movement. "It would have been stupid to do a large demo when you could have picked up a phone and made a couple of phone calls and gotten just the same results," commented Harrington.[164]

Implicit in this evaluation, however, is not simply a practical insistence on "doing what works," but also a transformed conception of the identity of the antagonist.[165] In place of the charges of genocide that activists had used in the early days of ACT UP to frame their critiques of the research establishment, these activists were now often inclined to acknowledge the good intentions of researchers. "There's a new respect for the scientists," said Gregg Gonsalves in an interview in the gay magazine the *Advocate:* "There is more of a willingness to focus on the problems that the scientists are really facing rather than what we once thought of as the scientists' malice." If so, Anthony Fauci has certainly endorsed the change of heart. He told the same reporter: "I have to admit it's gratifying that people who are highly qualified—and most of the activists that I have gotten to know are—have come around to support us. . . . In the late '80s we were getting pushed around to put people in clinical trials for drugs that we really didn't think were very promising anyway. . . . Now that we are in agreement about the need for basic research, maybe we will have better drugs and vaccines one day."[166]

Is this co-optation? Or is it well-advised realism that is the fruit of (sometimes bitter) experience? Garance Franke-Ruta's reflections suggest the ways in which the acquisition of the "realistic" perspective of the educated participant in science can constrain utopian imaginings, even as it paves the way for a more focused and sober activism: "When ACT UP started, people didn't know as much, and demanded much more. And there was something in ACT UP initially that was really wonderful, which was that out of ignorance of what is possible, you are sometimes able to do the impossible—whereas once you know what is possible and what is not possible, you let that define what it is that you're willing to ask for. *So the more we learned, in some ways the less we were able to ask for,* until eventually we knew so much that we felt—we feel—like sometimes we don't know that we can ask for anything [emphasis added]."[167]

There is, of course, virtue in self-doubt and critical reflection. Scientists, too, could be heard reporting their own. "I think we got a little bit too cocky too early," a Princeton molecular biologist told the *New York Times* in 1994, describing the need to refocus on basic research.[168] Such sentiments are a useful antidote to hubris and to a surplus of faith in what science can accomplish. Over the course of less than a decade and a half, researchers had vastly expanded the knowledge about AIDS, while treatment activists had garnered their own expertise and reshaped the conduct and contours of biomedical research. In the end, however, neither activists nor scientists could force a cure into being, no matter how committed their efforts or how sophisticated their interventions.

CONCLUSION

CREDIBLE KNOWLEDGE, HIERARCHIES OF EXPERTISE, AND THE POLITICS OF PARTICIPATION IN BIOMEDICINE

Science and the Struggle for Credibility

To no small degree, the first decade and a half of AIDS research in the United States has been marked by the sustained lay invasion of the domain of scientific fact-making. What have been the dynamics of interventions by uncredentialed participants in biomedicine? What have been their consequences? These questions demand attention to the specific character of credibility struggles in AIDS research and to the techniques employed by representatives of the AIDS movement in establishing their collective voice within science. After summarizing this analysis, I will turn to an assessment both of the concrete effects of AIDS activism and its varied implications for future struggles in biomedicine and other scientific domains. I will conclude by arguing that this case is important for what it tells us about the power inherent in expertise and about the deep dilemmas confronting social movements that seek to "democratize" science and technology.

THE BOUNDARIES OF IMPURE SCIENCE

The production of biomedical knowledge about the causes of and treatments for AIDS cannot be understood except with reference to a scientific field that is unusually broad and public and the site of an extraordinary degree of contestation. The shifting dimensions and porous borders of this field are not predetermined by any essential characteristics of science; rather, they become evident to the analyst by means of tracing the rebounding pathways of influence and engagement.[1] That crucial debates about AIDS are resolved through credibility struggles within a field of this sort is readily demonstrated by the dynamics of the causation controversies described in part one. An initial process of closure by virologists (the "black-boxing" of the HIV hypothesis) was strengthened through ratification by biomedical institutions, public health organizations and governmental bodies, the mainstream media, and grassroots AIDS organizations. Certainty about the causal role of HIV solidified before all details of the putatively required evidence were obtained, precisely because the hypothesis was plausible, the claimants were credible, and the viral hypothesis satisfied the interests of various players, both "insiders" and "outsiders." Dissenting voices were isolated until the appearance of Peter Duesberg with his impressive scientific credentials. Yet Duesberg's article in *Cancer Research* was ignored until it was taken up by a group of lay supporters who publicized the controversy. Mass media coverage then led directly to Duesberg's presentation of his arguments in the pages of *Science* and the *Proceedings of the National Academy of Sciences*. And these scientific publications, in turn, "proved" Duesberg's credibility to many laypeople and reporters while attracting the interest of other scientists such as Kary Mullis, Robert Root-Bernstein, and Walter Gilbert. It seems likely that without the sustained, interactive participation of scientists, the mass media, and voices within the AIDS movement, the controversy simply would not have achieved significance, either socially or scientifically, and the "black box" ("HIV causes AIDS") would never have been reopened for consideration.

Certainty and uncertainty about the efficacy of antiretroviral drugs (the subject of part two) are even more obviously collective products and outcomes of credibility struggles. Principal investigators of clinical trials have made claims and counterclaims. Government agencies and advisory bodies have assessed risks and benefits. Physicians have believed or disbelieved and have conveyed their assessments to patients.

Patients have complied with study protocols or disobeyed them and have demanded drugs or rejected them. Grassroots publications have bypassed the traditional pathways of publication in science, spreading information and opinions about treatments to patients around the world. Treatment activists have challenged the calculus of risks and benefits, and by becoming "lay experts" they have helped change the rules governing the kinds of evidence required to determine efficacy. It was in the nexus of interactions among these principals that facts were made, expertise constructed, and social order forged.

This analysis suggests the need for new approaches to the study of the politics of knowledge-making in scientific controversies with overtly public dimensions. Analysts of science and medicine should attend to the strategies pursued by lay actors in their attempts to speak credibly about science and medicine—how they frame arguments, how they disseminate scientific information, how they build their own expertise, and how they enlist supporters behind them. In particular, while the analysis of social movements has been commonplace elsewhere, it has been relatively underdeveloped in both the sociology of medicine and the sociology of science.[2] The case of AIDS activism suggests that social movements can pursue distinctive forms of participation in science and, conversely, that the engagement with science can shape such movements in powerful ways. An extended study of the relation between biomedicine and social movements could provide a deeper and more comprehensive analysis of the construction of medical knowledge and the transformation of medical practice.

CREDIBILITY AND THE
MANAGEMENT OF UNCERTAINTY

As players execute their moves within the field, they, as well as the audiences they play to, must assess the credibility of various claims-makers. Everyone looks to markers that seem to certify the trustworthiness and competence of claimants, yet these markers are highly variable and surprisingly unstable. According to Robert Gallo, Duesberg lacked credibility because he was a chemist with no medical training. Martin Delaney agreed with Gallo, but also portrayed Duesberg as someone who—unlike Joseph Sonnabend—had no personal ties to the communities afflicted by the epidemic and whose moral credibility was therefore suspect. For many journalists and people with AIDS or HIV, the cloud of suspicion that hung over Gallo following his dispute with Luc Montagnier cast doubt on any and all claims he put forward, while Duesberg seemed credible precisely because he was challenging an entrenched and untrustworthy orthodoxy. Treatment activists could speak credibly at ACTG meetings because they "knew their science," yet in other venues they could speak more credibly than the mainstream researchers because theirs was the voice of moral outrage. A long-term survivor like Michael Callen enjoyed credibility within the AIDS movement at least partly by virtue of staying alive: the markers of credibility were inscribed on his own body.

The scrutiny of individuals' tokens of credibility has not prevented the various parties from arriving at careful assessments of specific knowledge claims about the etiology of AIDS or the efficacy of antiretroviral drugs. But given the lack of unanimity about how to *interpret* the evidence—Are Koch's postulates the gold standard or aren't they? Is there a relevant animal model for AIDS or isn't there? Has the definitive clinical trial been performed or hasn't it?—it's not surprising that the varying assessments of credibility have focused so much on the *claimants,* and not just the *claims.*

Negotiations of credibility, in this sense, can be understood as mechanisms for the management and resolution of scientific uncertainty. One of the important findings of the sociology of scientific knowledge is that experiments do not, in the simple sense usually understood, "settle" scientific controversies. Nothing inherent in an experiment definitively establishes it as the "crucial" test of a hypothesis. Rather, scientists negotiate precisely what counts as evidence, which experiments represent a hypothesis adequately, and whether an instance of replication is a faithful recreation of a prior study.[3] Given the possibility of dispute on these points, uncertainty is often not just the cause of scientific controversy but its consequence.

The "interpretative flexibility" built into scientific findings was amply demonstrated, for example, by the initial reactions to the Concorde study—all of which seemed to follow predictably from the prior commitments of the actors. It wasn't so much that an inherent degree of uncertainty in the study sparked controversy about how to interpret it, as the fact that preexisting debate about AZT use in asymptomatics led various parties to endorse the study or to deconstruct it in different ways. Even a year later, Douglas Richman, one of the defenders of early intervention with antiretroviral drugs, would describe Concorde as a study with "no relation to reality": "Their data [are] perfectly true, it's just that they're irrelevant, and they're asking the wrong question." [4]

The notion that a "definitive" clinical trial can settle the question of drug efficacy or that a "definitive" epidemiological study can establish, once and for all, HIV's etiological role misses this fundamental point: a study's "definitiveness" is not given but is a negotiated outcome and one that may be actively resisted by some parties to the controversy. The extent to which closure is achieved, therefore, depends crucially on the capacity of actors to present themselves as credible representatives or interpreters of scientific experiments—to ensure that others trust their evaluations and will fall in line behind them.

PATHWAYS TO CREDIBILITY

If raw evidence alone does not resolve scientific controversies, and if the credibility of claims-makers must be invoked to give claims their force, what sorts of credibility are most potent? Certainly nothing in this study casts doubt on the supposition that the presentation of suitable and traditional credentials is the simplest and easiest route to establishing and maintaining credibility in biomedicine. Indeed, this is true not only in the construction of orthodox science but in the promotion of "heresy" as well. Even Sonnabend, a doctor with a history of scientific research, had no luck, after 1984, in gaining scientific support—or substantial extrascientific support—for his views. It took Duesberg's weightier status as a renowned molecular biologist and virologist to bring the causation controversy to general attention. (Hence, even those lay supporters of Duesberg who prided themselves on their iconoclasm typically pointed to Duesberg's impeccable credentials as an indicator of the legitimacy of dissent.)

Anyone doubting the power inherent in traditional markers of scientific accomplishment need only look to the example of Luc Montagnier, who (despite being rejected by both Duesberg and Gallo) was so frequently invoked as an ally for this or that side in debates about causation. Was Montagnier a dissident at heart? Had he undergone a conversion experience over time? Or was he just a mainstream researcher within a research community that was actually far more open to a range of views than the dissenters cared to admit? The multiple Montagniers who have been presented in the causation controversy are testament to the widespread recognition that Montagnier's support (or his perceived support) was a coin well worth possessing.

In a politicized and public controversy, however, credentials are a less sturdy indicator of credibility than they may first appear. One reason the media play such a crucial role in these stories is precisely because they transmit and construct meanings about what sort of expertise a credential entitles one to claim: "Media are likely to place greater emphasis on such credentials as awards (especially the Nobel Prize) and institutional affiliation and less emphasis on the scientist's disciplinary area of expertise," notes Rae Goodell.[5] Furthermore, the "anointing" of spokespersons by the media affects perceptions of credibility by constructing a parallel system of informal credentials. Media visibility, for example, has helped to cement the status of treatment activist leaders such as Mark Harrington and Martin Delaney, who are quoted routinely and regularly in publications such as the *New York Times* and not infrequently in the scientific press. Media designations of who counts as a spokesperson do not simply *mirror* the internal stratification of a social movement or a scientific community, but can even *construct* such hierarchies.[6]

Of course, Harrington would not have been quoted in *Science* or the *New York Times* in the first place had not ACT UP already succeeded in establishing itself as a credible player. These are perhaps the most interesting questions about credibility in the case of AIDS: What tactics do social movements pursue in order to marshal credibility in scientific controversies? How do movements that seek not to reject science but to transform it develop their capacity to make an impact "on the inside"? The case of AIDS treatment activism is instructive: it suggests that certain kinds of social movements, when pursuing distinctive strategies, can acquire credibility within specific domains of scientific practice. It matters that biomedicine is relatively more open to outside scrutiny than are other arenas of science and technology. But it also matters that activists have played their cards well.

First, activists imbibed and appropriated the languages and cultures of the biomedical sciences. By teaching themselves the vocabularies and conceptual schemes of virology, immunology, and biostatistics, activists have succeeded in forcing credentialed experts to deal with their arguments. Experts who maintained even nominal adherence to the notion that scientific arguments should be evaluated "without regard to person" have often found it difficult to dismiss such arguments simply on the basis of their "questionable" origin.[7] Second, activists have successfully established themselves as the voice of the clinical investigators' potential population of research subjects. Activists have thereby located themselves as an "obligatory passage point," and researchers and NIAID officials have had little choice but to engage them in discussion about trial protocols.[8] But activists also came forward as the bearers of privileged knowledge of patients' desires that would benefit researchers seeking to accrue subjects for their trials. Some researchers therefore came to welcome, or at least acknowledge benefits of, activist participation in the design of clinical trials.

Third, activists have gained credibility by yoking together moral (or political) arguments and methodological (or epistemological) arguments. For example, activists have contended that the inclusion of women and members of racial minority groups in clinical trials is both more ethical, insofar as it provides widespread access to experimental medications, and scientifically preferable by virtue of the fact that it produces more generalizable findings. Though activists' credibility in some arenas (such as the media) typically reflects their capacity to monopolize the moral high ground, their influence on scientific procedures owes more to their knack of translation between political and technical languages. Finally, activists have seized upon preexisting lines of cleavage within the biomedical establishment. In debates between biostatisticians and researchers, and between researchers and practicing physicians, activists have thrown their weight on one side or the other—sometimes tipping the balance.[9] In effect, activists have been able to "enroll allies" with the same result as that described by Bruno Latour in his analyses of scientists: they have strengthened their scientific claims against assault by bringing supporters on board.[10]

Once activists succeeded in establishing their credibility, they were able to gain representation on NIH and FDA advisory committees, institutional review boards at local hospitals and research centers, community advisory boards established by pharmaceutical companies, and—most recently—President Clinton's National Task Force on AIDS Drug Development. These strategic positions, in turn, have provided activists with an enhanced capacity to advance their arguments and augment their credibility. By introducing new "currencies" of credibility into circulation, and by successfully establishing a value for these currencies within the scientific field, activists have, in effect, transformed the field's mechanisms of operation—that is, they have transformed how biomedical knowledge gets made.[11]

The much greater leverage exerted by laypeople in AIDS treatment controversies than in the causation controversies reinforces the point that such successes are highly dependent on context. Although laypeople have played a crucial role in stoking the fires of the causation controversies, ultimately, lay actors have been far less capable of influencing debates about causation (a more insulated preserve of biomedicine) than those concerned with treatment (a more public and "applied" domain). Indeed, in the causation controversies, the rhetoric of "democracy" has been limited mostly to questions of academic freedom and the right of dissenting scientists to speak their piece. And even within the domain of treatment research, activists have been most successful when focused on clinical research as opposed to basic research, despite interesting recent moves by activists in the latter direction. The conduct and interpretation of clinical trials is the area where AIDS activists have made the most impact—where their tactics for obtaining credibility have proven most efficacious and where such credibility has proven most consequential in shifting the social construction of certainty.

This contribution to knowledge-making is, in the most direct sense, enabled by the activists' own vantage point: they (or the research subjects they represent) are implicated *within* the experimental apparatus—they are *part* of the experiment—and thus they have insights into how such experiments might be better conducted. To use Donna Haraway's term, activists can generate "situated knowledges": "partial, locatable, critical knowledges" produced by social actors on the basis of their position or location in society.[12] Like the environmental justice activists described by Giovanna Di Chiro, whose expertise is rooted in their very "living" and "breathing" at the epicenter of a toxic environment, AIDS activists have something to say simply because of where they stand.[13] This more immediate role of patients in clinical research, combined with the relatively greater accessibility of research methods to lay comprehension, explains the enhanced capacity of laypeople to intervene in debates about trial design and interpretation.

The Transformation of AIDS Research

CREDIT WHERE CREDIT IS DUE

That treatment activists have succeeded in establishing their scientific credibility and their cultural competence in biomedicine is widely acknowledged by a range of eminent researchers and government health officials. Although such testimonials appear sincere, they need not, of course, be taken entirely at face value. However, even the most cynical interpretation would suggest that these authorities see the activists as important enough to merit flattery. (This, too, is a credibility tactic that researchers can employ.) Anthony Fauci has made clear that "there are some [activists] who have no idea what the hell they're talking about," but he was nonetheless happy to grant that "there are some that are brilliant, and even more so than some of the scientists."[14] Robert Gallo has called Martin Delaney "one of the most impressive persons I've ever met in my life, bar none, in any field. . . . I'm not the only one around here who's said we could use him in the labs."[15] Gallo described the level of scientific knowledge attained by certain treatment activists as "unbelievably high": "It's frightening sometimes how much they know and how smart some of them are."[16] Prominent academic researchers also typically acknowledge the gradual acquisition of scientific competence on the part of key activists. "Mark Harrington is a perfect example," recalled Douglas Richman. "In the first meeting [of the Community Constituency Group] he got up and gave a lecture on CMV . . . that I would have punished a medical student for—in terms of its accuracy and everything else—and he's now become a very sophisticated, important contributor to the whole process."[17] Reflected John Phair, a former chair of the ACTG Executive Committee: "I would put them up against—in this limited area— many, many physicians, including physicians working [with] AIDS. They can be very sophisticated."[18]

Praise of treatment activists by biomedical authorities is one measure of the activists' acquisition of credibility. But real-world consequences speak louder: What difference has it made to have activists involved in issues of AIDS research and drug development? How has biomedical research been reconfigured as a result? Examples prove to be numerous: The arguments of AIDS activists have been published in scientific journals and presented at formal scientific conferences. Their publications have created new pathways for the dissemination of medical information. Their pressure has caused the prestigious journals to release findings faster to the press. Their voice and vote on review committees have helped determine which studies receive funding. Their efforts have led to changes in the very definition of "AIDS" to incorporate the HIV-related conditions that affect women. Their interventions have led to the establishment of new mechanisms for regulating drugs, such as expanded access and accelerated approval. Their arguments have brought about shifts in the balance of power between competing visions of how clinical trials should be conducted. Their close scrutiny has encouraged basic scientists to move compounds more rapidly into clinical trials. And their networking has brought different communities of scientists into cooperative relationships with one another, thereby changing patterns of informal communication within science. Though activists have never sought or established absolute jurisdiction over any contested scientific terrain, they have, to use Andrew Abbott's term, won the rights to an "advisory jurisdiction" analogous to the relation of the clergy to medicine or psychiatry. Of course, as Abbott notes, advisory jurisdictions are characteristically unstable, "sometimes a leading edge of invasion, sometimes the trailing edge of defeat."[19]

THE POLITICS OF ACCESS

Drug regulation is one arena where the sheer effect of activism would be hard to dispute. Activists were not the only ones calling for change in the FDA, but they were the key players in pushing for the approval of AIDS drugs at an earlier stage in the drug development pipeline. And although some procedures allowing early access to experimental therapies were already on the FDA's books, others, such as expanded access and accelerated approval, are new to medicine as a result of AIDS, and have resulted in the provision of such therapies to much larger groups of patients than had been the case in the past. (Expanded access has since been instituted for drugs treating other diseases, such as Alzheimer's, while a drug for multiple sclerosis has received accelerated approval.[20]) This book has not focused on drugs that treat or prevent opportunistic infections, but it is perhaps there that the significance of activist efforts has been felt most keenly: earlier access to anti-infective drugs, though not without risk, has meant a longer life and better quality of life for many people with AIDS and HIV.[21] In addition, activist efforts (for better or worse) propelled the adoption of interpretative mechanisms such as surrogate markers that, in turn, have hastened the approval process. Absent the AIDS activists, CD4 counts would not have been accepted as a surrogate marker of treatment efficacy in 1991; without the adoption of the CD4 marker, the AZT/ddC combination would not have been licensed in 1992.

Finally, activists have insisted on broadening the demographic characteristics of clinical trial participants, hence broadening access to experimental therapies. In fiscal year 1988, 82 percent of the new

subjects recruited into ACTG trials were white. By 1994, only 56 percent were white (26 percent were African-American, 16 percent were
Hispanic/Latino, and 2 percent were "other"). Over the same period,
the ratio of men to women in trials was reduced from about thirteen
to one to about five to one.[22] While activists cannot take all the credit
for the demographic diversification of trials, there can be little doubt
that politicization of the issue by activists brought about a climate in
which change became perceived as a necessity. The minutes of the
ACTG Executive Committee meetings recorded Daniel Hoth's exhor-
tations to investigators to diversify trials: on one occasion Hoth noted
that the ACTG was "under a great deal of political pressure to address
this issue successfully"; on another, he described a phone conversation
with the assistant secretary of health, "who had called to ask what the
ACTG was doing to increase minority participation."[23] These new
emphases at NIAID were matched by changes at the FDA: in March
1993 agency officials announced that, instead of excluding women
of childbearing age from trials, they would henceforth *insist on their
inclusion* in nearly all new drug applications. "We now believe that
there are ways to protect the fetus and to include women in studies at
the same time," David Kessler told the press.[24]

Beyond the very real concerns about risks to patients, the key criticism of expedited access to experimental therapies has focused on the
potential threat to the research process. If, for example, patients were
able to obtain drugs like ddI and ddC through expanded access programs, why would they bother to sign up for long-term clinical trials?
This criticism ignores the other reasons why patients might enroll in
trials—for example, altruism or the desire to obtain access to high-
quality medical care and intensive monitoring of their medical condition. But in the end, as Anthony Fauci notes, "the proof of the pudding
is that we were right. [Expanded access] hasn't hampered anything";
research subjects have enrolled and the trials have still been completed.[25]

"SITUATED KNOWLEDGES"
AND THE LURE OF SCIENCE

Besides drug regulation, the other arena in which the
hand of activism has most heavily been felt is the design and methodology of clinical trials. Here, activists have trained their attention on
a range of apparently narrow and technical questions: Was there truly

a scientific necessity to exclude potential research subjects with abnormal lab test values? Was there anything from a statistical standpoint that prevented patients from taking concomitant medications or being enrolled in more than one trial at a time? By raising these questions, activists, sometimes with support from biostatisticians, have helped bring changes to the world of AIDS trials, making the procedures that governed them more similar to those already in place for cancer trials. "The way I looked at it is that, when the wind is blowing hard, you can either bend or you can break," recalled former NCI and NIAID biostatistician Susan Ellenberg. "I think we bent a lot in terms of the way we normally do trials. I think we stood firm in terms of the most important principles. . . ." [26]

By pressing researchers to develop clinically relevant trials with designs that research subjects would find acceptable, activists have helped to ensure more rapid accrual of the required numbers of subjects and to reduce the likelihood of noncompliance on the part of those participating. And by working toward methodological solutions that satisfy, simultaneously, the procedural concerns of researchers and the ethical demands of the patient community, AIDS activists have, at least in specific instances, improved a tool for the production of knowledge in ways that even researchers acknowledge. In this sense, AIDS activists' efforts belie the commonplace notion that only the insulation of science from "external" pressures guarantees the production of secure and trustworthy knowledge.

In the aftermath of the Concorde trial, with its implication that changes in CD4 counts are not, as activists had maintained, an adequate surrogate marker for antiviral drug efficacy, there were suggestions that AIDS activists had muddied the waters of knowledge in their haste to see drugs approved. Activist insistence on the use of surrogate markers had "set back AIDS research for ten years," researcher and Antiviral Advisory Committee member Donald Abrams grumbled with some hyperbole in late 1993. [27] Yet any such assessment must consider the larger picture. Absent the activists, what sort of knowledge strategies would have been pursued? Pristine studies addressing less-than-crucial questions? Methodologically unimpeachable trials that failed to recruit or maintain patients? Inevitably, there are risks inherent in the interruption of the status quo. But these must be weighed against all the other attendant risks, including those that might have followed from letting normal science take its leisurely course while an epidemic raged.

In their critiques of "pure" or "clean" or "elegant" science, and in their invocation of the "real world" and "pragmatic" decision making, AIDS activists have emphasized the *local* and *contextual* character of usable scientific knowledge. In the mainstream conception of science epitomized by the randomized clinical trial, true knowledge is produced through abstraction and the transcendence of particularities. In the alternative conception that develops out of activist critiques, reliable knowledge is produced through close attention to the concrete social, moral, and political context: better science comes about *because of* the focus on individual patients and their needs, desires, and expectations. This alternative conception of science is willing to surrender claims to universal validity in exchange for knowledge that bears some local and circumscribed utility.[28]

At the same time, as some of the treatment activists have moved "inward" to cooperate closely with researchers and have become increasingly sensitized to the logic of biomedical research, their conceptions of the scientific process have turned in a more conventionally positivist direction. This development has led to cleavages within the movement about how to approach the politics of knowledge. "I've seen a lot of treatment activists get seduced by the power, get seduced by the knowledge, and end up making very conservative arguments," contends Michelle Roland, formerly active with ACT UP in San Francisco. "They understand the science and the methodology, they can make intelligent arguments, and it's like, 'Wait a minute . . . okay, you're smart. We accept that. But what's your role?'"[29] Ironically, insofar as activists start thinking like scientists and not like patients, the ground for their unique contributions to the science of clinical trials may be in jeopardy of erosion. ACTG researcher John Phair notes that activists "have given us tremendous insight into the feasibility of certain studies" but adds that "some of the activists have gotten very sophisticated, and then [they] forget that the idea might not sell" to the community of patients.[30]

Can one be both activist and scientist? Is the notion of a "lay expert" a contradiction in terms?[31] There are no simple answers here, nor should we expect there to be. But arguably, it was not possible for key treatment activists to become authorities on clinical trials and sit on the ACTG committees without, in some sense, growing closer to the worldview of the researchers—and without moving a bit away from their fellow activists engaged in other pursuits. It is no surprise that activists with this degree of intellectual sophistication are themselves reflexively engaged in the consideration of precisely such issues.

Michelle Roland commented on the differentiation of activism in intriguing terms: "I hold on to the very strong belief that the only way that I'm going to do really good work is if there are people who *do not* know what I know—[people] who are always coming from that very emotional, very bottom-line place, to keep reminding me about that place."[32]

TRIALS AND TRUTH-MAKING

In the end, it remains somewhat unclear precisely what approaches to, or conceptions of, science activists would like to promote. Are AIDS activists really just trying to "clean up" science by eliminating "biases" that academic researchers are introducing? Or to supplant "clean science" with something that answers to different epistemological and ethical aspirations? It may be the tension between these conflicting and ambiguously defined goals, more than anything else, that characterizes the activist engagement with the AIDS research effort. The attempt to wrestle with such ambiguities is apparent in activists' views of the randomized clinical trial as a technology for producing knowledge. Generally speaking, activists have rejected a narrow, positivist conception of the clinical trial as a controlled laboratory experiment, pure and simple. But not many of them are prepared to replace the randomized clinical trial with an entirely different method of assessing drugs.[33]

By contrast, in her analysis of controversial cancer trials, Evelleen Richards concludes with a call to curtail our reliance on the randomized clinical trial. Since the notion of a "definitive" clinical trial, she claims, is a myth that primarily serves the interest of professional legitimation, it would be better "to learn to live with the reality of uncertainty" and to introduce political, ethical, and subjective criteria into the evaluation of treatments. This "implies a more prominent role for non-experts, for patients and the public at large, in the processes of assessment and decision making. . . ."[34] Quite similarly, AIDS activists have emphasized the artifactual and historical character of the clinical trials methodology, and they have placed a spotlight on the perception of the patient as a genuine participant in clinical research and not just the object of study. Yet—perhaps especially as they have become enculturated into the biomedical research process—most AIDS treatment activists share with doctors and researchers a profound investment in the belief that the truth about treatments is, in principle, knowable through *some* application of the scientific method. Though many in the AIDS movement have at particular moments argued in favor of tolerating uncertainty as the necessary trade-off for access to experimental drugs, in the end few activists, and perhaps few people with AIDS or HIV infection, are sanguine about the prospect of "[living] with the reality of uncertainty." This is not surprising, since activists and people with AIDS and HIV are confronted daily by a burning need to know whether given treatments "work" or not. The activist critique of the randomized clinical trial unseats that methodology from the pinnacle on which it is sometimes placed, but it also assumes (I think rightly) a greater role for such trials than analysts such as Richards would recommend.

Just how radical, then, *is* the critique of science offered by AIDS treatment activists? The question is hard to answer, especially as positions shift over time and vary significantly between individuals and groups. But what sparks the ambivalence between radical and reformist perspectives on science are just these painful ironies that vex efforts to influence clinical practice. On one hand, engagement with clinical research has always been driven by the dictates of expediency and dire need: activists have no time for the leisurely pursuit of truth; they'll settle for today's best guess. Yet on the other hand, treatment activists—particularly the New Yorkers with the Treatment Action Group, but to some extent nearly all of them—have increasingly become *believers* in science (however understood), and they desperately want clinical trials to generate usable knowledge that can guide medical practice. "My doctors and I make decisions in the dark with every pill I put in my mouth," complains David Barr, and this is not an easy way to live.[35]

Insofar as activists want to rely on the knowledge generated by clinical trials, they must wrestle with the consequences of their own interventions. Do such actions enhance activists' capacity to push clinical research in the directions they choose? Or do activists and researchers alike become subject to the unintended effects of their words and deeds, trapped within evolving systems whose trajectories no one really controls? Here is a worst-case scenario of the spiraling effects of community-based interventions in the construction of belief in antiviral drugs—a caricature sketch, to be sure, but one that combines elements from a number of cases: Drug X performs well in preliminary studies, and a NIAID official is quoted as saying that X is a promising drug. The grassroots treatment publications write that X is the up-and-coming thing; soon everyone in the community wants access to

X, and activists are demanding large, rapid trials to study it. Everyone wants to be in the trial, because they believe that X will help them; but researchers want to conduct the trial *in order to determine* whether X has any efficacy. Those who cannot get into the trial demand expanded access, while others begin importing X from other countries or manufacturing it in clandestine laboratories. As X becomes more prevalent and emerges as the de facto standard of care, physicians begin to suggest to patients that they get hold of it however they can. Meanwhile, participants in the clinical trial of X who fear they are receiving a placebo or an inferior drug mix and match their pills with those of other participants. When the trial's investigators report potential treatment benefits, activists push for accelerated approval of X, leaving the final determination of X's efficacy to postmarketing studies. But who then wants to sign up for those studies, when everyone now believes that the drug *works*, since, after all, the FDA has licensed it and any doctor can prescribe it?

In seeking to control this troubling escalation, the recent moves on the part of TAG activists to extricate themselves from the "hype cycle" seem particularly important. "One disturbing but inevitable result of the urgency engendered by the AIDS crisis," wrote Mark Harrington in late 1993, "is that both researchers and community members tend to invest preliminary trials with more significance than they can possibly bear." [36] To the extent that activists can develop a critique of this phenomenon and communicate the *relative uncertainty* of such trials to the broader public of HIV-infected persons, it may be possible to imagine a clinical trials process that more fully reflects the interests of those who are most in need of answers. [37]

On the other hand, the turn toward positivism in the statements of some TAG members—the emphasis on "rigor," "objectivity," and "rule-following" as the guarantors of success [38]—seems not only inadequate but inconsistent with the goal of not making more of trial results than we ought. As the earlier optimism about finding solutions to AIDS has given way to disappointment or resignation, it is understandable that some activists would find the lure of "good science" vastly preferable to the subordination of scientific judgment to the exigencies of the moment, however profound. The trick, though, is to encourage trials that are both ethical and well designed *without* reifying the method so as to suggest that such trials will provide degrees of certitude that they simply cannot provide. As Brian Wynne has suggested, the solution cannot be to further the myth that clinical knowledge-production is a fully rule-bound enterprise. Rather, the only way forward is to open the "black box" of clinical research, expose the uncertainty and the value choices, and then convince people of the considerable importance of participating in such research *even after* they understand just how messy it truly is and how bounded is the usability of the knowledge produced by it.[39]

The Legacy of AIDS Activism

THE REFASHIONING
OF PATIENTS AND DOCTORS

The impact of the AIDS movement on biomedical institutions in the United States has been impressive and conspicuous. At the same time, as Alberto Melucci has noted, social movements often have a "hidden efficacy" which becomes apparent only over time: by challenging cultural codes and conventions, they suggest to the broader society "that alternative frameworks of meaning are possible and that the operational logic of power apparatuses is not the only possible 'rationality.'"[40] Given the diverse influences that AIDS activism has already begun to exert, it seems likely that the movement will engender just this kind of shift in systems of meaning.

For instance, it has rapidly become something of a cliché to say that the doctor-patient relationship will never be the same in the wake of AIDS. As Stanford AIDS researcher Thomas Merigan reflected, "The doctor isn't the same doctor [as] when I started in practice. . . . The doctor in the past was somebody who made your decisions for you and held your hand; and . . . you would just believe in him."[41] Granted, models of interaction between doctors and patients have diversified considerably in recent decades: AIDS provides a convenient frame for summarizing changes that were already in the works. What is perhaps the significant effect of AIDS, then, is that a more cooperative model has become normative (at least in medical rhetoric) and has been incorporated into medical school curriculums.[42] This changed conception of the doctor-patient relationship has also been linked explicitly to an emergent understanding of the appropriate researcher-subject relationship. Patients have a "participant's interest" in clinical research that extends beyond the mere protection of their "rights" as "human subjects"; communities have a stake in the review of research protocols that is not satisfied by the token request for their "input."[43]

"Having our patients or our research subjects ask—or demand—to have an active voice in what we do and how we do it may be challenging, time-consuming, and even unpleasant," comments UCSF's Robert Wachter, one of the organizers of the International AIDS Conference in 1990. "It is also undeniably right."[44]

On first glance it may be surprising, but on reflection it seems predictable that one of the ways in which AIDS treatment activists are changing the character of medical relationships is by deciding, in some cases, to pursue careers in medicine. Two of the activists interviewed for this book, Michelle Roland and Rebecca Smith, had already proceeded from ACT UP to medical school; a third, Garance Franke-Ruta, aspires to the "medical school class of 2000." "I was always interested in medicine," Roland recalls, "but I did *not* want to go to medical school"; "I did not *like* doctors, I thought they were arrogant, I thought they were just not pleasant people, I thought their values were fucked up—and I did not like Western medicine. I, at that point, wouldn't take aspirin for a headache. You know, I was one of those people." Ironically, it was Roland's experiences with ACT UP that made her recognize "that medical training was going to give me the power that I wanted [in order] to influence health care," and "that I was going to be a much more powerful advocate and a much more intelligent advocate if I understood what I was arguing about, and if I understood what the people I was arguing with believed...."[45] Smith, meanwhile, has sought to use her activist experience to improve the medical curriculum at her university by increasing students' exposure to the statistical principles underlying clinical trials.[46]

NEW VOICES ON THE MEDICAL HORIZON

The AIDS movement has encouraged individual patients to seek new ways of relating to their health-care providers and vice versa. But it has also inspired a range of *organized* challenges to biomedicine, some of which have developed into full-fledged social movements. Certainly, the history of medical self-help groups—ranging from the most reformist to the most radical—long precedes AIDS activism.[47] But the past few years in the United States have seen a marked upsurge of health-related activism of a distinctive type: the formation of groups that construct identities in relation to particular disease categories and assert political and scientific claims on the basis of these new identities. With its assimilation of the critiques put forward by the feminist health movement, the AIDS movement was a beneficiary of "social movement spillover"; now its own tactics and understandings have begun to serve as a "master frame" for a new series of challengers.[48]

Most notably patients with breast cancer but also those suffering from chronic fatigue, multiple chemical sensitivity, prostate cancer, mental illness, Lyme disease, Lou Gehrig's disease, Alzheimer's, and a host of other conditions have displayed a new militancy and demanded a voice in how their conditions are conceptualized, treated, and researched.[49] These groups have criticized not only the quality of their care but the ethics of clinical research ("Are placebo controls acceptable?") and the assignment of control over research directions ("Who decides which presentations belong on a conference program?"). While not every such group derives its approaches directly from AIDS activism, the tactics and political vocabulary of organizations like ACT UP would seem, at a minimum, to be "in the wind."[50] (Could one imagine, before the AIDS activist repudiation of "victimhood," people with muscular dystrophy denouncing the Jerry Lewis Telethon as an "annual ritual of shame" and chanting "Power, not pity" before the news cameras?[51]) To date, none of these constituencies has engaged in epistemological interventions that approach, in their depth or extent, AIDS treatment activists' critiques of the methodology of clinical trials. But Bernadine Healy, then director of the NIH, expressed it well in 1992 when she told a reporter: "The AIDS activists have led the way. . . . [They] have created a template for all activist groups looking for a cure."[52]

Breast cancer activism is an intriguing instance of this new wave, because the links to AIDS activism have been so explicit and so readily acknowledged. In 1991, more than 180 U.S. advocacy groups came together to form the National Breast Cancer Coalition. "They say they've had it with politicians and physicians and scientists who 'there, there' them with studies and statistics and treatments that suggest the disease is under control," read a prominent account in the *New York Times Sunday Magazine*.[53] In its first year of operation, the coalition convinced Congress to step up funding for breast cancer research by $43 million, an increase of almost 50 percent. "The next year, armed with data from a seminar they financed, the women asked for, wheedled, negotiated and won a whopping $300 million more."[54] The debt to AIDS activism was widely noted by activists and commentators alike. "They showed us how to get through to the Government," said a Bay Area breast cancer patient and organizer. "They took on an archaic system and turned it around while we have been quietly dying."[55] Another activist described how she met with the staff of *AIDS Treatment News* to learn the ropes of the drug development and regulatory systems.[56] In 1994, ACT UP/Golden Gate participated with San Francisco–based Breast Cancer Action in a "funeral procession"–style protest against the Genentech Corporation to demand access to a monoclonal antibody with potential efficacy against the disease.[57]

Gracia Buffleben, a "48-year-old heterosexual housewife and nurse" who joined Breast Cancer Action after her own diagnosis with cancer, was initially astonished by the expertise of the AIDS activists: "It was unbelievable to me that somebody could have the depth of knowledge that they had and not have a scientific background or a medical background."[58] For her part, Brenda Lein of ACT UP/Golden Gate was dismayed by how easily manipulated the breast cancer activists could be at first, in the absence of the sort of expertise about drug development that AIDS activists had acquired. She described attending an early meeting between cancer activists and pharmaceutical company representatives where the drug company scientists "were just *snowing them over* left and right—blatantly lying to them: 'No, you can't have access to protocols,' 'Oh, we don't share that information, it's confidential.'"[59] Lein worried, in 1993, about breast cancer activists "putting the cart before the horse": they appeared to be imitating the outward forms of AIDS treatment activism—"The AIDS folks have community advisory boards, we want that too!"—without first developing the knowledge base that had made those institutions meaningful. But increasingly, breast cancer activists were stepping back to learn the science and to educate themselves about clinical trial design—even to attend oncology sessions at the ACTG meetings.[60]

Of course, it would be rash to assume that AIDS activism has created an automatic receptiveness on the part of scientists or doctors to health movements of this sort, and that the next round of activists can simply step up to the counter and claim their rewards. A more likely scenario is that AIDS activism will usher in a new wave of democratization struggles in the biomedical sciences and health care—struggles that may be just as hard fought as those of the past fifteen years. It is worth remembering, too, how difficult this sort of activism is to sustain: organizing a social movement is arduous enough without having to learn oncology in your spare time. In 1994, Mark Harrington was happy that his term on the ACTG's Community Constituency Group had expired; he cited the "incredible amount of work" involved in preparing for scientific meetings: "There are enormous faxes and Federal Express boxes, and there are four to six conference calls a month." More profoundly, one of the challenges for any movement that would follow in the footsteps of AIDS treatment activism is how to sustain, over an extended period, what Harrington describes as "a lasting culture of information, advocacy, intervention, and resistance." Asked Harrington: "How can we foster this culture that is probably going to need to continue for longer than all of us may? This becomes a very important issue, and one that we didn't consider in the first few years. . . ."[61]

EXPERTISE AND DEMOCRACY

"If citizens ought to be empowered to participate in determining their society's basic structure," writes Richard Sclove, "and technologies are an important species of social structure, it follows that technological design and practice should be democratized."[62] There is a growing, international body of literature suggesting means by which science and technology can be brought further under popular control—studies of "science shops" that bring researchers into collaboration with citizens, "science courts" that invite laypeople to pass judgment on political controversies with scientific dimensions, and citizen boards to assess technological risks.[63] Yet there is also good cause to recognize the extraordinary difficulty of eradicating hierarchies founded on knowledge-possession—hierarchies that can cut across social movements just as easily as they can divide "laypeople" from "experts." This, too, is a dilemma that will confront future groups that seek to democratize biomedical knowledge-making or other domains of science and technology.

In the goals of democratizing science and building "lay expertise," at least three distinct difficulties are interwoven. First, the practices of science by their nature presuppose specialization: no one can know everything; everyone must therefore acknowledge that others speak with authority—at least *some* others, *some* of the time. To participate in science, then, means inevitably to *cede* authority over most of its domains at the same time that one constitutes expertise over a particular one. Even AIDS treatment activists tend to specialize among themselves and construct a division of expert labor: some study vaccine development, others follow immunology, still others "adopt" a particular drug and track its development. In this way, activists become essential to one another, since all must trust that the others have done their homework and know what they're talking about. Understood in these terms, "democratization" of science is inevitably a partial and uneven process and one that, ironically, proceeds hand in hand with the consolidation of new relationships of trust and authority.

The second difficulty confronted by social movements that seek to democratize the practices of knowledge-making is that there may be tension between participation in the construction of scientific knowledge and the requirements of movement-building. While inarguably successful in important ways and according to various criteria, the shift "inward" and "backward" by key treatment activist groups has made it harder for them to frame issues for the media or a broader public, to recruit new members, and to maintain a broad-based and socially diverse movement. The ways of representing natural and social reality that activists develop in their role as "lay experts" may differ significantly from the representations that they elaborate in street demonstrations and other, more conventional, activist venues. And the tactics of "expertification" that have ensured the activists' credibility before the research establishment may be, at least to some degree, in conflict with the goal of ensuring movement leaders' credibility in the eyes of the communities that the movement seeks to represent.

Issues of professionalization and hierarchy—and risks of co-optation—are not, of course, unique to AIDS activism.[64] Other movements, such as the environmental movement, have struggled over "insider" and "outsider" strategies and the relative merits of professionalized activism when interacting with credentialed experts.[65] Few are the cases, however, of movements so fundamentally *dependent* on their adversaries as is the AIDS movement, and it is this binding of need and antagonism that has accentuated the complexities of the interaction and brought them into sharper relief. The experience of AIDS treatment activism suggests that confronting highly technical domains of science can have a wide range of effects upon the internal and external dynamics of a social movement. Even when activists deliberately erode the boundaries between "science" and "politics," they may find that the tactics and tools that facilitate their engagement with scientific elites are at variance with other movement goals and may distance them from some of their "lay" compatriots who perceive them then as "experts." Such developments can lead to profound internal struggles to determine a movement's very identity, as well as how it communicates its messages and what it sets out to accomplish.

The third problem is that knowledge hierarchies are rarely "accidental" in their origins: They tend both to build upon and reinforce social cleavages based on other markers of difference—class, formal education, race, gender, sexuality, and nationality. When the power of expert knowledge within a social movement overlaps with other systems of hierarchy, the results can be problematic for the movement, even if the new experts work entirely in good faith for the benefit of all. The interweaving of expertise with diverse forms of power is evident to those who become positioned on the margins. It is apparent, in another way, to "border people"—as Garance Franke-Ruta (a white woman) refers to the position of herself and Moisés Agosto (a Puerto Rican gay man) inside TAG, an organization that is predominantly composed of white gay men.[66] As an "outsider" who believed in the importance of treatment activism for communities of color, Agosto found he had to fight his way into a position of access and influence— to break into the tight circles that the first generation of treatment activists had constructed between themselves, government health officials, academic researchers, and pharmaceutical companies. Wearing two hats, Agosto took a staff position with the National Minority AIDS Council but remained active with TAG, becoming a member of its board. However, once he found himself appointed to the National Task Force on AIDS Drug Development, Agosto confronted an ironic challenge from the grassroots: "People have come to me and said, 'Well, we lost you. You're on the inside now with the Task Force.'"[67]

Agosto rightly observes that his options have not been foreclosed: "I can [still] go and scream in the streets if I feel I have to." But he cannot entirely escape the metamorphosis of identity that follows from engagements with power and knowledge. The fact that various dimensions of social hierarchy, such as those constructed in relation to racial difference, crisscross and intertwine with the politics of expertise only complicates the story and imbues it with added poignancy. These considerations suggest the true dimensions of the problem: it is unlikely that knowledge-making practices can be substantially democratized, except when efforts to do so are carried out in conjunction with other social struggles that challenge other, entrenched systems of domination.[68]

This broadening of perspectives would set heady goals for a movement more immediately concerned with the concrete business of saving lives. But even the most "professionalized," "expert" activists pursuing "insider" strategies have seen precisely these deeper purposes as the motivation for their efforts. "If AIDS activists ever leave any legacy other than their own bodies," wrote Gregg Gonsalves and Mark Harrington in 1992, "it will be, among other things, a movement for national health care and the democratization of research."[69] Certainly the genuine progress that has been made in the struggle to democratize biomedicine is not negated by the failure to realize it in full, any more than the medical advances in the fight to keep people with AIDS alive are belied by the failure to eradicate the epidemic. In the meantime, the struggle continues on multiple fronts, and AIDS activists' strategies for engaging with medical science continue to provoke controversy and provide inspiration.

METHODOLOGICAL APPENDIX

Sources

I generated the analysis in this book from a range of sources that I treated as primary data: first, published instances of claims-making found in scientific and medical journal articles, mass media news reports, articles in the gay and lesbian press, activist documents and publications, and government documents; second, extensive interviews with more than thirty of the principals in the story (researchers, activists, and government officials); and third, conferences, meetings, forums, demonstrations, and other public events that I attended. My fundamental analytical strategy has been to bring into critical juxtaposition contemporaneous records from different "social worlds." The sources that I have considered document the positions that actors have taken and the claims they have advanced; these sources are also, in themselves, important arenas of struggle. My assumption is that each of these different sources engages in a different calculus of credibility—that, for example, the *New York Times* version of reality is not the same as the *Gay Community News* version. Bringing them into common focus reveals the different regimes of credibility assessment, just as it exposes the stratification of credibility that inevitably becomes manifest when different social worlds collide. Of course, published sources tell only part of the story—sometimes, in their linearity and smoothness, finished documents *conceal* the story—and it is in that regard that interviews with the participants in events have helped me to describe those events in a more satisfactory way and to provide needed context.

In some cases, as in my reconstruction of the controversy surrounding Peter Duesberg, my strategy has tended toward the exhaustive, and I have unearthed sources from less influential publications as well as better-known ones. In other cases, the enormity of the source materials available has necessitated certain strategic choices. With regard to scientific and medical journals, popular impressions coincide with evidence from citation analyses in suggesting that *Science, Nature,* the *New England Journal of Medicine, Lancet,* the *Journal of the American Medical Association (JAMA),* and the *Annals of Internal Medicine* are the most generally significant, influential, and credible in the world of biomedical research.[1] In studying debates in the mass media, I have relied almost entirely on influential print sources, such as the *New York Times,* the *Los Angeles Times,* and the *Washington Post,* as well as *Time, Newsweek,* and, where appropriate to the story, the British press. My material from the gay press derives mainly, though not entirely, from those newspapers and magazines with some fair degree of national circulation, particularly the *Advocate* (California), *Gay Community News* (Boston), and the *New York Native,* but also a number of local newspapers and magazines. In terms of treatment publications (which I cite heavily in part two), I make most use of *AIDS Treatment News* (San Francisco), *PI Perspectives* (San Francisco), *Treatment Issues* (New York City), the *ACT UP/New York Treatment & Data Digest,* and *TAGline* (New York City).

Symmetry and the Study of Scientific Controversies

How can scientific controversies best be reconstructed? One of the guiding principles of the sociology of scientific knowledge is the so-called principle of symmetry, which proposes that the researcher invoke the same types of causes or apply the same conceptual tools to explain "true" and "false" beliefs.[2] This principle represents a crucial break with a more traditional approach, which begins by accepting the views of dominant scientists and then sets itself the task of explaining why the other side in the controversy (creationists, say, or anti-fluoridationists) might be so deluded as to persist in its errors. In the traditional approach, "social explanations are selectively applied to the side without authoritative scientific backing."[3] By contrast, contemporary sociologists of scientific knowledge insist on employing a common conceptual apparatus to explore the knowledge claims and social factors on both (or all) sides of a controversy. In my view, a symmetric analysis is not necessarily a "neutral" analysis, either in intent or in effect. But it is, potentially, the most fair-minded way to approach knowledge controversies, and one that requires the investigator to bend over backwards to consider the arguments of scientific "underdogs."[4]

Archeology and Genealogy

Without suggesting any strict allegiance, I would also characterize my method as having affinities with modes of investigation employed in the work of Michel Foucault. First, my analysis is "archeological" in that it seeks to focus attention on the *conditions of possibility* of different forms of knowledge in different places at different times. Such an analysis concerns itself with a recovery of the immanent rules of what is sayable and unsayable, thinkable and unthinkable.[5] Second, my account is "genealogical" insofar as it aims to disrupt any assumptions of a smooth path of development of knowledge about AIDS over time. A genealogical analysis rejects teleological accounts in order to emphasize shifts and discontinuities. By the logic of genealogy, contemporary knowledge about AIDS cannot be inferred in some automatic fashion from earlier moments in the epidemic, nor was early thinking about the epidemic predictive of a pathway to the present. Rather, without denying the links from one moment to the next, we must be attentive to gaps, breaks, and transmutations in the trajectory of knowledge development.

Finally, the notion of genealogy is consistent with my "democratic" approach to claims-making—my strategy of attending to the claims of an activist reported in the gay press in the same way that I note those of a famous scientist writing in the pages of *Nature*. Genealogical research, in Foucault's words, "[entertains] the claims to attention of local, discontinuous, disqualified, illegitimate knowledges against the claims of a unitary body of theory which would filter, hierarchise and order them in the name of some true knowledge and some arbitrary idea of what constitutes a science and its objects."[6] The recovery of these "subjugated," "local," or "situated" knowledges and their juxtaposition with formal, accredited knowledge is essential to a full understanding of the relations of power and the formation of knowledge in a given society at a given time.[7]

Content Analysis

The remainder of this appendix provides details concerning the design of the two content analyses reported in chapter 2— the analysis of scientific journal articles that cited Gallo's 1984 paper (see tables 1, 2, and 3) and the analysis of references to causation in the *New York Times* (see table 4).[8]

SCIENTIFIC JOURNAL ARTICLES

I selected key scientific and medical journals for the period 1984–1986 using the *Science Citation Index Journal Citation Reports*,[9] which rank journals annually based on the number of citations to the articles they publish. Three highly prominent general science journals (*Science, Nature,* and the *Proceedings of the National Academy of Sciences*) and two highly prominent medical journals (the *New England Journal of Medicine* and *Lancet*) ranked within the top ten for all three years.[10] Two other prominent medical journals (the *Annals of Internal Medicine* and *Journal of the American Medical Association*) ranked only within the top fifty but ranked near the top of the subset of journals designated as "Medicine, General and Internal";[11] moreover, these journals account for a high percentage of publications specifically about AIDS, according to several studies.[12] Therefore, I selected these seven publications for the content analysis.

Next, I identified all articles published in these journals in 1984, 1985, or 1986 that cited Gallo's paper, using the 1984–1987 issues of the *Science Citation Index*.[13] I retrieved and photocopied the selected articles and then screened them for "meatiness" using an algorithm developed for this purpose by Garfield.[14] This algorithm selects for communications (articles, letters, and so on) reporting substantive research while eliminating items likely to have minimal impact. Items failing to achieve the threshold level identified by Garfield (such as short letters) I excluded from consideration. This yielded a total population of 244 articles, which I included in the content analysis.[15]

I then coded each article for three pieces of information:

1. In the sentence containing the citation of Gallo's article,[16] what kind of causal claim is made?

   Explicit unqualified reference to the virus as the cause (These include, for example, "The cause of AIDS has been found to be HTLV-III"; "HIV, the virus that causes AIDS . . ."; "HIV is the primary etiological agent in AIDS"; and so on.)

   Implicit unqualified reference to the virus as the cause (The virus is referred to as "the AIDS virus.")

   Qualified reference to the virus as the cause (These include "HIV, the putative agent in AIDS . . ."; "HIV is believed to cause AIDS"; "The bulk of the evidence suggests [or strongly suggests] that AIDS is caused by HTLV-III"; or the use of words such as "etiologically linked," "associated," and so on.)

   Implicit reference to the possibility that the virus may not be the cause (I included this coding possibility for the sake of logical completeness, but no articles were coded as such; therefore I excluded it in my subsequent analysis.)

   Explicit reference to the possibility that the virus may not be the cause (These include references to the lack of evidence, to other hypotheses, to the need for cofactors, and so on.)

   Article not cited in conjunction with a causal claim (Some authors cited the Gallo paper simply to establish a different point about HTLV-III.)

2. Are any of the thirteen coauthors of the Gallo article included among the coauthors of the article in question?[17]

3. Are additional articles cited to support the causal claim? (Here I distinguished between articles that cited only Gallo or that cited Gallo along with earlier or roughly concurrent articles [1983 and 1984] by the Gallo, Montagnier, or Levy groups and those articles that also cited subsequent articles by any authors [1985 and 1986].)

I then tabulated data by journal. However, due to the small numbers, I have reported results only for the full population (the seven journals combined).[18]

NEW YORK TIMES ARTICLES

I performed a database search to identify and retrieve all articles from July 1, 1984, to December 31, 1986, that included the word "AIDS" and any of the following terms: "HIV," "HTLV," "LAV," and "virus." I excluded letters to the editor, indexes, and substantively irrelevant articles. For the second half of 1984, I subjected the entire population of articles to content analysis. Due to the explosion in reporting about AIDS after 1984, for subsequent six-month time periods, I selected samples of the full article population. Samples consisted of every fifth article, in chronological order, beginning with a randomly selected number from one to five. This procedure yielded a total sample of 115 articles.

I then coded these articles according to causal claims made anywhere in the body of the article:

Only unqualified references to the virus as cause (The virus is identified, without qualifiers, as the cause of AIDS, one or more times in the article; no qualified references appear anywhere in the article.)

Only qualified references to the virus as cause (Qualified references ["Most scientists believe that AIDS is caused by a virus called HTLV-III"; "HIV, the virus believed to cause AIDS"; and so on] appear one or more times in the article; no unqualified references appear anywhere in the article.)

Mixed qualified and unqualified references (Both qualified and unqualified references appear in the article.)

Implicit claim that the virus is the cause (This was usually indicated by references to the "AIDS virus" in the absence of any other qualified or unqualified causal claims.)

Explicit references to the possibility that the virus may not be the cause (This included articles about alternative etiological hypotheses.)

No causal claim (No qualified or unqualified references and no use of the phrase "AIDS virus"; this proved to characterize only a very small percentage of the articles.)

On the basis of this coding procedure, I then tabulated and reported data for each of the time periods studied.

NOTES

Introduction

1. Elizabeth Pincus, "Harvard Medical Establishment Ripped by ACT UP/ Boston," *Gay Community News*, 11 September 1988, 1.

2. On credibility in science, see Steven Shapin, "Cordelia's Love: Credibility and the Social Studies of Studies," *Perspectives on Science* 3, no. 3 (1995): 255–275; Steven Shapin, *A Social History of Truth: Civility and Science in Seventeenth-Century England* (Chicago: Univ. of Chicago Press, 1994); Barry Barnes and David Edge, "Science as Expertise," in *Science in Context: Readings in the Sociology of Science,* ed. Barry Barnes and David Edge (Cambridge, Mass.: Massachusetts Institute of Technology Press, 1982), 233–249; Bruno Latour and Steve Woolgar, *Laboratory Life: The Construction of Scientific Facts* (Princeton, N.J.: Princeton Univ. Press, 1986), chapter 5; Brian Martin, *Scientific Knowledge in Controversy: The Social Dynamics of the Fluoridation Debate* (Albany: State Univ. of New York Press, 1991), chapter 4; Susan Leigh Star, *Regions of the Mind: Brain Research and the Quest for Scientific Certainty* (Stanford: Stanford Univ. Press, 1989), 138–144; Rob Williams and John Law, "Beyond the Bounds of Credibility," *Fundamenta Scientiae* 1 (1980): 295–315. My conception of credibility bears an affinity to Susan Cozzens's definition of scientific power as enrollment capacity plus legitimacy. See Susan E. Cozzens, "Autonomy and Power in Science," in *Theories of Science in Society,* ed. Susan E. Cozzens and Thomas F. Gieryn (Bloomington: Indiana Univ. Press, 1990), 164–184, esp. 168–174.

3. See Michel Foucault, *Discipline and Punish: The Birth of the Prison* (New York: Vintage Books, 1979), 26.

4. Adele E. Clarke, "Controversy and the Development of Reproductive Science," *Social Problems* 37 (February 1990): 18–37, esp. 30.

5. On the historical constitution of the expert/lay divide, see Steven Shapin, "Science and the Public," in *Companion to the History of Modern Science,* ed. R. C. Olby et al. (London and New York: Routledge, 1990), 990–1007.

6. See Jürgen Habermas, *Toward a Rational Society: Student Protest, Science, and Politics* (Boston: Beacon Press, 1970), 62–80.

7. Dorothy Nelkin, "The Political Impact of Technical Expertise," *Social Studies of Science* 5 (February 1975): 35–54, quote from 54. See also Steven Brint, *In an Age of Experts: The Changing Role of Professionals in Politics and Public Life* (Princeton, N.J.: Princeton Univ. Press, 1994), 15.

8. U.S. opinion polls suggest that public confidence in science and medicine declined in the 1960s and 1970s and stabilized in the 1980s. However, these declines were no more marked than those for most other professions, all of which suffered from a "confidence gap" during this time. See Seymour Martin Lipset and William Schneider, *The Confidence Gap: Business, Labor, and Government in the Public Mind* (New York: Free Press, 1983).

9. For summaries of various critiques of science, see Robert N. Proctor, *Value-Free Science? Purity and Power in Modern Knowledge* (Cambridge, Mass.: Harvard Univ. Press, 1991, 232–261); Stanley Aronowitz, *Science as Power* (Minneapolis: Univ. of Minnesota Press, 1988), chapter 1; Sandra Harding, *The Science Question in Feminism* (Ithaca: Cornell Univ. Press, 1986).

10. Foucault, *Discipline and Punish*; Jean Baudrillard, *Selected Writings* (Stanford, Calif.: Stanford Univ. Press, 1988); Jean-François Lyotard, *The Postmodern Condition: A Report on Knowledge* (Minneapolis: Univ. of Minnesota Press, 1984).

11. Harry Collins and Trevor Pinch, *The Golem: What Everyone Should Know about Science* (Cambridge, England: Cambridge Univ. Press, 1993), 142.

12. For a recent discussion, see Charles E. Rosenberg, "Disease and Social Order in America: Perceptions and Expectations" in *AIDS: The Burdens of History*, ed. Elizabeth Fee and Daniel M. Fox (Berkeley: Univ. of California Press, 1988), 12–32.

13. Paul Starr, *The Social Transformation of American Medicine* (New York: Basic Books, 1982), 4. In Jürgen Habermas' terms, doctors stand at the boundary between "system" and "lifeworld."

14. Ibid., esp. 9–13, 59.

15. Ibid., 336.

16. See, for example, John Ehrenreich, ed., *The Cultural Crisis of Modern Medicine* (New York: Monthly Review Press, 1978); Barbara and John Ehrenreich, *The American Health Empire* (New York: Vintage Books, 1971).

17. Jay Katz, *The Silent World of Doctor and Patient* (New York: Free Press, 1984), xv.

18. David J. Rothman, *Strangers at the Bedside* (New York: Basic Books 1991), 85–100.

19. Stephen O. Murray and Kenneth W. Payne, "Medical Policy without Scientific Evidence: The Promiscuity Paradigm and AIDS," *California Sociologist* 11 (winter-summer 1988): 13–54, esp. 14.

20. Yaron Ezrahi, "The Authority of Science in Politics," in *Science and Values: Patterns of Tradition and Change*, ed. Arnold Thackray and Everett Mendelsohn (New York: Humanities Press, 1974), 215–251, quote from 220. See also Yaron Ezrahi, *The Descent of Icarus: Science and the Transformation*

of Contemporary Democracy (Cambridge, Mass.: Harvard Univ. Press, 1990).

21. Steven Shapin and Simon Schaffer, *Leviathan and the Air-Pump: Hobbes, Boyle, and the Experimental Life* (Princeton, N.J.: Princeton Univ. Press, 1985), 336, 343.

22. Thomas F. Gieryn, "Boundary Work and the Demarcation of Science from Non-Science: Strains and Interests in Professional Ideologies of Scientists," *American Sociological Review* 48 (December 1983): 781–795; Thomas F. Gieryn, "Boundaries of Science," in *Handbook of Science and Technology Studies,* ed. Sheila Jasanoff et al. (Thousand Oaks, Calif.: Sage, 1995), 393–443.

23. Philip J. Hilts, "Does Anybody Want to Lead N.I.H. If Job Lasts Only till Next Election?" *New York Times,* 8 September 1989, A-12. Wyngaarden had just stepped down as director of the NIH a few months before.

24. For defenses of scientific autonomy, see Robert K. Merton, "Science and the Social Order" in: Robert K. Merton, *The Sociology of Science: Theoretical and Empirical Investigations* (Chicago: Univ. of Chicago Press, 1973), esp. 257–60 (this article dates from 1938); Edward A. Shils, *The Torment of Secrecy: The Background and Consequences of American Security Policies* (New York: Free Press, 1956), 176–191. Subsequent, more skeptical scholarship has proposed that the defense of professional autonomy can serve to disguise the pursuit of professional power. However, for a critical perspective on science that in the end returns to an endorsement of scientific autonomy as the guarantor of progress, see Pierre Bourdieu, "The Specificity of the Scientific Field and the Social Conditions of the Progress of Reason," *Social Science Information* 14 (December 1975): 19–47.

25. On the AIDS activist repudiation of the "victim" designation, see Max Navarre, "Fighting the Victim Label," in *AIDS: Cultural Analysis, Cultural Activism,* ed. Douglas Crimp (Cambridge, Mass.: Massachusetts Institute of Technology Press, 1988), 143–146.

26. Susan E. Cozzens and Edward J. Woodhouse, "Science, Government, and the Politics of Knowledge," in *Handbook of Science and Technology Studies,* ed. Sheila Jasanoff et al. (Thousand Oaks, Calif.: Sage, 1995), 533–553, quote from 538.

27. Michael Bury, "The Sociology of Chronic Illness: A Review of Research and Prospects," *Sociology of Health & Illness* 13 (December 1991): 451–468.

28. See Mark A. Chesler, "Mobilizing Consumer Activism in Health Care: The Role of Self-Help Groups," *Research in Social Movements, Conflicts and Change* 13 (1991): 275–305; Miriam J. Stewart, "Expanding Theoretical Conceptualizations of Self-Help Groups," *Social Science and Medicine* 31 (May 1990): 1057–1066; and the special issue of the *American Journal of Community Psychology* 19 (October 1991).

29. Gerald E. Markle and James C. Petersen, eds., *Politics, Science, and Cancer: The Laetrile Phenomenon* (Boulder, Colo.: Westview Press, 1980).

30. Sheryl Burt Ruzek, *Feminist Alternatives to Medical Control* (New York: Praeger, 1978), 144. See also Rima D. Apple, ed., *Women, Health, and*

Medicine in America: A Historical Handbook (New Brunswick, N.J.: Rutgers Univ. Press, 1990 (including the extensive bibliography); Elizabeth Fee, ed., *Women and Health: The Politics of Sex in Medicine* (Farmingdale, N.Y.: Baywood, 1982); Boston Women's Health Book Collective, *Our Bodies, Ourselves: A Book by and for Women* (New York: Simon & Schuster, 1973).

31. Hilary Arksey, "Expert and Lay Participation in the Construction of Medical Knowledge," *Sociology of Health & Illness* 16 (September 1994): 448–468.

32. Rainald von Gizycki, "Cooperation between Medical Researchers and a Self-Help Movement: The Case of the German Retinitis Pigmentosa Society," in *The Social Direction of the Public Sciences,* ed. Stuart Blume et al. (Dordrecht, Holland: D. Reidel, 1987), 75–88.

33. Initially the syndrome was defined with reference to "risk groups," such as gay men, hemophiliacs, injection drug users, and (for a while) Haitians. More recently, as AIDS increasingly becomes a disease of the poor, there is a growing tendency to define the affected population by race or class.

34. Erving Goffman, *Stigma: Notes on the Management of Spoiled Identity* (Englewood Cliffs, N.J.: Prentice-Hall, 1963).

35. On the importance of "resource mobilization" for social movements, see William A. Gamson, *The Strategy of Social Protest,* 2d ed. (Belmont, Calif.: Wadsworth, 1990); J. D. McCarthy and M. N. Zald, "Resource Mobilization and Social Movements: A Partial Theory," *American Journal of Sociology* 82 (May 1977): 1212–1241. For an analysis comparing the mobilization to confront the epidemic by lesbian and gay communities with that of African-American communities, see Cathy Jean Cohen, "Power, Resistance and the Construction of Crisis: Marginalized Communities Respond to AIDS" (Ph.D. diss., University of Michigan, 1993).

36. John D'Emilio, *Sexual Politics, Sexual Communities: The Making of a Homosexual Minority in the United States, 1940–1970* (Chicago: Univ. of Chicago Press, 1983); Dennis Altman, *The Homosexualization of America* (Boston: Beacon Press, 1982); Barry D. Adam, *The Rise of a Gay and Lesbian Movement* (Boston: Twayne Publishers, 1987).

37. Jeffrey Escoffier, "The Politics of Gay Identity," *Socialist Review,* July-October 1985, 119–153.

38. See Ronald Bayer, *Homosexuality and American Psychiatry: The Politics of Diagnosis* (New York: Basic Books, 1981). On medicalization and demedicalization more generally, see Peter Conrad and Joseph W. Schneider, *Deviance and Medicalization: From Badness to Sickness* (St. Louis: C. V. Mosby, 1980).

39. See Jackie Winnow, "Lesbians Evolving Health Care: Cancer and AIDS," *Feminist Review,* summer 1992, 68–77; Amber Hollibaugh, "Lesbian Denial and Lesbian Leadership in the AIDS Epidemic: Bravery and Fear in the Construction of a Lesbian Geography of Risk," in *Women Resisting AIDS: Feminist Strategies of Empowerment,* ed. Beth E. Schneider and Nancy E. Stoller (Philadelphia: Temple Univ. Press, 1995), 219–230; Nancy Stoller, "Lesbian Involvement in the AIDS Epidemic: Changing Roles and Generational Differences," in *Women Resisting AIDS* (above), 270–285; Gena

Corea, *The Invisible Epidemic: The Story of Women and AIDS* (New York: HarperCollins, 1992).

40. David S. Meyer and Nancy Whittier, "Social Movement Spillover," *Social Problems* 41 (May 1994): 277–298.

41. On "micro-mobilization contexts" and their role in social movement organizing, see D. McAdam, J. D. McCarthy, and M. N. Zald, "Social Movements," in *Handbook of Sociology,* ed. Neil Smelser (Newbury Park, Calif.: Sage, 1988), 695–737, esp. 709–716; Clarence Y. H. Lo, "Communities of Challengers in Social Movement Theory," in *Frontiers in Social Movement Theory,* ed. Aldon D. Morris and Carol McClurg Mueller (New Haven: Yale Univ. Press, 1992), 224–247. Those suffering from diseases more randomly distributed in the population have had only the hospital itself as a micro-mobilization context; see Chesler, "Mobilizing Consumer Activism."

42. Pierre Bourdieu, *The Logic of Practice* (Stanford, Calif.: Stanford Univ. Press, 1990), 122–134. On the cultural roots of social movements, see also Doug McAdam, "Culture and Social Movements," in *New Social Movements: From Ideology to Identity,* ed. Enrique Laraña, Hank Johnston, and Joseph R. Gusfield (Philadelphia: Temple Univ. Press, 1994), 36–57.

43. See Antonio Gramsci, *Selections from the Prison Notebooks* (New York: International Publishers, 1971), 3–23.

44. See Dorothy Nelkin, *The Creation Controversy: Science or Scripture in the Schools* (New York: W. W. Norton, 1982), esp. 178–179.

45. For an analysis of the varying attitudes that social movements take toward experts and the various ways they approach them, see John Gaventa, "The Powerful, the Powerless, and the Experts: Knowledge Struggles in an Information Age," in *Voices of Change: Participatory Research in the United States and Canada,* ed. Peter Park et al. (Westport, Conn.: Bergin & Garvey, 1993), 21–40.

46. Phil Brown, "Popular Epidemiology and Toxic Waste Contamination: Lay and Professional Ways of Knowing," *Journal of Health and Social Behavior* 33 (September 1992): 267–281, quote from 269. For other relevant examples, see Giovanna Di Chiro, "Defining Environmental Justice: Women's Voices and Grassroots Politics," *Socialist Review,* October-December 1992, 93–130; Diana Dutton, "The Impact of Public Participation in Biomedical Policy: Evidence from Four Case Studies," in *Citizen Participation in Science Policy,* ed. James C. Petersen (Amherst: Univ. of Massachusetts Press, 1984), 147–181.

47. Cozzens and Woodhouse, "Science, Government, and the Politics of Knowledge," 547.

48. Ronald Bayer, "AIDS and the Gay Movement: Between the Specter and the Promise of Medicine," *Social Research* 52 (autumn 1985): 581–606.

49. The sociology of scientific knowledge is an important field within the broader domain known variously as science studies, science and technology studies, social studies of science, and so on. For some recent overviews and introductions to the sociology of scientific knowledge and/or the broader arena, see Steven Shapin, "Here and Everywhere: Sociology of Scientific Knowledge," *Annual Review of Sociology* 21 (1995): 289–321; Sheila

Jasanoff et al., eds., *Handbook of Science and Technology Studies* (Thousand Oaks, Calif.: Sage, 1995); Adele E. Clarke and Joan H. Fujimura, "What Tools? Which Jobs? Why Right?" in *The Right Tools for the Job: At Work in Twentieth-Century Life Sciences,* ed. Adele E. Clarke and Joan H. Fujimura (Princeton, N.J.: Princeton Univ. Press, 1992), 3–44; Collins and Pinch, *Golem;* Susan E. Cozzens and Thomas F. Gieryn, "Introduction: Putting Science Back in Society," in *Theories of Science in Society,* ed. Susan E. Cozzens and Thomas F. Gieryn (Bloomington: Indiana Univ. Press, 1990), 1–14; Karin D. Knorr-Cetina and Michael Mulkay, "Introduction: Emerging Principles in Social Studies of Science," in *Science Observed: Perspectives on the Social Study of Science,* ed. Karin D. Knorr-Cetina and Michael Mulkay (London: Sage, 1993), 1–17; Andrew Pickering, "From Science as Knowledge to Science as Practice," in *Science as Practice and Culture,* ed. Andrew Pickering (Chicago: Univ. of Chicago Press, 1992), 1–26.

50. Shapin, "Here and Everywhere," 305.

51. See note 2 above.

52. Bruno Latour, *Science in Action* (Cambridge, Mass: Harvard Univ. Press, 1987). For an extension of this model to the construction of expertise, see Alberto Cambrosio, Camille Limoges, and Eric Hoffman, "Expertise as a Network: A Case Study of the Controversy over the Environmental Release of Genetically Engineered Organisms," in *The Culture and Power of Knowledge: Inquiries into Contemporary Societies,* ed. Nico Stehr and Richard V. Ericson (Berlin: Walter de Gruyter, 1992), 341–361.

53. See, in particular, Shapin, *Social History of Truth.*

54. Barry Barnes, *About Science* (Oxford: Basil Blackwell, 1985), 83.

55. Harry Collins, *Changing Order: Replication and Induction in Scientific Practice,* 2d ed. (Chicago: Univ. of Chicago Press, 1992), 130.

56. Shapin, *Social History of Truth,* 17; see also 52, n. 44.

57. See Stephen P. Turner, "Forms of Patronage," in *Theories of Science in Society,* ed. Susan E. Cozzens and Thomas F. Gieryn (Bloomington: Indiana Univ. Press, 1990), 185–211.

58. Shapin, *Social History of Truth,* 416. Shapin borrows the phrase "access points" from Anthony Giddens, *The Consequences of Modernity* (Stanford, Calif.: Stanford Univ. Press, 1989), 83.

59. Turner, "Forms of Patronage"; Chandra Mukerji, *A Fragile Power: Scientists and the State* (Princeton, N.J.: Princeton Univ. Press, 1989).

60. Naomi Aronson, "Science as a Claims-Making Activity," in *Studies in the Sociology of Social Problems,* ed. Joseph W. Schneider and John I. Kitsuse (Norwood, N.J.: Ablex Publishing, 1984), 1–30.

61. Gieryn, "Boundary Work"; Gieryn, "Boundaries of Science." On this point more generally, see Andrew Abbott, *The System of Professions: An Essay on the Division of Expert Labor* (Chicago: Univ. of Chicago Press, 1988).

62. Dorothy Nelkin, "Managing Biomedical News," *Social Research* 52 (autumn 1985): 625–646.

63. Barnes and Edge, "Science as Expertise"; Nelkin, "Political Impact of Technical Expertise."

64. Brian Wynne, "Between Orthodoxy and Oblivion: The Normalisation

of Deviance in Science," in *On the Margins of Science: The Social Construction of Rejected Knowledge,* ed. Roy Wallis (Keele, England: Univ. of Keele Press, 1979), 67–84, quote from 79.

65. Shapin, "Cordelia's Love," 260.

66. Collins, *Changing Order,* 142–145.

67. For critiques of Collins in this regard, see Brian Wynne, "Public Uptake of Science: A Case for Institutional Reflexivity," *Public Understanding of Science* 2 (1993): 321–337; Hilary Arksey, "Expert and Lay Participation in the Construction of Medical Knowledge," *Sociology of Health & Illness* 16 (September 1994): 448–468; Evelleen Richards, "(Un)boxing the Monster," *Social Studies of Science* 26 (May 1996): 323–356.

68. Harry M. Collins and Trevor J. Pinch, "The Construction of the Paranormal: Nothing Unscientific is Happening," in *On the Margins of Science: The Social Construction of Rejected Knowledge,* ed. Roy Wallis (Keele, England: Univ. of Keele Press, 1979), 237–270.

69. Wynne, "Public Uptake of Science," 331.

70. Quoted in Adele Clarke and Theresa Montini, "The Many Faces of RU486: Tales of Situated Knowledges and Technological Contestations," *Science, Technology & Human Values* 18 (winter 1993): 42–78, quote from 45.

71. Latour, *Science in Action,* 175–176.

72. Gieryn, "Boundary Work"; Gieryn, "Boundaries of Science."

73. Adele Clarke, "A Social Worlds Adventure: The Case of Reproductive Science," in *Theories of Science in Society,* ed. Susan E. Cozzens and Thomas F. Gieryn (Bloomington: Indiana Univ. Press, 1990), 15–42, quote from 18 (I have removed the emphasis on the word "activities" that appeared in the original text). See also Elihu M. Gerson, "Scientific Work and Social Worlds," *Knowledge: Creation, Diffusion, Utilization* 4 (March 1983): 357–377; Joan H. Fujimura, "The Molecular Biological Bandwagon in Cancer Research: Where Social Worlds Meet," *Social Problems* 35 (June 1988), 261–283; Susan Leigh Star and James R. Griesemer, "Institutional Ecology, 'Translations' and Boundary Objects: Amateurs and Professionals in Berkeley's Museum of Vertebrate Zoology, 1907–39," *Social Studies of Science* 19 (August 1989): 387–420.

74. On boundary objects in science, see Star and Griesemer, "Institutional Ecology, 'Translations' and Boundary Objects."

75. Bourdieu, *Logic of Practice;* Pierre Bourdieu, "The Genesis of the Concepts of *Habitus* and of *Field,*" *Sociocriticism* 2 (December 1985), 11–24. Fields are defined in terms of "objective relations between positions" that correlate with "the structure of the distribution of species of power (or capital) whose possession commands access to the specific profits that are at stake in the field" (Pierre Bourdieu and Loïc J. D. Wacquant, *An Invitation to Reflexive Sociology* [Chicago: Univ. of Chicago Press, 1992], 97).

76. In the end, however, Bourdieu's specific conception of the *scientific* field is unduly narrow: Bourdieu portrays scientific practice as something carried out in a world of laboratories, universities, and peer-reviewed journals but apparently not in a world of foundations, defense departments, and private industries, let alone activist movements and the mass media. Thus,

ironically, his own depiction of the scientific field would be inappropriate for
an analysis of the production of scientific knowledge in the AIDS epidemic.
Nevertheless, in conceptualizing my work, I find his general theoretical per-
spective on fields to be useful, as is his understanding of the scientific field as
"the locus of a competitive struggle, in which the *specific* issue at stake is the
monopoly of *scientific authority.*" See Bourdieu, "Specificity of the Scientific
Field," 19 (emphasis in the original); Pierre Bourdieu, "Animadversiones in
Mertonem," in *Robert K. Merton: Consensus and Controversy,* ed. Jon Clark,
Celia Modgil, and Sohan Modgil (London: Falmer Press, 1990), 297–301;
Pierre Bourdieu, "The Peculiar History of Scientific Reason," *Sociological Fo-*
rum 6 (March 1991): 3–26. For a critique of Bourdieu's conception of science,
see Karin D. Knorr-Cetina, "Scientific Communities or Transepistemic Arenas
of Research? A Critique of Quasi-Economic Models of Science," *Social Stud-*
ies of Science 12 (February 1982): 101–130.

77. Dorothy Nelkin, "Controversies and the Authority of Science," in *Sci-*
entific Controversies: Case Studies in the Resolution and Closure of Disputes
in Science and Technology, ed. H. Tristram Engelhardt Jr. and Arthur L.
Caplan (Cambridge, England: Cambridge Univ. Press, 1987), 283–293.

78. James M. Jasper and Dorothy Nelkin, *The Animal Rights Crusade:*
The Growth of a Moral Protest (New York: Free Press, 1992).

79. Lily M. Hoffman, *The Politics of Knowledge: Activist Movements in*
Medicine and Planning (Albany: State Univ. of New York Press, 1989); Kelly
Moore, "Doing Good While Doing Science: The Origins and Consequences
of Public Interest Science Organizations in America, 1945–1990" (Ph.D. diss.,
University of Arizona, 1993); Rob Kling and Suzanne Iacono, "The Mobiliza-
tion of Support for Computerization: Computerization Movements," *Social*
Problems 35 (June 1988): 226–243.

80. Bart Simon, "Post-Closure Cold Fusion and the Survival of a Research
Community: An Hauntology for the Scientific Afterlife" (Ph.D. diss., University of California, San Diego, forthcoming). Other studies of the relation between activism and science include Brian Balogh, *Chain Reaction: Expert De-*
bate and Public Participation in American Commercial Nuclear Power, 1945–
1975 (Cambridge, England: Cambridge Univ. Press, 1991); Brown, "Popular
Epidemiology"; Joske Bunders and Loet Leydesdorff, "The Causes and Con-
sequences of Collaborations between Scientists and Non-Scientist Groups," in
The Social Direction of the Public Sciences, ed. Stuart Blume et al. (Dordrecht,
Holland: D. Reidel, 1987), 331–347; Cozzens and Woodhouse, "Science,
Government, and the Politics of Knowledge"; Jacqueline Cramer, Ron Eyer-
man, and Andrew Jamison, "The Knowledge Interests of the Environmental
Movement and Its Potential for Influencing the Development of Science," in
The Social Direction of the Public Sciences (above), 89–115; Di Chiro, "De-
fining Environmental Justice"; Dutton, "Impact of Public Participation"; Deb-
bie Indyk and David Rier, "Grassroots AIDS Knowledge: Implications for the
Boundaries of Science and Collective Action," *Knowledge: Creation, Diffu-*
sion, Utilization 15 (September 1993): 3–43; Robert W. Rycroft, "Environmentalism and Science: Politics and the Pursuit of Knowledge," *Knowledge:*
Creation, Diffusion, Utilization 13 (December 1991): 150–169; von Gizycki,

"Cooperation between Medical Researchers and a Self-Help Movement"; and the essays in James C. Petersen, ed., *Citizen Participation in Science Policy* (Amherst: Univ. of Massachusetts Press, 1984).

81. But see James C. Petersen and Gerald E. Markle, "Expansion of Conflict in Cancer Controversies," *Research in Social Movements, Conflicts and Change* 4 (1981): 151–169; Moore, "Doing Good While Doing Science"; Indyk and Rier, "Grassroots AIDS Knowledge."

82. See, for example, Bert Klandermans, "The Formation and Mobilization of Consensus," *International Social Movement Research* 1 (1988): 173–196; Bert Klandermans and Sidney Tarrow, "Mobilization into Social Movements: Synthesizing European and American Approaches," *International Social Movement Research* 1 (1988): 1–38.

83. See, for example, Alberto Melucci, *Nomads of the Present: Social Movements and Individual Needs in Contemporary Society* (Philadelphia: Temple Univ. Press, 1989); Verta Taylor and Nancy E. Whittier, "Collective Identity in Social Movement Communities: Lesbian Feminist Mobilization," in *Frontiers in Social Movement Theory*, ed. Aldon D. Morris and Carol McClurg Mueller (New Haven: Yale Univ. Press, 1992), 104–129; William A. Gamson, "The Social Psychology of Collective Action," in *Frontiers in Social Movement Theory* (above), 53–76; Joshua Gamson, "Must Identity Movements Self-Destruct? A Queer Dilemma," *Social Problems* 42 (August 1995): 390–407; Arlene Stein, "Sisters and Queers: The Decentering of Lesbian Feminism," *Socialist Review*, January-March 1992, 33–55; Hank Johnston, Enrique Laraña, and Joseph R. Gusfield, "Identities, Grievances, and New Social Movements," in *New Social Movements: From Ideology to Identity*, ed. Enrique Laraña, Hank Johnston, and Joseph R. Gusfield (Philadelphia: Temple Univ. Press, 1994), 3–35.

84. See Todd Gitlin, *The Whole World Is Watching: Mass Media in the Making and Unmaking of the New Left* (Berkeley: Univ. of California Press, 1980), 6; David A. Snow et al., "Frame Alignment Processes: Micromobilization and Movement Participation," *American Sociological Review* 51 (August 1986): 464–481; David A. Snow and Robert D. Benford, "Ideology, Frame Resonance, and Participant Mobilization," *International Social Movement Research* 1 (1988): 197–217; Robert D. Benford and Scott A. Hunt, "Dramaturgy and Social Movements: The Social Construction and Communication of Power," *Sociological Inquiry* 62 (February 1992): 36–55; William A. Gamson, "Political Discourse and Collective Action," *International Social Movements Research* 1 (1988): 219–244; Hugh Mehan and John Wills, "MEND: A Nurturing Voice in the Nuclear Arms Debate," *Social Problems* 35 (October 1988): 363–383.

85. Petersen and Markle, "Expansion of Conflict," 153. On resource mobilization more generally, see W. Gamson, *Strategy of Social Protest;* McCarthy and Zald, "Resource Mobilization and Social Movements."

86. Indyk and Rier, "Grassroots AIDS Knowledge."

87. See, for example, Carl Boggs, *Social Movements and Political Power: Emerging Forms of Radicalism in the West* (Philadelphia: Temple Univ. Press, 1986); Jean Cohen, "Strategy or Identity: New Theoretical Paradigms and

Contemporary Social Movements," *Social Research* 52 (winter 1985): 663–716; Barbara Epstein, *Political Protest and Cultural Revolution: Nonviolent Direct Action in the 1970s and 1980s* (Berkeley: Univ. of California Press, 1991); Jürgen Habermas, "New Social Movements," *Telos* 49 (fall 1981): 33–37; H. Kriesi, "New Social Movements and the New Class in the Netherlands," *American Journal of Sociology* 94 (March 1989): 1078–1116; Melucci, *Nomads of the Present;* Claus Offe, "New Social Movements: Challenging the Boundaries of Institutional Politics," *Social Research* 52 (winter 1985): 817–868; Alain Touraine, "An Introduction to the Study of Social Movements," *Social Research* 52 (winter 1985): 749–787; the essays in Aldon D. Morris and Carol McClurg Mueller, eds., *Frontiers in Social Movement Theory* (New Haven: Yale Univ. Press, 1992); and the essays in Enrique Laraña, Hank Johnston, and Joseph R. Gusfield, eds., *New Social Movements: From Ideology to Identity* (Philadelphia: Temple Univ. Press, 1994).

That sociology of science has not engaged with the literature on new social movements is, however, less surprising than the fact that the AIDS movement has been ignored by those who study new social movements. For exceptions, see Joshua Gamson, "Silence, Death, and the Invisible Enemy: AIDS Activism and Social Movement 'Newness,'" *Social Problems* 36 (October 1989): 351–365; C. Cohen, "Power, Resistance and the Construction of Crisis"; Gilbert Elbaz, "The Sociology of AIDS Activism, the Case of ACT UP/New York, 1987–1992" (Ph.D. diss., City University of New York, 1992).

88. Alvin W. Gouldner, *The Future of Intellectuals and the Rise of the New Class* (New York: Oxford Univ. Press, 1979).

89. Habermas, "New Social Movements," 33.

90. Johnston, Laraña, and Gusfield, "Identities, Grievances, and New Social Movements," 6–9.

91. David M. Halperin, *Saint Foucault: Toward a Gay Hagiography* (New York: Oxford Univ. Press, 1995), 27. See also Simon Watney, *Policing Desire: Pornography, AIDS and the Media* (Minneapolis: Univ. of Minnesota Press, 1987).

92. Jean Comaroff, "Medicine: Symbol and Ideology," in *The Problem of Medical Knowledge,* ed. Peter Wright and Andrew Treacher (Edinburgh: Edinburgh Univ. Press, 1982), 49–68, quote from 51.

93. Melucci, *Nomads of the Present,* 125.

94. On medicine and the body, see Bryan S. Turner, *Medical Power and Social Knowledge* (London: Sage, 1987); David Armstrong, *Political Anatomy of the Body: Medical Knowledge in Britain in the Twentieth Century* (Cambridge, England: Cambridge Univ. Press, 1983); Deborah Lupton, *Medicine as Culture: Illness, Disease and the Body in Western Societies* (London: Sage, 1994), chapter 2.

95. Jim Eigo, "How AIDS Will Change the Way We Test Drugs" (paper presented at the annual conference of the American Academy for the Advancement of Science, Washington, D.C., 17 February, 1991), tape recorded proceedings.

96. Jean Cohen, "Strategy or Identity," 694.

97. W. Gamson, "Social Psychology of Collective Action," 60. On collec-

tive identity, see also the citations in note 83. Within science studies, it is Brian Wynne who has most forcefully insisted that the construction and renegotiation of a social identity is what gives rise to "the unacknowledged reflexive capability of laypeople in articulating responses to scientific expertise" ("Misunderstood Misunderstandings: Social Identities and Public Uptake of Science," *Public Understanding of Science* 1 [July 1992]: 281–304, quote from 301).

98. J. Gamson, "Silence, Death, and the Invisible Enemy," 355, 358.

99. For Foucault's understanding of new social movements as those movements that resist normalization, see Michel Foucault, "The Subject and Power," in *Michel Foucault: Beyond Structuralism and Hermeneutics*, ed. Hubert Dreyfus and Paul Rabinow (Chicago: Univ. of Chicago Press, 1983), 211–212.

100. Pierre Bourdieu, "Symbolic Power," *Critique of Anthropology* 4 (summer 1979): 77–85.

101. See, for example, H. M. Collins, "Certainty and the Public Understanding of Science: Science on Television," *Social Studies of Science* 17 (November 1987): 689–713; Thomas F. Gieryn and Anne E. Figert, "Ingredients for a Theory of Science in Society: O-Rings, Ice Water, C-Clamp, Richard Feynman, and the Press," in *Theories of Science in Society*, ed. Susan E. Cozzens and Thomas F. Gieryn (Bloomington: Indiana Univ. Press, 1990), 67–97; Rae Goodell, "The Role of the Mass Media in Scientific Controversies," in *Scientific Controversies: Case Studies in the Resolution and Closure of Disputes in Science and Technology*, ed. H. Tristram Engelhardt Jr. and Arthur L. Caplan (Cambridge, England: Cambridge Univ. Press, 1987), 585–597; Anne Karpf, *Doctoring the Media: The Reporting of Health and Medicine* (London: Routledge, 1988); Nelkin, "Managing Biomedical News."

102. David Phillips et al., "Importance of the Lay Press in the Transmission of Medical Knowledge to the Scientific Community," *New England Journal of Medicine* 325 (17 October 1991): 1180–1183, quote from 1183.

103. Klandermans, "Formation and Mobilization of Consensus," 186.

104. On the capacity of the gay and lesbian press, as an alternative-media institution, to be more resistant to the automatic ratification of medical authority, see Matthew Paul McAllister, "Medicalization in the News Media: A Comparison of AIDS Coverage in Three Newspapers" (Ph.D. diss., University of Illinois at Urbana-Champaign, 1990), 97–106. On alternative media in general, see Nina Eliasoph, "Routines and the Making of Oppositional News," *Critical Studies in Mass Communication* 5 (December 1988): 313–334.

105. See Indyk and Rier, "Grassroots AIDS Knowledge"; Katherine Bishop, "Underground Press Leads Way on AIDS Advice," *New York Times*, 16 December 1991, A-16.

106. See Stephen Hilgartner, "The Dominant View of Popularization: Conceptual Problems, Political Uses," *Social Studies of Science* 20 (August 1990): 519–539.

107. Indyk and Rier, "Grassroots AIDS Knowledge," 15.

108. Abbott, *System of Professions*, 323. On the professions, see also Burton J. Bledstein, *The Culture of Professionalism: The Middle Class and the*

372 NOTES TO PAGES 23–24

Development of Higher Education in America (New York: W. W. Norton, 1976); Magali Sarfatti Larson, *The Rise of Professionalism: A Sociological Analysis* (Berkeley: Univ. of California Press, 1977). On the medical profession in particular, see also Charles L. Bosk, *Forgive and Remember: Managing Medical Failure* (Univ. of Chicago Press, 1979); Eliot Freidson, *Profession of Medicine: A Study of the Sociology of Applied Knowledge* (Chicago: Univ. of Chicago Press, 1988); Starr, *Social Transformation of American Medicine.*

109. Foucault, *Discipline and Punish;* Michel Foucault, *The History of Sexuality* (Vol. 1: An Introduction) (New York: Vintage Books, 1980).

110. Eliot Freidson, "The Impurity of Professional Authority," in *Institutions and the Person,* ed. Howard S. Becker et al. (Chicago: Aldine, 1968), 25–34.

111. On the "art" vs "science" distinction in medicine, see Deborah R. Gordon, "Clinical Science and Clinical Expertise: Changing Boundaries between Art and Science in Medicine," in *Biomedicine Examined,* ed. M. Lock and D. R. Gordon (Dordrecht, Holland: Kluwer Academic Publishing, 1988), 257–295. On the related distinction between the "applied" knowledge of the practitioner and the "formal" knowledge of the academic, see Eliot Freidson, *Professional Powers: A Study of the Institutionalization of Formal Knowledge* (Chicago: Univ. of Chicago Press, 1986).

112. For a mission statement in that regard, see Monica J. Casper and Marc Berg, "Constructivist Perspectives on Medical Work: Medical Practices and Science and Technology Studies," *Science, Technology, & Human Values* 20 (autumn 1995): 395–407.

113. Snow and Benford have noted that social movements first diagnose problems and attribute blame or causality, then offer a prognosis by specifying solutions, strategies, tactics, and targets ("Ideology, Frame Resonance, and Participant Mobilization," 197–217). Abbott, in his study of the professions, identified the "sequence of diagnosis, inference, and treatment" as "the essential cultural logic of professional practice" (Abbott, *System of Professions,* 40). Michael Schudson used equivalent terms to describe the professional orientation of news reporters in their packaging of social reality in the form of stories (Michael Schudson, *Discovering the News: A Social History of American Newspapers* [New York: Basic Books, 1978]).

114. Gitlin, *The Whole World Is Watching,* 6; see also Erving Goffman, *Frame Analysis: An Essay on the Organization of Experience* (New York: Harper & Row, 1974), 10–11.

115. Gitlin, *Whole World Is Watching,* 28.

116. Charles E. Rosenberg, "Framing Disease: Illness, Society, and History (Introduction)," in *Framing Disease: Studies in Cultural History,* ed. Charles E. Rosenberg and Janet Golden (New Brunswick, N.J.: Rutgers Univ. Press, 1992), xiii–xxvi. Although she has used a different vocabulary, Susan Sontag is also fundamentally concerned with the "framing of disease" and "disease as frame"; see *Illness as Metaphor* (New York: Farrar, Straus and Giroux, 1978) and *AIDS and Its Metaphors* (New York: Farrar, Straus and Giroux, 1989).

117. Joel Best, "Introduction: Typification and Social Problems Construc-

tion," in *Images of Issues: Typifying Contemporary Social Problems,* ed. Joel Best (New York: Aldine de Gruyter, 1989), xv–xxii. See also Joseph W. Schneider and John I. Kitsuse, eds., *Studies in the Sociology of Social Problems* (Norwood, N.J.: Albex, 1984); Joseph R. Gusfield, *The Culture of Public Problems* (Chicago: Univ. of Chicago Press, 1981).

118. See note 84 above.

119. Snow and Benford, "Ideology, Frame Resonance, and Participant Mobilization," 198.

120. David A. Snow and Robert D. Benford, "Master Frames and Cycles of Protest," in *Frontiers in Social Movement Theory,* ed. Aldon D. Morris and Carol McClurg Mueller (New Haven: Yale Univ. Press, 1992), 133–155.

121. Clearly there are unexplored affinities here between the conceptions of mobilization, representation, and collective identity formation that have been developed in the study of social movements and parallel concepts in science studies. One obvious example is Latour's notion of "enrollment" (*Science in Action*). Another is Shapin's analysis of how the constitution of personal and collective scientific identities was a crucial step in the creation of modern scientific organizations and methods and a prerequisite for the production of credible scientific knowledge (*Social History of Truth,* 42–64, 126 ff). See also Brian Wynne's analysis of collective identity in "Misunderstood Misunderstandings."

122. Shapin, "Cordelia's Love," 260.

123. Cf. Paul Starr's observation that authority rests on the "twin supports of dependence and legitimacy": "When one is weak, the other may take over . . ." (*Social Transformation of American Medicine,* 10).

124. See Latour's discussion of the stripping away of "modalities" (qualifiers) in the construction of scientific facts in *Science in Action,* 22 ff.

125. F. Barré-Sinoussi et al., "Isolation of a T-Lymphotropic Retrovirus from a Patient at Risk for Acquired Immune Deficiency Syndrome (AIDS)," *Science* 220 (20 May 1983): 868–870; Robert C. Gallo et al., "Frequent Detection and Isolation of Cytopathic Retroviruses (HTLV-III) from Patients with AIDS and at Risk for AIDS," *Science* 224 (4 May 1984): 500–502; Jay A. Levy et al., "Isolation of Lymphocytopathic Retroviruses from San Francisco Patients with AIDS," *Science* 225 (24 August 1984): 840–842.

126. The phrase is from Cindy Patton, *Inventing AIDS* (New York: Routledge, 1990), chapter 3.

127. Peter Duesberg, "Retroviruses as Carcinogens and Pathogens: Expectations and Reality," *Cancer Research* 47 (1 March 1987): 1199–1220; quote from 1215.

128. P. H. Duesberg, "The Role of Drugs in the Origin of AIDS," *Biomedicine & Pharmacotherapy* 46 (January 1992): 10.

129. Jon Cohen, "The Duesberg Phenomenon," *Science* 266 (9 December 1994): 1642–1649.

130. Manfred Eigen, "The AIDS Debate," *Naturwissenschaften* 76 (August 1989): 341–350; Luis Benitez Bribiesca, "¿Son En Verdad Los VIH Los Agentes Causales Del SIDA?" *Gaceta Médica de México* 127 (January–February 1991): 75–84.

131. Joel N. Shurkin, "The AIDS Debate: Another View," *Los Angeles Times*, 18 January 1988, II-4; Philip M. Boffey, "A Solitary Dissenter Disputes Cause of AIDS," *New York Times*, 12 January 1988, C-3; Neville Hodgkinson, "Experts Mount Startling Challenge to Aids Orthodoxy," *Sunday Times* (London), 26 April 1992, 1.

132. National Public Radio (segment reported by Mike Hornwick, Canadian Broadcasting Corporation), *NPR Weekend Edition*, 16 May 1992; Gary Null, "AIDS: A Man-Made Plague?" *Penthouse*, January 1989, 160.

133. "Who Are the HIV Heretics?: Discussion Paper #5" (Project Inform, San Francisco, 3 June, 1992, photocopy); Celia Farber, "AIDS: Words from the Front." *Spin*, January 1988, 43–44, 73.

134. See chapters 3 and 4 for many examples.

135. See, for instance, Tom Bethell, "Heretic," *American Spectator*, May 1992, 18–19.

136. Peter H. Duesberg and Bryan J. Ellison, "Peter H. Duesberg and Bryan J. Ellison Respond," *Heritage Foundation Policy Review*, fall 1990, 81–83 (letter to the editor).

137. From the public forum at the VIII International Conference on AIDS Update, San Francisco, 10 August 1992 (author's field notes).

138. Latour, *Science in Action*, chapter 1.

139. Collins, *Changing Order*, 162.

140. See Henry Frankel, "The Continental Drift Debate," in *Scientific Controversies: Case Studies in the Resolution and Closure of Disputes in Science and Technology*, ed. H. Tristram Engelhardt Jr. and Arthur L. Caplan (Cambridge, England: Cambridge Univ. Press, 1987), 203–248.

141. Jad Adams, "Paradigm Unvisited," *Heritage Foundation Policy Review*, fall 1990, 75–76 (letter to the editor).

142. On closure in scientific controversies, see H. Tristram Engelhardt Jr. and Arthur L. Caplan, eds., *Scientific Controversies: Case Studies in the Resolution and Closure of Disputes in Science and Technology* (Cambridge, England: Cambridge Univ. Press, 1987); Harry Collins, "The Seven Sexes: A Study in the Sociology of a Phenomenon, or the Replication of Experiments in Physics," *Sociology* 9 (May 1975): 205–224; Peter Galison, *How Experiments End* (Chicago: Univ. of Chicago Press, 1987).

143. Jason DeParle, "Rush, Rash, Effective, Act-Up Shifts AIDS Policy," *New York Times*, 3 January 1990, B-1.

144. Albert R. Jonsen and Jeff Stryker, eds., *The Social Impact of AIDS in the United States* (Washington, D.C.: National Academy Press, 1993), 89–90.

145. Gregg Gonsalves and Mark Harrington, "AIDS Research at the NIH: A Critical Review. Part I: Summary" (Treatment Action Group, New York, 1992, photocopy), 1.

146. See Gregg Gonsalves, "Basic Research on HIV Infection: A Report from the Front" (Treatment Action Group, New York, 1993, photocopy); Martin Delaney, "The Evolution of Community-Based Research" (Plenary Address at the IX International Conference on AIDS), Berlin, 8 June 1993.

147. There is an emergent literature in science studies on the history, functions, and controversies surrounding the randomized clinical trial. See Harry

Milton Marks, "Ideas as Reforms: Therapeutic Experiments and Medical Practice, 1900–1980" (Ph.D. diss., Massachusetts Institute of Technology, 1987); Evelleen Richards, "The Politics of Therapeutic Evaluation: The Vitamin C and Cancer Controversy," *Social Studies of Science* 18 (1988), 653–701; Evelleen Richards, *Vitamin C and Cancer: Medicine or Politics?* (New York: St. Martin's, 1991); Anni Dugdale, "Devices and Desires: Constructing the Intrauterine Device, 1908–1988" (Ph.D. diss., Univ. of Wollongong, Australia, 1995); Marcia Lynn Meldrum, "'Departing from the Design': The Randomized Clinical Trial in Historical Context, 1946–1970" (Ph.D. diss., State University of New York at Stony Brook, 1994); J. Rosser Matthews, *Quantification and the Quest for Medical Certainty* (Princeton: Princeton Univ. Press, 1995); Caroline Jean Acker, "Addiction and the Laboratory: The Work of the National Research Council's Committee on Drug Addiction, 1928–1939," *Isis* 86 (June 1995): 167–193; Alan Yoshioka, "British Clinical Trials of Streptomycin, 1946–51" (Ph.D. diss., Imperial College, forthcoming).

148. See Robert M. Veatch, *The Patient as Partner: A Theory of Human-Experimentation Ethics* (Bloomington: Indiana Univ. Press, 1987), 6–7, 211.

149. Meldrum, *Departing from the Design,* 384–386.

150. The latter phrase is borrowed from Richards, "Politics of Therapeutic Evaluation."

151. Douglas Richman, interview by author, tape recording, San Diego, 1 June 1994.

152. Shapin, "Cordelia's Love," 262.

153. On the denaturalization of research materials, see Adele E. Clarke, "Research Materials and Reproductive Science in the United States, 1910–1940," in *Physiology in the American Context, 1850–1940,* ed. Gerald L. Geison (Bethesda, Md.: American Physiological Society, 1987), 323–350. On the destabilization of technologies, see Ronald Kline and Trevor Pinch, "Taking the Black Box Off Its Wheels: The Social Construction of the Car in the Rural United States" (manuscript, Cornell University, 2 February 1995). On the tactic of revealing the "artifactual and conventional" status of the beliefs of one's opponents in scientific controversies, see Shapin and Schaffer, *Leviathan and the Air-Pump,* 7.

154. See Jack P. Lipton and Alan M. Hershaft, "On the Widespread Acceptance of Dubious Medical Findings," *Journal of Health and Social Behavior* 26 (December 1985): 336–351.

155. Sheila Jasanoff, *The Fifth Branch: Science Advisers as Policymakers* (Cambridge, Mass.: Harvard Univ. Press, 1990), chapter 8; Henk J. H. W. Bodewitz, Henk Buurma, and Gerard H. de Vries, "Regulatory Science and the Social Management of Trust in Medicine," in *The Social Construction of Technological Systems: New Directions in the Sociology and History of Technology,* ed. Wiebe E. Bijker, Thomas P. Hughes, and Trevor J. Pinch (Cambridge, Mass.: Massachusetts Institute of Technology Press, 1987), 243–259; John Abraham, "Distributing the Benefit of the Doubt: Scientists, Regulators, and Drug Safety," *Science, Technology, & Human Values* 19 (autumn 1994): 493–522; Brian Wynne, "Unruly Technology: Practical Rules, Impractical Discourses and Public Understanding," *Social Studies of Science,* 18

(1988), 147–167, esp. 162–63; Theodore M. Porter, *Trust in Numbers: The Pursuit of Objectivity in Science and Public Life* (Princeton, N.J.: Princeton Univ. Press, 1995), 203–216.

156. Jasanoff, *The Fifth Branch,* 76–83. On the adversarial culture of regulation in the United States, see Sheila Jasanoff, "Cross-National Differences in Policy Implementation," *Evaluation Review* 15 (February 1991): 103–119.

157. Randy Shilts, *And the Band Played On: Politics, People, and the AIDS Epidemic* (New York: St. Martin's, 1987). Shilts died of AIDS in 1994.

158. Steve Connor and Sharon Kingman, *The Search for the Virus,* 2d ed. (London: Penguin Books, 1989).

159. C. Self, W. Filardo, and W. Lancaster, "Acquired Immunodeficiency Syndrome (AIDS) and the Epidemic Growth of Its Literature," *Scientometrics* 17 (July 1989): 49–60; I. N. Sengupta and Lalita Kumari, "Bibliometric Analysis of AIDS Literature," *Scientometrics* 20 (1991): 297–315; Jonathan Elford, Robert Bor, and Pauline Summers, "Research into HIV and AIDS between 1981 and 1990: The Epidemic Curve," *AIDS* 5 (December 1991): 1515–1519; John S. Lyons et al., "A Systematic Analysis of the Quantity of AIDS Publications and the Quality of Research Methods in Three General Medical Journals," *Evaluation and Program Planning* 13 (1990): 73–77.

160. Henry Small and Edwin Greenlee, "A Co-Citation Study of AIDS Research," in *Scholarly Communication and Bibliometrics,* ed. Christine L. Borgman (Newbury Park, Calif.: Sage, 1990), 166–193.

161. See Indyk and Rier, "Grassroots AIDS Knowledge."

162. Dennis Altman, *AIDS in the Mind of America* (Garden City, N.J.: Anchor Press, 1986); Cindy Patton, *Sex and Germs: The Politics of AIDS* (Boston: South End Press, 1985).

163. Patton, *Inventing AIDS;* Dennis Altman, *Power and Community: Organizational and Cultural Responses to AIDS* (London: Taylor & Francis, 1994).

164. Paula A. Treichler, "AIDS: An Epidemic of Signification," in *AIDS: Cultural Analysis, Cultural Activism,* ed. Douglas Crimp (Cambridge, Mass.: Massachusetts Institute of Technology Press, 1988), 31–70; "AIDS, Gender, and Biomedical Discourse: Current Contests for Meaning," in *AIDS: The Burdens of History,* ed. Elizabeth Fee and Daniel M. Fox (Berkeley: Univ. of California Press, 1988), 190–266; "How to Have Theory in an Epidemic: The Evolution of AIDS Treatment Activism," in *Technoculture,* ed. Constance Penley and Andrew Ross (Minneapolis: Univ. of Minnesota Press, 1991), 57–106; "AIDS, HIV, and the Cultural Construction of Reality," in *The Time of AIDS: Social Analysis, Theory, and Method,* ed. Gilbert Herdt and Shirley Lindenbaum (Newbury Park, Calif.: Sage, 1992), 65–98.

165. Sontag, *AIDS and Its Metaphors;* Watney, *Policing Desire,* Simon Watney, "The Spectacle of AIDS," in *AIDS: Cultural Analysis, Cultural Activism,* ed. Douglas Crimp (Cambridge, Mass.: Massachusetts Institute of Technology Press, 1988), 71–86; Emily Martin, *Flexible Bodies: Tracking Immunity in American Culture—From the Days of Polio to the Age of AIDS* (Boston: Beacon Press, 1994); John Nguyet Erni, *Unstable Frontiers: Technomedicine and the Cultural Politics of "Curing" AIDS* (Minneapolis: Univ.

of Minnesota Press, 1994); Allan M. Brandt, "AIDS and Metaphor: Toward
the Social Meaning of Epidemic Disease," *Social Research* 55 (autumn 1988):
413–432; Sander Gilman, "AIDS and Syphilis: The Iconography of Disease,"
in *AIDS: Cultural Analysis, Cultural Activism,* ed. Douglas Crimp (Cambridge, Mass.: Massachusetts Institute of Technology Press, 1988), 87–107;
Laurence J. Ray, "AIDS as a Moral Metaphor: An Analysis of the Politics of
the 'Third Epidemic,'" *Archives Européennes de Sociologie* 30 (June 1989):
243–273; Alfred J. Fortin, "AIDS, Surveillance and Public Policy: The Politics
of Medical Discourse" (Ph.D. diss., University of Hawaii, 1989).

166. Watney, *Policing Desire;* Edward Albert, "AIDS and the Press: The
Creation and Transformation of a Social Problem," in *Images of Issues: Typi-
fying Contemporary Social Problems,* ed. Joel Best (New York: Aldine de
Gruyter, 1989), 39–54; David C. Colby and Timothy E. Cook, "Epidemics and
Agendas: The Politics of Nightly News Coverage of AIDS," *Journal of Health
Politics, Policy and Law* 16 (summer 1991): 215–249; James Kinsella, *Cov-
ering the Plague: AIDS and the American Media* (New Brunswick, N.J.: Rutg-
ers Univ. Press, 1989); McAllister, *Medicalization in the News Media;* Claudine
Herzlich and Janine Pierret, "The Construction of a Social Phenomenon: AIDS
in the French Press," *Social Science & Medicine* 29 (June 1989): 1235–1242;
Ivan Emke, "Speaking of AIDS in Canada: The Texts and Contexts of Official,
Counter-Cultural and Mass Media Discourses Surrounding AIDS" (Ph.D.
diss., Carleton University, Ottawa, Ontario, 1991); W. Russell Neuman, Mar-
ion R. Just, and Ann N. Crigler, *Common Knowledge: News and the Construction of Political Meaning* (Chicago: Univ. of Chicago Press, 1992).

167. C. Cohen, "Power, Resistance and the Construction of Crisis";
Corea, *Invisible Epidemic;* Elbaz, "Sociology of AIDS Activism"; J. Gamson,
"Silence, Death, and the Invisible Enemy"; Beth E. Schneider and Nancy E.
Stoller, eds., *Women Resisting AIDS: Feminist Strategies of Empowerment*
(Philadelphia: Temple Univ. Press, 1995); Maxine Wolfe, "The AIDS Coali-
tion to Unleash Power, New York (ACT UP NY): A Direct Action Political
Model of Community Research for AIDS Prevention," in *AIDS Prevention
and Services: Community Based Research,* ed. J. Van Vugt (Westport, Conn.:
Bergin Garvey, forthcoming); Ernest Quimby and Samuel R. Friedman, "Dy-
namics of Black Mobilization against AIDS in New York City," *Social Prob-
lems* 36 (October 1989): 403–415; Douglas Crimp and Adam Rolston, *AIDS
Demographics* (Seattle: Bay Press, 1990); Ty Geltmaker, "The Queer Nation
Acts Up: Health Care, Politics, and Sexual Diversity in the County of Angels,"
Society and Space 10 (December 1992): 609–650.

168. On women, see ACT UP/New York Women and AIDS Book Group,
Women, AIDS, and Activism (Boston: South End Press, 1990); Schneider and
Stoller, *Women Resisting AIDS;* Corea, *Invisible Epidemic;* Cindy Patton, *Last
Served: Gendering the HIV Pandemic* (London: Taylor & Francis, 1994). On
African-Americans, see C. Cohen, "Power, Resistance, and the Construction
of Crisis"; Harlon L. Dalton, "AIDS in Blackface," *Daedalus* 118 (summer
1989): 205–227; Evelynn Hammonds, "Race, Sex, AIDS: The Construction of
'Other,'" *Radical America,* November-December 1986, 28–36; Quimby and
Friedman, "Dynamics of Black Mobilization against AIDS." On Haitians, see

Paul Farmer, *AIDS and Accusation: Haiti and the Geography of Blame* (Berkeley: Univ. of California Press, 1992). On prostitutes, see Valerie Jenness, *Making It Work: The Prostitutes' Rights Movement in Perspective* (New York: Aldine de Gruyter, 1993). On injection drug users, see Don C. Des Jarlais, Samuel R. Friedman, and Jo L. Sotheran, "The First City: HIV among Intravenous Drug Users in New York City," in *AIDS: The Making of a Chronic Disease,* ed. Elizabeth Fee and Daniel M. Fox (Berkeley: Univ. of California Press, 1992), 279–295.

169. Charles L. Bosk and Joel E. Frader, "AIDS and Its Impact on Medical Work: The Culture and Politics of the Shop Floor," *Milbank Quarterly* 68, suppl. 2 (1990): 257–279; Mary-Rose Mueller, "Science in the Community: The Redistribution of Medical Authority in Federally Sponsored Treatment Research for AIDS" (Ph.D. diss., University of California at San Diego, 1995); Robert M. Wachter, *The Fragile Coalition: Scientists, Activists, and AIDS* (New York: St. Martin's, 1991); Robert M. Wachter, "The Impact of the Acquired Immunodeficiency Syndrome on Medical Residency Practice," *New England Journal of Medicine* 314 (16 January 1986): 177–180; Rosenberg, "Disease and Social Order in America."

170. For example, Charles Perrow and Mauro F. Guillén, *The AIDS Disaster* (New Haven: Yale Univ. Press, 1990); Ronald Bayer, *Private Acts, Social Consequences: AIDS and the Politics of Public Health* (New York: Free Press, 1989); David L. Kirp and Ronald Bayer, eds., *AIDS in the Industrialized Democracies: Passions, Politics, and Policies* (New Brunswick, N.J.: Rutgers Univ. Press, 1992); Sandra Panem, *The AIDS Bureaucracy* (Cambridge, Mass.: Harvard Univ. Press, 1988); Daniel M. Fox, "AIDS and the American Health Polity: The History and Prospects of a Crisis of Authority," in *AIDS: The Burdens of History,* ed. Elizabeth Fee and Daniel M. Fox (Berkeley: Univ. of California Press, 1988), 316–343; Michaël Pollak, Geneviève Paicheler, and Janine Pierret, *AIDS: A Problem for Sociological Research* (London: Sage, 1992); David L. Kirp et al., *Learning by Heart: AIDS and Schoolchildren in America's Communities* (New Brunswick, N.J.: Rutgers, 1989).

171. For example, Rose Weitz, *Life with AIDS* (New Brunswick, N.J.: Rutgers Univ. Press, 1991); Steven Seidman, "Transfiguring Sexual Identity: AIDS and the Contemporary Construction of Homosexuality," *Social Text* 19/20 (fall 1988): 187–205; Peter Conrad, "The Social Meaning of AIDS," *Social Policy* (summer 1986), 51–56; Eric Gilder, "The Process of Political *Praxis:* Efforts of the Gay Community to Transform the Social Signification of AIDS," *Communication Quarterly* 37 (winter 1989): 27–38; Richard Poirier, "AIDS and Traditions of Homophobia," *Social Research* 55 (autumn 1988): 461–475.

172. Murray and Payne, "Medical Policy without Scientific Evidence"; Stephen O. Murray and Kenneth W. Payne, "The Social Classification of AIDS in American Epidemiology," *Medical Anthropology* 10 (March 1989): 115–128; Gerald M. Oppenheimer, "In the Eye of the Storm: The Epidemiological Construction of AIDS," in *AIDS: The Burdens of History,* ed. Elizabeth Fee and Daniel M. Fox (Berkeley: Univ. of California Press, 1988), 267–300.

173. Joan H. Fujimura and Danny Y. Chou, "Dissent in Science: Styles of Scientific Practice and the Controversy over the Cause of AIDS," *Social Sci-*

ence and Medicine 38 (April 1994): 1017–1036. This article provides an intriguing analysis of the use of competing "styles of scientific practice" in the causation controversy. While offering an overview of the public dimensions of the Duesberg controversy, the authors have not placed those dimensions in the foreground where I believe they belong—as essential to the very constitution of the scientific controversy and the dynamics of its unfolding. On the AIDS causation controversy, see also Treichler, "AIDS, HIV, and the Cultural Construction of Reality."

174. Peter S. Arno and Karyn L. Feiden, *Against the Odds: The Story of AIDS Drug Development, Politics and Profits* (New York: HarperCollins, 1992); Jonathan Kwitny, *Acceptable Risks* (New York: Poseidon Press, 1992); Bruce Nussbaum, *Good Intentions: How Big Business and the Medical Establishment Are Corrupting the Fight Against AIDS* (New York: Atlantic Monthly Press, 1990); Wachter, *The Fragile Coalition;* Harold Edgar and David J. Rothman, "New Rules for New Drugs: The Challenge of AIDS to the Regulatory Process," *The Milbank Quarterly* 68, suppl. 1 (1990): 111–142; Corea, *Invisible Epidemic;* Mueller, "Science in the Community"; Jonsen and Stryker, *Social Impact of AIDS,* chapter 4; Meurig Horton, "Bugs, Drugs and Placebos: The Opulence of Truth, or How to Make a Treatment Decision in an Epidemic," in *Taking Liberties: AIDS and Cultural Politics,* ed. Erica Carter and Simon Watney (London: Serpent's Tail, 1989), 161–181; Arthur D. Kahn, *AIDS: The Winter War* (Philadelphia: Temple Univ. Press, 1993); William Francis Patrick Crowley III, "Gaining Access: The Politics of AIDS Clinical Drug Trials in Boston" (undergraduate thesis, Harvard College, 1991). Another book on this subject is being published as this one goes to press: Elinor Burkett, *The Gravest Show on Earth: America in the Age of AIDS* (New York: Houghton Mifflin, 1995).

175. On vaccine development, see Christine Grady, *The Search for an AIDS Vaccine: Ethical Issues in the Development and Testing of a Preventive HIV Vaccine* (Bloomington: Indiana Univ. Press, 1995); P. Lurie et al., "Ethical, Behavioral, and Social Aspects of HIV Vaccine Trials in Developing Countries," *Journal of the American Medical Association* 271 (January 1994): 295–301.

Chapter 1

1. Dominique Lapierre, *Beyond Love,* trans. Kathryn Spink (New York: Warner Books, 1991), 51–54; Randy Shilts, *And the Band Played On: Politics, People, and the AIDS Epidemic* (New York: St. Martin's, 1987), 42–67.

2. "*Pneumocystis* Pneumonia—Los Angeles," *Morbidity and Mortality Weekly Report* 30 (5 June 1981): 250–252.

3. "Kaposi's Sarcoma and *Pneumocystis* Pneumonia among Homosexual Men—New York City and California," *Morbidity and Mortality Weekly Report* 30 (3 July 1981): 305–308.

4. Lawrence K. Altman, "Rare Cancer Seen in 41 Homosexuals," *New York Times,* 3 July 1981, A-20.

5. Lawrence Mass, "Cancer in the Gay Community," *New York Native,* 27 July 1981, 1, 21, 30.

6. Michael S. Gottlieb et al., "*Pneumocystis Carinii* Pneumonia and Mucosal Candidiasis Found in Previously Healthy Homosexual Men," *New England Journal of Medicine* 305 (10 December 1981): 1425–1431; Henry Masur et al., "An Outbreak of Community-Acquired *Pneumocystis Carinii* Pneumonia," *New England Journal of Medicine* 305 (10 December 1981): 1431–1438; Frederick P. Siegal et al., "Severe Acquired Immunodeficiency in Male Homosexuals, Manifested by Chronic Perianal Ulcerative Herpes Simplex Lesions," *New England Journal of Medicine* 305 (10 December 1981): 1439–1444; David T. Durack, "Opportunistic Infections and Kaposi's Sarcoma in Homosexual Men," *New England Journal of Medicine* 305 (10 December 1981): 1465–1467; Centers for Disease Control Task Force on Kaposi's Sarcoma and Opportunistic Infections, "Special Report: Epidemiologic Aspects of the Current Outbreak of Kaposi's Sarcoma and Opportunistic Infections," *New England Journal of Medicine* 306 (28 January 1982): 248–252.

7. Helper T cells go by various names, including T4 cells and CD4 cells, the latter term referring to the CD4 molecule that serves as the receptor site by which other entities bind to the cell. Colloquially, in discussions of AIDS, these cells are often simply called T cells, and I shall do the same except when it is important to distinguish the helper T cells from other varieties of T cells. Increasingly, however, laypeople who are "in the know" use the term "CD4" to demonstrate their linguistic competence. In the later chapters of the book, I adopt that term as well.

8. Siegal et al., "Severe Acquired Immunodeficiency in Male Homosexuals," 1441.

9. Robert O. Brennan and David T. Durack, "Gay Compromise Syndrome," *Lancet* 2 (December 1981): 1338–1339 (letter to the editor).

10. Masur et al., "Outbreak of Community-Acquired *Pneumocystis Carinii* Pneumonia."

11. Durack, "Opportunistic Infections and Kaposi's Sarcoma in Homosexual Men," 1466.

12. Matt Clark and Mariana Gosnell, "Diseases That Plague Gays," *Newsweek,* 21 December 1981, 51–52.

13. Dennis Altman, *AIDS in the Mind of America* (Garden City: Anchor Press/Doubleday, 1986), 33–36, esp. 35; see also Cindy Patton, *Sex and Germs: The Politics of AIDS* (Boston: South End Press, 1985), 6–7.

14. On "normalization," see Michel Foucault, *Discipline and Punish: The Birth of the Prison* (New York: Vintage Books, 1979).

15. Gottlieb et al., for instance, reported in December 1981 that, of four patients, one had been monogamous for four years, two had several regular partners, and only one "was highly sexually active and frequented homosexual bars and bathhouses" ("*Pneumocystis Carinii* Pneumonia and Mucosal Candidiasis," 1429).

16. Irving Kenneth Zola, "Pathways to the Doctor: From Person to Patient," in *Perspectives in Medical Sociology,* ed. Phil Brown (Belmont, Calif.: Wadsworth, 1989), 223–238, quote from 234.

17. Eliot Freidson, *Profession of Medicine: A Study of the Sociology of Applied Knowledge* (Chicago: Univ. of Chicago Press, 1988), 270.

18. David Perlman, "Drug Users Started AIDS Epidemic, Doctor Says," *San Francisco Chronicle,* 18 October 1985, 28; Cindy Patton, *Inventing AIDS* (New York: Routledge, 1990), 27–28.

19. The currency of this term has been reported by Shilts, among others, and it was used in the *New York Times* (Shilts, *And the Band Played On,* 121; Lawrence K. Altman, "New Homosexual Disorder Worries Health Officials," *New York Times,* 11 May 1982, C1). However, as Murray and Payne have noted, few instances can be found in the published medical literature, suggesting that "GRID" never became institutionalized as a legitimate designation for the syndrome (Stephen O. Murray and Kenneth W. Payne, "Medical Policy without Scientific Evidence: The Promiscuity Paradigm and AIDS," *California Sociologist* 11 [winter-summer 1988]: 13–54, esp. 44, note 5). But see Michael S. Gottlieb et al., "Gay-Related Immunodeficiency (GRID) Syndrome: Clinical and Autopsy Observations" (abstract submitted to the Thirty-Ninth Annual National Meeting of the American Federation for Clinical Research, Washington, D.C., 7–10 May 1982), *Clinical Research* 30 (April 1982): 349A; M. Vogt et al., "GRID-Syndrome," *Deutsche Medizinische Wochenschrift* 107 (15 October 1982): 1539–1542.

20. On "framing," see Erving Goffman, *Frame Analysis: An Essay on the Organization of Experience* (New York: Harper & Row, 1974). On the framing of illnesses, see Charles E. Rosenberg, "Introduction: Framing Disease: Illness, Society, and History," in *Framing Disease: Studies in Cultural History,* ed. Charles E. Rosenberg and Janet Golden (New Brunswick, N.J.: Rutgers Univ. Press, 1992), xiii–xxvi.

21. See Gerald M. Oppenheimer, "In the Eye of the Storm: The Epidemiological Construction of AIDS," in *AIDS: The Burdens of History,* ed. Elizabeth Fee and Daniel M. Fox (Berkeley: Univ. of California Press, 1988), 279–280.

22. Shilts, *And the Band Played On,* 83, 104, 171.

23. Henry L. Kazal et al., "The Gay Bowel Syndrome: Clinico-Pathologic Correlation in 260 Cases," *Annals of Clinical and Laboratory Science* 6 (March-April 1976): 184–192; Yehudi M. Felman, "Examining the Homosexual Male for Sexually Transmitted Diseases," *Journal of the American Medical Association* 238 (7 November 1977): 2046–2047; Samuel Vaisrub, "Homosexuality—A Risk Factor in Infectious Disease," *Journal of the American Medical Association* 238 (26 September 1977): 14 (editorial); Alexander McMillan, "Gonorrhea in Homosexual Men: Frequency of Infection by Culture Site," *Sexually Transmitted Diseases* 5 (October-December 1978): 146–150; Richard R. Babb, "Sexually Transmitted Infections in Homosexual Men," *Postgraduate Medicine* 65 (March 1979): 215–218; Yehudi M. Felman, "Homosexual Hazards," *The Practitioner* 224 (November 1980): 1151–1156; Franklyn N. Judson, "Comparative Prevalence Rates of Sexually Transmitted Diseases in Heterosexual and Homosexual Men," *American Journal of Epidemiology* 112 (December 1980): 836–843; William M. Owen Jr., "Sexually Transmitted

Diseases and Traumatic Problems in Homosexual Men," *Annals of Internal Medicine* 92 (June 1980): 805–808; H. Hunter Handsfield, "Sexually Transmitted Diseases in Homosexual Men," *American Journal of Public Health* 71 (September 1981): 989–990 (editorial); R. R. Willcox, "Sexual Behaviour and Sexually Transmitted Disease Patterns in Male Homosexuals," *British Journal of Venereal Diseases* 57 (June 1981): 167–169.

24. See Steven Epstein, "Moral Contagion and the Medicalizing of Gay Identity: AIDS in Historical Perspective," *Research in Law, Deviance and Social Control* 9 (1988): 3–36.

25. Felman, "Homosexual Hazards."

26. Michel Foucault, *The History of Sexuality*, vol. 1 (New York: Vintage, 1980), 43; Jeffrey Escoffier, "The Politics of Gay Identity," *Socialist Review*, July-October 1985, 119–153; Jeffrey Weeks, *Sexuality and Its Discontents: Meanings, Myths and Modern Sexualities* (London: Routledge & Kegan Paul, 1985); Peter Conrad and Joseph W. Schneider, *Deviance and Medicalization: From Badness to Sickness* (St. Louis: C. V. Mosby, 1980).

27. For a history of "gay bowel syndrome" and its relation to essentialist conceptions of the gay male body, see Michael Scarce, "Urban Bums and Rough Rides: A Bad Case of Gay Bowel Syndrome" (master's thesis, Ohio State University, 1995). Clearly, there are important parallels here to the medical portrayal of gender and racial differences; see Deborah Lupton, *Medicine as Culture: Illness, Disease and the Body in Western Societies* (London: Sage, 1994).

28. Alan P. Bell and Martin S. Weinberg, *Homosexualities: A Study of Diversity among Men and Women* (New York: Simon and Schuster, 1978).

29. In fact, most of these blanket characterizations of gay male sexuality were based on studies of patients at clinics for treatment of sexually transmitted diseases. One study did attempt to recruit a large sample of homosexual men from the "gay community" at large by distributing questionnaires in a gay magazine and through gay organizations (William Darrow et al., "The Gay Report on Sexually Transmitted Diseases," *American Journal of Public Health* 71 [September 1981]: 1004–1011); but it is doubtful that the 1.5 percent response rate generated a representative sample of readers of the magazine or members of the organizations, let alone members of "the gay community," whatever its supposed locus and boundaries.

30. "Immunocompromised Homosexuals," *Lancet* 2 (12 December 1981): 1326 (editorial).

31. Murray and Payne, "Medical Policy without Scientific Evidence"; Stephen O. Murray and Kenneth W. Payne, "The Social Classification of AIDS in American Epidemiology," *Medical Anthropology* 10 (March 1989): 115–128.

32. Quoted in "Safe-Sex Comic Book for Gays Riles Senate," *San Francisco Chronicle*, 15 October 1987, A-7.

33. Jana L. Armstrong, "Causal Explanations of AIDS," in *The Meaning of AIDS: Implications for Medical Science, Clinical Practice, and Public Health Policy*, ed. Eric T. Juengst and Barbara A. Koenig (New York: Praeger, 1989), 12.

34. *Dorland's Illustrated Medical Dictionary,* 27th ed. (Philadelphia: W. B. Saunders Company, 1988), 285.

35. Charles Rosenberg, *The Cholera Years* (Chicago: Univ. of Chicago Press, 1962), 133–150.

36. Judith Walkowitz, *Prostitution and Victorian Society: Women, Class, and the State* (Cambridge, England: Cambridge Univ. Press, 1980), 56.

37. Joan Trauner, "The Chinese as Medical Scapegoats in San Francisco, 1870–1905," *California History,* spring 1978, 70–87.

38. Shilts, *And the Band Played On,* 149.

39. See Michael Bronski, "AIDing Our Guilt and Fear," *Gay Community News,* 9 October 1982, 8.

40. A publication called *BAPHRON,* the newsletter for the Bay Area chapter, is a useful source of information about the activities and concerns of this group.

41. See Dennis Altman, *The Homosexualization of America* (Boston: Beacon Press, 1982).

42. See D. Altman, *AIDS in the Mind of America;* Patton, *Sex and Germs;* Steven Petrow, Pat Franks, and Timothy R. Wolfred, eds., *Ending the HIV Epidemic: Community Strategies in Disease Prevention and Health Promotion* (Santa Cruz, Calif.: Network Publications, 1990).

43. Quoted in Lawrence Mass, "An Epidemic Q&A," *New York Native,* 21 June 1982, 11 (emphasis in the original).

44. "Update on Acquired Immune Deficiency Syndrome (AIDS)—United States," *Morbidity and Mortality Weekly Report* 31 (24 September 1982): 508.

45. Lawrence K. Altman, "AIDS Now Seen as a Worldwide Health Problem," *New York Times,* 29 November 1983, C-1.

46. Cristine Russell, "Body's Immune System Disease Seen Occurring Also in Equatorial Africa," *Washington Post,* 2 April 1983, A-7.

47. Victor Cohn, "Africa May Be the Origin of AIDS Disease," *Washington Post,* 27 November 1983, A-4.

48. Anthony S. Fauci, "The Syndrome of Kaposi's Sarcoma and Opportunistic Infections: An Epidemiologically Restricted Disorder of Immunoregulation," *Annals of Internal Medicine* 96 (June 1982): 777–779 (editorial).

49. "Opportunistic Infections and Kaposi's Sarcoma among Haitians in the United States," *Morbidity and Mortality Weekly Report* 31 (9 July 1982): 353–361.

50. "*Pneumocystis Carinii* Pneumonia among Persons with Hemophilia A," *Morbidity and Mortality Weekly Report* 31 (16 July 1982): 366.

51. Lawrence Mass, "A Major Meeting on the Epidemic," *New York Native,* 2 August 1982, 11, 12.

52. Allan M. Brandt, *No Magic Bullet: A Social History of Venereal Diseases in the United States Since 1880* (New York: Oxford Univ. Press, 1985), 4.

53. René Dubos, *Mirage of Health: Utopias, Progress, and Biological Change* (New York: Harper & Brothers, 1959), 86.

54. Judith S. Mausner and Shira Kramer, *Epidemiology—An Introductory*

384   NOTES TO PAGES 58–60

Text, 2d ed. (Philadelphia: W. Saunders, 1985), 27–34. For a critique of such approaches, see Sylvia Noble Tesh, _Hidden Arguments: Political Ideology and Disease Prevention Policy_ (New Brunswick, N.J.: Rutgers Univ. Press, 1990).

55. See, for example, Barbara Ellen Smith, "Black Lung: The Social Production of Disease," in _Perspectives in Medical Sociology,_ ed. Phil Brown (Prospect Heights, Ill: Waveland Press, 1992), 122–141.

56. Andrew Abbott, _The System of Professions: An Essay on the Division of Expert Labor_ (Chicago: Univ. of Chicago Press, 1988), 136, 193.

57. Harry Nelson, "Mysterious Fever Now an Epidemic," _Los Angeles Times,_ 31 May 1982, 1, 3, 20.

58. "'Homosexual Plague' Strikes New Victims," _Newsweek,_ 23 August 1982, 10.

59. "Possible Transfusion-Associated Acquired Immune Deficiency Syndrome (AIDS)—California," _Morbidity and Mortality Weekly Report_ 31 (10 December 1982): 652–654.

60. "Immunodeficiency among Female Sexual Partners of Males with Acquired Immune Deficiency Syndrome (AIDS)—New York," _Morbidity and Mortality Weekly Report_ 31 (7 January 1983): 697–698.

61. Catherine Macek, "Acquired Immunodeficiency Syndrome Cause(s) Still Elusive," _Journal of the American Medical Association_ 248 (24 September 1982): 1423–1431.

62. For biographical information on Sonnabend, see Bruce Nussbaum, _Good Intentions: How Big Business and the Medical Establishment Are Corrupting the Fight Against AIDS_ (New York: Atlantic Monthly Press, 1990), chapter 4.

63. Anne-Christine d'Adesky, "The Man Who Invented Safer Sex Returns," _Out,_ summer 1992, 29.

64. J. A. Sonnabend, "Promiscuity Is Bad for Your Health: AIDS and the Question of an Infectious Agent," _New York Native,_ 13 September 1982, 39.

65. On the importance of recruiting allies in scientific controversies, see Bruno Latour, _Science in Action_ (Cambridge, Mass.: Harvard Univ. Press, 1987), chapter 4.

66. Barry Adkins, "Looking at AIDS in Totality: A Conversation with Joseph Sonnabend," _New York Native,_ 7 October 1985, 22.

67. Latour has stressed that the effect of powerful scientific rhetoric is precisely to "isolate" opponents and make them feel "lonely"; see _Science in Action,_ 33, 44.

68. Adkins, "Looking at AIDS in Totality," 24.

69. Joseph Sonnabend, Steven S. Witkin, and David T. Purtilo, "Acquired Immunodeficiency Syndrome, Opportunistic Infections, and Malignancies in Male Homosexuals: A Hypothesis of Etiologic Factors in Pathogenesis," _Journal of the American Medical Association_ 249 (6 May 1983): 2370–2374. Reprinted in Irving J. Selikoff, Alvin S. Teirstein, and Shalom Z. Hirschman, eds., _Acquired Immune Deficiency Syndrome,_ vol. 437 of _Annals of the New York Academy of Sciences_ (New York: 1984); and in Helene M. Cole and George D. Lundberg, eds., _AIDS: From the Beginning_ (Chicago: American Medical Association, 1986).

70. Sonnabend, Witkin, and Purtilo, "Acquired Immunodeficiency Syndrome."

71. J. A. Sonnabend, "The Etiology of AIDS," *AIDS Research* 1 (1983): 1–12.

72. James J. Goedert et al., "Amyl Nitrite May Alter T Lymphocytes in Homosexual Men," *Lancet* 1 (20 February 1982): 412–415.

73. Mass, "Major Meeting on the Epidemic," 11.

74. Lawrence Mass, "The Epidemic Continues: Facing a New Case Every Day, Researchers Are Still Bewildered," *New York Native*, 29 March 1982, 1, 12–15.

75. Gordon Murray, "The 'Gay Disease' Epidemic," *Gay Community News*, 9 October 1982, 8.

76. Bronski, "AIDing Our Guilt," 9.

77. G. Murray, "'Gay Disease' Epidemic," 11.

78. Editors' note, *New York Native*, 8–21 November 1982, 22.

79. Peter Seitzman, "Good Luck, Bad Luck: The Role of Chance in Contracting AIDS," *New York Native*, 8–21 November 1982, 22.

80. Michael Callen and Richard Berkowitz, "We Know Who We Are: Two Gay Men Declare War on Promiscuity," *New York Native*, 8 November 1982, 23–29, quote from 23.

81. Charles Jurrist, "In Defense of Promiscuity: Hard Questions about Real Life," *New York Native*, 6 December 1982, 27, 29.

82. D. Altman, *AIDS in the Mind of America*, 40–47; Patton, *Sex and Germs*, 119–158.

83. Michael Lynch, quoted in D. Altman, *AIDS in the Mind of America*, 137.

84. Lawrence Mass, "The Case against Medical Panic," *New York Native*, 17 January, 1983, 25.

85. Callen and Berkowitz, "We Know Who We Are," 29.

86. Dennis Altman, "Legitimation through Disaster: AIDS and the Gay Movement," in *AIDS: The Burdens of History*, ed. Elizabeth Fee and Daniel M. Fox (Berkeley: Univ. of California Press, 1988), 301–315. On the role of community in social movement mobilization, see Clarence Y. H. Lo, "Communities of Challengers in Social Movement Theory," in *Frontiers in Social Movement Theory*, ed. Aldon D. Morris and Carol McClurg Mueller (New Haven: Yale Univ. Press, 1992), 224–247.

87. See, for example, Jean-Robert Leonidas and Nicole Hyppolite, "Haiti and the Acquired Immunodeficiency Syndrome," *Annals of Internal Medicine* 98 (June 1982): 1020–1021. More generally, see Paul Farmer, *AIDS and Accusation: Haiti and the Geography of Blame* (Berkeley: Univ. of California Press, 1992).

88. Cathy Jean Cohen, "Power, Resistance and the Construction of Crisis: Marginalized Communities Respond to AIDS" (Ph.D. diss., University of Michigan, 1993), 472, 484.

89. Ibid., 450–451.

90. Robert C. Gallo, "HIV—The Cause of AIDS: An Overview on Its Biology, Mechanisms of Disease Induction, and Our Attempts to Control It," *Journal of Acquired Immune Deficiency Syndromes* 1 (December 1988): 521.

91. John M. Coffin, "Introduction to Retroviruses," in *AIDS and Other Manifestations of HIV Infection*, 2d ed., ed. Gary P. Wormser (New York: Raven Press, 1992), 37–56; Steve Connor and Sharon Kingman, *The Search for the Virus*, 2d ed. (London: Penguin Books, 1989), 29.

92. Connor and Kingman, *Search for the Virus*, 29.

93. Robert Gallo, *Virus Hunting* (New York: Basic Books, 1991), 133.

94. Joan Fujimura, "Constructing 'Do-Able' Problems in Cancer Research: Articulating Alignments," *Social Studies of Science* 17 (May 1987): 257–293.

95. Gallo, *Virus Hunting*, 134.

96. Robert C. Gallo and Luc Montagnier, "AIDS in 1988," *Scientific American* 259 (October 1988): 40 ff.

97. Gallo, *Virus Hunting*, 148–149.

98. John Crewdson, "The Great AIDS Quest (Part 1: Science under the Microscope)," *Chicago Tribune*, 19 November 1989, C-1.

99. Jacques Leibowitch, *A Strange Virus of Unknown Origin* (New York: Ballantine Books, 1985), esp. chapter 1.

100. Quoted in Crewdson, "The Great AIDS Quest (Part 1)."

101. Ibid.; Connor and Kingman," *Search for the Virus, 33*.

102. Robert C. Gallo et al., "Isolation of Human T-Cell Leukemia Virus in Acquired Immune Deficiency Syndrome (AIDS)," *Science* 220 (20 May 1983): 865–867; F. Barré-Sinoussi et al., "Isolation of a T-Lymphotropic Retrovirus from a Patient at Risk for Acquired Immune Deficiency Syndrome (AIDS)," *Science* 220 (20 May 1983): 868–870.

103. Crewdson, "The Great AIDS Quest (Part 1)."

104. Jay Levy, interview by author, tape recording, San Francisco, 16 December 1993.

105. Gallo, *Virus Hunting*, 170.

106. Crewdson, "The Great AIDS Quest (Part 1)."

107. In November 1993, the Office of Research Integrity of the Department of Health and Human Services concluded a four-year investigation by dropping all accusations of scientific misconduct against Gallo. Gallo declared himself "completely vindicated," but the office said it was "acting reluctantly" in response to the adoption of a new, more stringent definition of what constitutes misconduct in science. See Philip J. Hilts, "Misconduct Charges Dropped against AIDS Virus Scientist," *New York Times*, 13 November 1993, A-1.

108. Lawrence K. Altman, "Federal Official Says He Believes Cause of AIDS Has Been Found," *New York Times*, 22 April 1984, 1.

109. Shilts, *And the Band Played On*, 451.

110. Lawrence K. Altman, "New U.S. Report Names Virus That May Cause AIDS," *New York Times*, 24 April 1984, C-1.

111. Levy, interview.

112. Connor and Kingman, *Search for the Virus*, 41.

113. Shilts, *And the Band Played On*, 451.

114. John Crewdson, "The Great AIDS Quest (Part 4: 'Could You Patent the Sun?')," *Chicago Tribune*, 19 November 1989, C-7.

115. "A Viral Competition over AIDS," *New York Times*, 26 April 1984, 22 (editorial).

116. Crewdson, "The Great AIDS Quest (Part 4)."

117. Robert C. Gallo et al., "Frequent Detection and Isolation of Cytopathic Retroviruses (HTLV-III) from Patients with AIDS and at Risk for AIDS," *Science* 224 (4 May 1984): 500–502.

118. Ibid., 502.

119. Gallo, "HIV—The Cause of AIDS," 523.

120. In one of the other papers, Gallo and his colleagues reported finding *antibodies* to the virus in three of five asymptomatic IV drug users and six of seventeen asymptomatic homosexual men. Again, there was no knowledge at that point about whether these individuals would develop AIDS. Moreover, the presence of antibodies to the virus was somewhat weaker evidence than the presence of the virus itself (M. G. Sarngadharan et al., "Antibodies Reactive with Human T-Lymphotropic Retroviruses [HTLV-III] in the Serum of Patients with AIDS," *Science* 224, 4 May 1984, 506–508).

121. Robert Gallo, interview by author, tape recording, Bethesda, Md., 3 November 1994.

122. Gallo, *Virus Hunting*, 277–280; Alfred S. Evans, "Does HIV Cause AIDS? An Historical Perspective," *Journal of Acquired Immune Deficiency Syndromes* 2 (April 1989): 107–113.

123. Richard M. Krause, "Koch's Postulates and the Search for the AIDS Agent," *Reviews of Infectious Diseases* 6 (March-April 1984): 272, 278. The original talk was presented at the International Congress for Infectious Diseases, Vienna, Austria, August 24–27, 1983.

124. Lawrence K. Altman, "How AIDS Researchers Strive for Virus Proof," *New York Times*, 23 October 1984, C-3.

125. James E. D'Eramo, "Federal Health Officials Announce Cause of AIDS," *New York Native*, 7 May 1984, 8.

126. Nathan Fain, "Researchers Track Down Virus They Believe Is AIDS' Cause," *Advocate*, 29 May 1984, 8–9.

127. Mausner and Kramer, *Epidemiology—An Introductory Text*, 185.

128. Jay A. Levy et al., "Isolation of Lymphocytopathic Retroviruses from San Francisco Patients with AIDS," *Science* 225, 24 August 1984, 840–842.

129. Levy, interview.

130. Levy et al., "Isolation of Lymphocytopathic Retroviruses," 225.

131. See, for example, Flossie Wong-Staal and Robert C. Gallo, "The Family of Human T-Lymphotropic Leukemia Viruses: HTLV-I as the Cause of Adult T Cell Leukemia and HTLV-III as the Cause of Acquired Immunodeficiency Syndrome," *Blood* 65 (February 1985), 253–263.

132. John Coffin et al., "Human Immunodeficiency Viruses," *Science* 232 (9 May 1986): 697 (letter to the editor).

133. On the stabilization of HIV, see also Paula A. Treichler, "AIDS: An Epidemic of Signification," in *AIDS: Cultural Analysis, Cultural Activism*, ed. Douglas Crimp (Cambridge, Mass.: Massachusetts Institute of Technology Press, 1988), 31–70, esp. 57.

134. Steven Seidman, "Transfiguring Sexual Identity: AIDS and the Contemporary Construction of Homosexuality," *Social Text* 19/20 (fall 1988): 187–205.

135. On struggles over the ownership of social problems, see Joseph R.

Gusfield, *The Culture of Public Problems* (Chicago: Univ. of Chicago Press, 1981).

136. On courtesy stigmas in AIDS, see Peter Conrad, "The Social Meaning of AIDS," *Social Policy* (summer 1986), 53. On the role of lesbians, see Amber Hollibaugh, "Lesbian Denial and Lesbian Leadership in the AIDS Epidemic: Bravery and Fear in the Construction of a Lesbian Geography of Risk," in *Women Resisting AIDS: Feminist Strategies of Empowerment,* ed. Beth E. Schneider and Nancy E. Stoller (Philadelphia: Temple Univ. Press, 1995), 219–230; Nancy Stoller, "Lesbian Involvement in the AIDS Epidemic: Changing Roles and Generational Differences," in *Women Resisting AIDS,* 270–285.

Chapter 2

1. Jonathan Elford, Robert Bor, and Pauline Summers, "Research into HIV and AIDS between 1981 and 1990: The Epidemic Curve," *AIDS* 5 (December 1991): 1515–1519, esp. 1516.

2. C. Self, W. Filardo, and W. Lancaster, "Acquired Immunodeficiency Syndrome (AIDS) and the Epidemic Growth of Its Literature," *Scientometrics* 17 (July 1989): 49–60, esp. 55. The increasing importance of AIDS research within biomedicine and scientific research as a whole is suggested by the "maps" of scientific research patterns generated by co-citation analysis, a quantitative technique that constructs linkages between articles that have been jointly cited by other researchers. See Henry Small and Edwin Greenlee, "A Co-Citation Study of AIDS Research," in *Scholarly Communication and Bibliometrics,* ed. Christine L. Borgman (Newbury Park, Calif.: Sage, 1990), 166–193.

3. See the semilogarithmic graph in I. N. Sengupta and Lalita Kumari, "Bibliometric Analysis of AIDS Literature," *Scientometrics* 20 (January 1991): 301.

4. The following figures are from Elford et al., "Research into HIV and AIDS," 1517, and are based on the indexing schema used in the Medline database of the National Library of Medicine.

5. "New AIDS Virus Found Different from First," *New York Times,* 18 December 1986, B-31.

6. Paula A. Treichler, "AIDS, HIV, and the Cultural Construction of Reality," in *The Time of AIDS: Social Analysis, Theory, and Method,* ed. Gilbert Herdt and Shirley Lindenbaum (Newbury Park, Calif.: Sage, 1992), 65–98, quote from 76.

7. Robert C. Gallo et al., "Frequent Detection and Isolation of Cytopathic Retroviruses (HTLV-III) from Patients with AIDS and at Risk for AIDS," *Science* 224 (4 May 1984): 500–502.

8. On the transformation of scientific facts into taken-for-granted knowledge, see, for example, Bruno Latour, *Science in Action* (Cambridge, Mass.: Harvard Univ. Press, 1987), 42–43. Montagnier's 1983 paper, initially almost ignored but increasingly recognized as the first report of the discovery of HIV, ended up being cited even more often than Gallo's 1984 paper: Montagnier's

paper was cited 147 times in 1984, 366 times in 1985, 416 times in 1986, and 399 times in 1987. My content analysis focuses on Gallo's 1984 paper only: For my purposes, it was more important to study citations of Gallo's work, since he has tended to receive credit for confirming that the virus causes AIDS, than to study citations of Montagnier's work, since he has tended to be credited instead for the discovery of the virus (see Small and Greenlee's conclusions on this point, "Co-Citation Study of AIDS Research," 185). In practice, my content analysis revealed that the two papers were very frequently co-cited, often along with Levy's 1984 article in *Science*. See also Alison Rawling, "The AIDS Virus Dispute: Awarding Priority for the Discovery of the Human Immunodeficiency Virus (HIV)," *Science, Technology, & Human Values* 19 (summer 1994): 342–360.

9. A chi-square test using the data in table 1 (comparing the five categories over the three years) confirms that the shift is highly statistically significant ($\chi^2 = 68.5$, df $= 8$, $p < .001$).

10. Council on Scientific Affairs of the Division of Scientific Activities of the American Medical Association, "Acquired Immunodeficiency Syndrome: Commentary," *Journal of the American Medical Association* 252 (19 October 1984): 2039.

11. James W. Curran et al., "The Epidemiology of AIDS: Current Status and Future Prospects," *Science* 229 (September 1985): 1352.

12. Gerald V. Quinnan Jr. et al., "Mechanisms of T-Cell Functional Deficiency in the Acquired Immunodeficiency Syndrome," *Annals of Internal Medicine* 103 (November 1985): 710.

13. "AIDS and HTLV Type III," *Lancet* 1 (5 May 1984): 1031 (editorial note); "The Cause of AIDS?" *Lancet* 1 (12 May 1984): 1053–1054 (editorial), quote from 1054.

14. Robert S. Klein et al., "Oral Candidiasis in High-Risk Patients as the Initial Manifestation of the Acquired Immunodeficiency Syndrome," *New England Journal of Medicine* 311 (9 August 1984): 354.

15. Arthur J. Ammann, "Etiology of AIDS," *Journal of the American Medical Association* 252 (14 September 1984): 1281–1282 (letter to the editor).

16. This was confirmed by performing separate chi-squares (on the five citation categories vs. the two authorship categories) for each of the three years reported in table 2. In each case, the differences between articles without an author from the Gallo group and articles with such an author were not statistically significant (1984: $\chi^2 = 5.5$, df $= 4$, $p < .30$; 1985: $\chi^2 = 1.7$, df $= 4$, $p < .80$; 1986: $\chi^2 = 1.2$, df $= 4$, $p < .90$).

17. Françoise Barré-Sinoussi et al., "Isolation of Lymphadenopathy-Associated Virus (LAV) and Detection of LAV Antibodies from US Patients with AIDS," *Journal of the American Medical Association* 253 (22–29 March 1985): 1737.

18. Luc Montagnier, "Lymphadenopathy-Associated Virus: From Molecular Biology to Pathogenicity," *Annals of Internal Medicine* 103 (November 1985): 693.

19. Chi-square tests were performed separately for the 1985 and 1986

data. Data from table 3 were combined into 2×2 tables: explicit unqualified references vs. all other references (combined); and those citing early papers vs. those citing later research. In 1985 there was no statistically significant difference between those citing early papers and those citing later research, in terms of the tendency to make explicit unqualified references ($\chi^2 = .0028$, df $= 1$, $p < .95$). Similarly, in 1986, the difference was not statistically significant ($\chi^2 = 1.84$, df $= 1$, $p < .20$).

20. This shift is highly significant statistically, as confirmed by a chi-square test of the "Citations of early papers" column (the four citation categories in 1985 vs. the four categories in 1986): $\chi^2 = 332.4$, df $= 3$, $p < .001$.

21. Samuel Broder and Robert C. Gallo, "A Pathogenic Retrovirus (HTLV-III) Linked to AIDS," *New England Journal of Medicine* 311 (15 November 1984): 1292–1297; Flossie Wong-Staal and Robert C. Gallo, "Human T-Lymphotropic Retroviruses," *Nature* 317 (3–9 October 1985): 395–403.

22. S. Zaki Salahuddin et al., "Isolation of Infectious Human T-Cell Leukemia/Lymphotropic Virus Type III (HTLV-III) from Patients with Acquired Immunodeficiency Syndrome (AIDS) or AIDS-Related Complex (ARC) and from Healthy Carriers: A Study of Risk Groups and Tissue Sources," *Proceedings of the National Academy of Sciences* 82 (August 1985), 5530–5534.

23. Ibid., 5533.

24. Flossie Wong-Staal and Robert C. Gallo, "The Family of Human T-Lymphotropic Leukemia Viruses: HTLV-I as the Cause of Adult T Cell Leukemia and HTLV-III as the Cause of Acquired Immunodeficiency Syndrome," *Blood* 65 (February 1985): 253–263.

25. This study, coauthored by Gallo, was reported in Harvey J. Alter et al., "Transmission of HTLV-III Infection from Human Plasma to Chimpanzees: An Animal Model for AIDS," *Science* 226 (2 November 1984), 549–552.

26. Wong-Staal and Gallo, "The Family of Human T-Lymphotropic Leukemia Viruses," 259.

27. See, for example, the summary of the evidence in S. Harada, Y. Koyanagi, and N. Yamamoto, "Infection of HTLV-III/LAV in HTLV-I-Carrying Cells MT-2 and MT-4 and Application in a Plaque Assay," *Science* 229 (9 August 1985): 563–566.

28. For example, CDC researcher Paul Feorino and his coauthors, reporting on an early transfusion study in *Science* in July 1984, noted that "the ultimate proof that LAV or any other virus is the cause of AIDS requires studies that cumulatively fulfill the modern equivalent of Koch's postulates." See P. M. Feorino et al., "Lymphadenopathy-Associated Virus Infection of a Blood Donor-Recipient Pair with Acquired Immunodeficiency Syndrome," *Science* 225 (6 July 1984): 70–71.

29. Wong-Staal and Gallo, "The Family of Human T-Lymphotropic Leukemia Viruses," 259.

30. Jeffrey Laurence et al., "Lymphadenopathy-Associated Viral Antibody in AIDS," *New England Journal of Medicine* 311 (15 November 1984), 1269–1273.

31. Harada et al., "Infection of HTLV-III/LAV," 563.

32. See "Chimp Finally Shows AIDS Symptoms," *Science* 270 (13 October 1995): 223.

33. Donald P. Francis et al., "Infection of Chimpanzees with Lymph-adenopathy-Associated Virus," *Lancet* 2 (1 December 1984): 1276–1277 (letter to the editor).

34. For an early example, see Jerome E. Groopman et al., "Virologic Studies in a Case of Transfusion-Associated AIDS," *New England Journal of Medicine* 311 (29 November 1984): 1419.

35. Paul M. Feorino et al., "Transfusion-Associated Acquired Immunodeficiency Syndrome," *New England Journal of Medicine* 312 (16 May 1985): 1293–1296.

36. H. W. Jaffe et al., "Transfusion-Associated AIDS: Serologic Evidence of Human T-Cell Leukemia Virus Infection in Donors," *Science* 223 (23 March 1984): 1309–1311.

37. The crucial differences are (1) that Feorino and his co-researchers actually isolated the virus, instead of simply assaying for antibodies; and (2) that Feorino and his associates found the virus more consistently both in donors and recipients than Jaffe and his associates had found antibodies in either group. In fact, buried in the paper by Jaffe et al. was the admission that they could find HTLV-I antibodies in only three of the eight transfusion *recipients* for whom serum samples were available (p. 1310).

38. Robert C. Gallo, "AIDS: Words from the Front," interview by Anthony Liversidge and Celia Farber, *Spin*, February 1988, 56.

39. S. Pahwa et al., "Influence of the Human T-Lymphotropic Virus/Lymphadenopathy-Associated Virus on Functions of Human Lymphocytes: Evidence for Immunosuppressive Effects and Polyclonal B-Cell Activation by Banded Viral Preparations," *Proceedings of the National Academy of Sciences* 82 (December 1985): 8198–8202.

40. R. F. Wykoff, E. R. Pearl, and F. T. Saulsbury, "Immunologic Dysfunction in Infants Infected through Transfusion with HTLV-III," *New England Journal of Medicine* 312 (31 January 1985): 294–296.

41. On bandwagons in science, see Joan H. Fujimura, "The Molecular Biological Bandwagon in Cancer Research: Where Social Worlds Meet," *Social Problems* 35 (June 1988): 261–283.

42. H. M. Collins, "Certainty and the Public Understanding of Science: Science on Television," *Social Studies of Science* 17 (November 1987): 692.

43. "Revision of Case Definition of Acquired Immunodeficiency Syndrome for National Reporting—United States," *Morbidity and Mortality Weekly Report* 34 (28 June 1985): 373–375.

44. Antibody-negative patients could still be included, however, if they had a positive result on another test (such as a viral culture) or if they had a low ratio of helper T cells to suppressor T cells. Moreover, the CDC continued to count as AIDS cases patients with diseases included on the list who had simply never been tested for HIV antibodies.

45. Karen Wright, "Mycoplasmas in the AIDS Spotlight," *Science* 248 (11 May 1990): 682–683.

46. Lawrence K. Altman, "AIDS Findings Made by a Virus Expert," *New York Times*, 3 August 1986, 1.

47. Wright, "Mycoplasmas in the AIDS Spotlight," 683.

48. See Shyh-Ching Lo et al., "Enhancement of HIV-1 Cytocidal Effects

in CD4+ Lymphocytes by the AIDS-Associated Mycoplasma," *Science* 251 (1 March 1991): 1074–1076.

49. On the role of the news media as a "reflexive" institution whose "accounts are embedded in the very reality that they characterize, record, or structure," see Gaye Tuchman, *Making News: A Study in the Construction of Reality* (New York: Free Press, 1978), 189.

50. See the Methodological Appendix for details concerning article selection and coding.

51. The term "the AIDS virus" was actually used most often in the second half of 1985, which was also when news coverage of AIDS soared following the announcement that Rock Hudson suffered from the syndrome.

52. The trend over time toward implicit etiological claims-making, shown in table 4 ,was found to be highly significant statistically. (Implicit claims were compared to all other claims combined, over the five time periods [a 2×5 table] [$\chi^2 = 31.1$, df$= 4$, $p < .001$].)

53. Judy Glass, "L.I. Cases of AIDS Reported on Rise," *New York Times*, 3 June 1984, Section 11, p. 1.

54. Lawrence Altman, "How AIDS Researchers Strive for Virus Proof," *New York Times*, 23 October 1984, C-3.

55. Lawrence K. Altman, "AIDS Immunization Tested on Humans," *New York Times*, 17 December 1986, A-1.

56. Chuck Frutchey, letter, 10 December 1984, included in "AIDS: An Infection Control and General Information Packet for Health Care Providers" (San Francisco: San Francisco Bay Area Chapter of the Association for Practitioners in Infection Control and the San Francisco AIDS Foundation, 1984).

57. Dennis Altman, *AIDS in the Mind of America* (Garden City, N.J.: Anchor Press, 1986), 182.

58. Paul Cameron, "Homosexuality: A Deathstyle, Not a Lifestyle," *Moral Majority Report*, September 1983, 7.

59. D. Altman, *AIDS in the Mind of America*, 64.

60. See, for example, the leaflet "AIDS Is Germ Warfare by the U.S. Gov't against Gays and Blacks!" (San Francisco: Information Network against War & Fascism, n.d. [circa 1987], photocopy); James Brooke, "In Cradle of AIDS Theory, a Defensive Africa Sees a Disguise for Racism," *New York Times*, 19 November 1987, B-13; Tom Curtis, "The Origin of AIDS," *Rolling Stone*, 19 March 1992, 54; Tom Curtis, "Did a Polio Vaccine Experiment Unleash AIDS in Africa?" *Washington Post*, 5 April 1992, C-3 (op-ed); Charles Gilks, "AIDS, Monkeys and Malaria," *Nature* 354 (28 November 1991): 262 (commentary); Red Jackson, "Hitler's Labs Created AIDS Virus," *Sun*, 3 January 1989, 7; Robert Lederer, "Chemical-Biological Warfare, Medical Experiments, and Population Control," *Covert Action Information Bulletin*, summer 1987, 33–42; Robert Lederer, "Origin and Spread of AIDS: Is the West Responsible?" *Covert Action Information Bulletin*, summer 1987, 43–54; Brian Martin, "Peer Review and the Origin of AIDS—A Case Study in Rejected Ideas," *BioScience* 43 (October 1993): 624–627 (roundtable discussion); Gary Null, "AIDS: A Man-Made Plague?" *Penthouse*, January 1989, 160; Louis Pascal, *What Happens When Science Goes Bad. The Corruption*

of Science and the Origin of AIDS: A Study in Spontaneous Generation, working paper no. 9, University of Wollongong, Australia: Science and Technology Analysis Research Programme, December 1991; "Soviets Say CIA Created AIDS to Use in Biological Warfare," *San Francisco Examiner,* 31 October 1985, A-9; Pearce Wright, "Smallpox Vaccine 'Triggered Aids Virus,'" *London Times,* 11 May 1987, 1.

61. Susan M. Blake and Elaine Bratic Arkin, *AIDS Information Monitor: A Summary of National Public Opinion Surveys on AIDS: 1983 through 1986* (Washington, D.C.: American Red Cross, 1983).

62. Of course, the danger was that, by encouraging people at risk for AIDS to take the test, AIDS organizations might make a quarantine more *feasible* simply by identifying more people who carried the virus. For this reason, the pros and cons of "taking the test" were fiercely debated in gay communities in the mid-1980s, and many groups (particularly on the East Coast, where suspicions ran higher) promoted the message "Don't take the test." Other groups rallied behind the idea of anonymous testing, which provided people with test results while protecting their identities. Eventually, a consensus in favor of anonymous testing materialized among the AIDS organizations, but not until the tests were shown to be relatively accurate, and never fully until the advent of "early intervention" therapies in the late 1980s.

63. See Cindy Patton, *Inventing AIDS* (New York: Routledge, 1990), 42.

64. D. Altman, *AIDS in the Mind of America,* 153.

65. For a somewhat contrasting perspective, see Patton, *Inventing AIDS,* 42.

66. Nathan Fain, "The Proof Is In on a Virus," *Advocate,* 4 September 1984, 8–9.

67. Christine Guilfoy, "HTLV-III Test Availability Elicits Mixed Response," *Gay Community News,* 27 April 1985, 3.

68. John Lauritsen and Hank Wilson, *Poppers & AIDS,* 2d ed. (San Francisco: Committee to Monitor Poppers, 1985).

69. John Lauritsen, "The Drugs Connection," *Gay Community News,* 12 October 1986, 5 (op-ed).

70. For representative criticism of Ortleb by an AIDS activist, see Douglas Crimp, "How to Have Promiscuity in an Epidemic," in *AIDS: Cultural Analysis, Cultural Activism,* ed. Douglas Crimp (Cambridge, Mass.: Massachusetts Institute of Technology Press, 1988), 237–270, esp. 238. The best analysis of the role of the *Native* in covering AIDS is provided by James Kinsella in chapter 2 of *Covering the Plague: AIDS and the American Media* (New Brunswick, N.J.: Rutgers Univ. Press, 1989).

71. J. A. Sonnabend and S. Saadoun, "What Does a Positive Test Mean?" *New York Native,* 24 September–7 October 1984, 19–20.

72. Barry Adkins, "Looking at AIDS in Totality: A Conversation with Joseph Sonnabend," *New York Native,* 7 October 1985, 24.

73. James E. D'Eramo, "Discovering the Cause of AIDS: An Interview with Dr. Robert C. Gallo," *New York Native,* 27 August 1984, 17, 18.

74. Jane Teas, "Could AIDS Agent Be a New Variant of African Swine Fever Virus?" *Lancet* 1 (23 April 1983): 923 (letter to the editor).

75. J. Colaert et al., "African Swine Fever Virus Antibody Not Found in AIDS Patients," *Lancet* 1 (14 May 1983): 1098 (letter to the editor); Emmanuel Arnoux et al., "AIDS and African Swine Fever," *Lancet* 2 (9 July 1983): 110 (letter to the editor).

76. Council on Scientific Affairs of the Division of Scientific Activities of the American Medical Association, "Acquired Immunodeficiency Syndrome: Commentary."

77. Jane Teas, "An AIDS Odyssey," *New York Native*, 17 December 1984, 15.

78. Ibid.

79. Kinsella, *Covering the Plague*, 38-44; D. Altman, *AIDS in the Mind of America*, 52.

80. See Kinsella's account in *Covering the Plague*, 41-42.

81. Lawrence K. Altman, "Studies Fail to Link AIDS with Swine Fever," *New York Times*, 19 September 1985, B-15.

82. Crimp, "How to Have Promiscuity in an Epidemic," 238.

83. Helene M. Cole and George D. Lundberg, eds., *AIDS: From the Beginning* (Chicago: American Medical Association, 1986).

84. Institute of Medicine, National Academy of Sciences, *Confronting AIDS: Directions for Public Health, Health Care, and Research* (Washington, D.C.: National Academy Press, 1986), quote from viii. For an extended critique of the report, see Alfred J. Fortin, "AIDS, Surveillance and Public Policy: The Politics of Medical Discourse" (Ph.D. diss., University of Hawaii, 1989).

85. Institute of Medicine, National Academy of Sciences, *Confronting AIDS*, 40.

86. Ibid., 195.

87. Ibid., 177-259.

88. John Lauritsen, "Caveat Emptor: The Report of the National Academy of Sciences on AIDS Is Filled with Misinformation," *New York Native*, 9 March 1987, 32.

Chapter 3

1. Joan Hideko Fujimura, "Bandwagons in Science: Doable Problems and Transportable Packages as Factors in the Development of the Molecular Genetic Bandwagon in Cancer Research" (Ph.D. diss., University of California at Berkeley, 1986).

2. This includes sixty-nine published in the 1970s (twenty with Duesberg as first author) and fifty-nine in the 1980s (eighteen as first author). Medline dates back to 1965. (In some cases, Medline does not include references to book chapters or to foreign journals, so it may understate an author's publication history.)

3. See Eugene Garfield, *Citation Indexing—Its Theory and Application in Science, Technology, and Humanities* (New York: John Wiley & Sons, 1979), esp. 244 ff. For a skeptical perspective on the use of citation counts, see David

Edge, "Quantitative Measures of Communication in Science: A Critical Review," *History of Science* 17 (June 1979): 102–134.

4. Duesberg was born in 1936, Gallo in 1937. Duesberg received his Ph.D. in 1963, the same year that Gallo received his medical degree.

5. Robert Teitelman, "The Baffling Standoff in Cancer Research," *Forbes,* 15 July 1985, 110.

6. Peter H. Duesberg, "Activated Proto-Onc Genes: Sufficient or Necessary for Cancer?" *Science* 228 (10 May 1985): 669–677.

7. Peter H. Duesberg, "Retroviruses as Carcinogens and Pathogens: Expectations and Reality," *Cancer Research* 47 (1 March 1987): 1199–1220, quotes from 1199–1200.

8. Peter Duesberg, interview by author, tape recording, Berkeley, Calif., 28 September 1992.

9. Duesberg, "Retroviruses as Carcinogens and Pathogens," 1212–1213.

10. Ibid., 1215.

11. See Bruno Latour, *Science in Action* (Cambridge, Mass.: Harvard Univ. Press, 1987), 40–41.

12. John Lauritsen, "First Things First: Some Thoughts on the 'AIDS Virus' and AZT," *New York Native,* 1 June 1987, 1, 14–16 (cover story).

13. This was a section heading in Lauritsen's article (ibid., 14). For debates surrounding the safety and efficacy of AZT, see part two of this book.

14. Latour, "Science in Action," 44.

15. Lauritsen, "First Things First," 14–15.

16. John Lauritsen, "Saying No to HIV: An Interview with Prof. Peter Duesberg, Who Says, 'I Would Not Worry about Being Antibody Positive,'" *New York Native,* 6 July 1987, 1, 17–25 (cover story), quote from 24.

17. Ibid., 21.

18. Ibid.

19. James Kinsella, *Covering the Plague: AIDS and the American Media* (New Brunswick, N.J.: Rutgers Univ. Press, 1989), 46.

20. Charles Shively, "AIDS and Genes," *Gay Community News,* 4 October 1987, 3, 13, 14.

21. Katie Leishman, "AIDS and Insects," *The Atlantic,* September 1987, 56–72, quote from 71.

22. "Channel 4 Programme Challenges Established Theories on Aids," *Origin Universal News Services,* 12 November 1987.

23. Peter Duesberg, "A Challenge to the AIDS Establishment," *Bio/Technology* 5 (November 1987): 1244.

24. See, for example, Duesberg's brief appearance as a quotable authority in John Crewdson, "Weak Immune System May Open AIDS Door," *Chicago Tribune,* 20 December 1987, 1.

25. Lori Kenschaft, "Why Look at HIV?" *Gay Community News,* 20 December 1987, 3. See also "Scientist Disputes HIV Theory of AIDS," *Bay Area Reporter,* 24 December 1987, 16.

26. Celia Farber, "AIDS: Words from the Front," *Spin,* January 1988, 43–44, 73.

27. Duesberg was referring to an incident that had occurred in August the

previous year, when arsonists set fire to the Florida home of three antibody-positive hemophiliac brothers after the family waged a successful legal battle to keep the boys from being excluded from public school. See David L. Kirp et al., *Learning by Heart: AIDS and Schoolchildren in America's Communities* (New Brunswick, N.J.: Rutgers, 1989), 1–4.

28. Farber, "AIDS: Words from the Front," 73.

29. William Booth, "A Rebel without a Cause of AIDS," *Science* 239 (25 March 1988): 1485.

30. Peter H. Duesberg, "In Pursuit of Harmless Viruses: The Last Stand of the Microbe Hunters," *Raum & Zeit* 1, no. 5 (1990): 4–8, quote from 6.

31. Ibid., 5, 7–8.

32. Pierre Bourdieu, "The Specificity of the Scientific Field and the Social Conditions of the Progress of Reason," *Social Science Information* 14 (December 1975): 19–47, esp. 30.

33. Duesberg, "In Pursuit of Harmless Viruses," 1.

34. Joe Nicholson, "AIDS Experts on Wrong Track: Top Doc," *New York Post*, 7 January 1988, 9.

35. Phillip M. Boffey, "A Solitary Dissenter Disputes Cause of AIDS," *New York Times*, 12 January 1988, C-3.

36. Joel N. Shurkin, "The AIDS Debate: Another View," *Los Angeles Times*, 18 January 1988, II-4.

37. Anthony Liversidge and Celia Farber, "AIDS: Words from the Front," *Spin*, February 1988, 56–57, 67, 70.

38. Booth, "A Rebel without a Cause of AIDS," 1485.

39. Liversidge and Farber, "AIDS: Words from the Front," 57, 67.

40. Ibid., 57.

41. Ibid., 67.

42. Quote of the Week, *Gay Community News*, 27 December 1987, 2.

43. Evidence on progression from a state of asymptomatic HIV infection to an AIDS diagnosis came primarily from combined retrospective and longitudinal studies of gay men whose blood samples were taken initially for hepatitis B vaccine trials in the early 1980s but were subsequently analyzed for HIV antibodies. As time passed, more and more of these HIV-infected men developed AIDS, leading scientists to boost upward both their predictions of the percentage of infected people who would eventually sicken and their assessments of the mean time between infection and the onset of illness.

44. David Perlman, "Positive AIDS Tests for Half of Gays in Study," *San Francisco Chronicle*, 1 January 1986.

45. These developments are discussed in detail in part two of this book.

46. Randy Shilts, "Theory That AIDS Is a 'Super Syphilis,'" *San Francisco Chronicle*, 13 January 1988, A-7.

47. Caden Gray, "Biologist Brings Message to Castro," *San Francisco Sentinel*, 15 January 1988, 7.

48. Roger Rapaport, "Dissident Scientist's AIDS Theory Angers Colleagues," *Oakland Tribune*, 31 January 1988, B-4.

49. Ann Giudici Fettner, "Dealing with Duesberg: Bad Science Makes Strange Bedfellows," *Village Voice*, 2 February 1988, 25.

50. Quote of the Week, *Gay Community News*, 7 February 1988, 2.

51. Fettner, "Dealing with Duesberg," 25.

52. Jack Anderson, "AIDS Researcher Won't Confront Alternate Theory," *Newsday*, 9 February 1988, 64.

53. Booth, "Rebel without a Cause of AIDS," 1486.

54. Philip M. Boffey, "Reagan Names 12 to Panel on AIDS," *New York Times*, 24 July 1987, A-12.

55. Drew Hopkins, "Peter Duesberg and the Media," *Christopher Street*, April 1988, 59.

56. Katie Leishman, "The AIDS Debate That Isn't," *Wall Street Journal*, 26 February 1988, 14 (op-ed).

57. My account of the AmFAR forum is based primarily on the summary prepared from a transcript and published as: Harold S. Ginsberg, "Scientific Forum on AIDS: A Summary (Does HIV Cause AIDS?)," *Journal of Acquired Immune Deficiency Syndromes* 1 (April 1988): 165–172.

58. Quoted in Kathleen McAuliffe, "The Etiology of AIDS," *AIDS Targeted Information Newsletter* 2 (May 1988): 1–3 (editorial).

59. Ginsberg, "Scientific Forum on AIDS," 168.

60. Michael Specter, "Panel Rebuts Biologist's Claims on Cause of AIDS," *Washington Post*, 10 April 1988, A-4.

61. Ginsberg, "Scientific Forum on AIDS," 169.

62. Ibid., 170.

63. Ibid., 172.

64. Ann Giudici Fettner, "Duesberg's AIDS Theories Get Scrutiny from Peers," *San Francisco Sentinel*, 15 April 1988, 6; John Lauritsen, "Kangaroo Court Etiology," *New York Native*, 9 May 1988, 14–19.

65. An exception was Michael Specter's article in the *Washington Post*, a short but hard-hitting piece that left little doubt about Specter's opinion that Duesberg had lost the debate (Specter, "Panel Rebuts Biologist's Claims").

66. William Booth, "Duesberg Gets His Day in Court," *Science* 240 (15 April 1988): 279.

67. Rebecca Ward, "Mainstream Scientists Confront Unorthodox View of AIDS," *Nature* 332 (14 April 1988): 574.

68. Peter Duesberg, "AIDS and the 'Innocent' Virus," *New Scientist*, 28 April 1988, 34–35.

69. "And Yet It Kills," *New Scientist*, 14 April 1988, 17 (editorial).

70. Harvey Bialy, letter to Daniel Koshland, 2 March 1988.

71. W. Blattner, R. C. Gallo, and H. M. Temin, "Blattner and Colleagues Respond to Duesberg," *Science* 241 (29 July 1988): 514–517, quote from 517.

72. Robert Gallo, interview by author, tape recording, Bethesda, Md., 3 November 1994.

73. W. Blattner, R. C. Gallo, and H. M. Temin, "HIV Causes AIDS," *Science* 241 (29 July 1988): 515.

74. Peter Duesberg, "Duesberg's Response to Blattner and Colleagues," *Science* 241 (29 July 1988): 515–516, quote from 516.

75. Drew Hopkins, "Peter Duesberg and the Media," *Christopher Street*,

April 1988, 52–59; Thomas Ryan, "AIDS as Career," *Christopher Street*, May 1988, 28–35.

76. Rex Wockner, "Dissident Scientists Battle AIDS Dogmas," *In These Times*, 4 May 1988, 5.

77. "Alternative Therapy" (segment by Spencer Michels, KQED San Francisco), *MacNeil/Lehrer News Hour*, 3 May 1988.

78. Jack Anderson, "Doubts Raised about Virus as a Cause of AIDS," *Newsday*, 27 June 1988, 54.

79. Jeff Miller, "AIDS Heresy," *Discover*, June 1988, 63.

80. "Alternative Therapy."

81. Ryan, "AIDS as Career," 32.

82. Robert C. Gallo, "HIV—The Cause of AIDS: An Overview on Its Biology, Mechanisms of Disease Induction, and Our Attempts to Control It," *Journal of Acquired Immune Deficiency Syndromes* 1 (December 1988): 521–535, quotes from 523.

83. Institute of Medicine, National Academy of Sciences, *Confronting AIDS: Update 1988* (Washington, D.C.: National Academy Press, 1988), vi.

84. Ibid., 33.

85. Presidential Commission on the Human Immunodeficiency Virus Epidemic, *Report of the Presidential Commission on the Human Immunodeficiency Virus Epidemic, Submitted to the President of the United States, June 24, 1988* (Washington, D.C., 1988), xvii.

86. William Booth, "AIDS Paper Raises Red Flag at PNAS," *Science* 243 (10 February 1989): 733.

87. Evelleen Richards, *Vitamin C and Cancer: Medicine or Politics?* (New York: St. Martin's, 1991), 90–91, 178–180.

88. Peter H. Duesberg, "Human Immunodeficiency Virus and Acquired Immunodeficiency Syndrome: Correlation but Not Causation," *Proceedings of the National Academy of Sciences* 86 (February 1989): 755–764.

89. Peter H. Duesberg, "AIDS Epidemiology: Inconsistencies with Human Immunodeficiency Virus and with Infectious Disease," *Proceedings of the National Academy of Sciences* 88 (February 1991): 1575–1579.

90. Booth, "AIDS Paper Raises Red Flag," 733.

91. Anthony Liversidge, "*PNAS* Publication of AIDS Article Spurs Debate over Peer Review," *The Scientist*, 3 April 1989, 1, 4, 5, 19.

92. For a discussion of debates about causation at the conference that took place in Montreal the previous year, see Paula A. Treichler, "AIDS, HIV, and the Cultural Construction of Reality" in *The Time of AIDS: Social Analysis, Theory, and Method,* ed. Gilbert Herdt and Shirley Lindenbaum (Newbury Park, Calif.: Sage, 1992), 65–98.

93. Montagnier presented his case formally in: M. Lemaître et al., "Protective Activity of Tetracycline Analogs against the Cytopathic Effect of the Human Immunodeficiency Viruses in CEM Cells," *Research in Virology* 141 (January-February 1990): 5–16.

94. Philip J. Hilts, "Evidence Is Said to Increase on Microbe's Role in AIDS," *New York Times*, 22 June 1990, A-18.

95. Michael Miller, "Doctors Offer Witch's Brew of Alternative Aids

Treatments," *Reuters Library Report,* 22 June 1990. This report carried a San Francisco dateline.

96. "The AIDS Catch" (documentary produced and directed by Joan Shenton, shown on Channel 4, British television), Meditel Productions, 5 March 1990.

97. Jad Adams, *AIDS: The HIV Myth* (New York: St. Martin's, 1989).

98. "The AIDS Catch."

99. Peter H. Duesberg and Bryan J. Ellison, "Is the AIDS Virus a Science Fiction? Immunosuppressive Behavior, Not HIV, May Be the Cause of AIDS," *Heritage Foundation Policy Review,* summer 1990, 40–51.

100. Bryan Ellison, interview by author, Berkeley, Calif., 1 October 1992.

101. Adam Meyerson, "Is HIV the Cause of AIDS?" *Heritage Foundation Policy Review,* fall 1990, 70 (editor's introduction to a special letters section).

102. Duesberg and Ellison, "Is the AIDS Virus a Science Fiction?" 41.

103. Ibid., 43.

104. Institute of Medicine, National Academy of Sciences, *Mobilizing against AIDS* (Cambridge, Mass.: Harvard Univ. Press, 1989), app. B. First printed in the *Morbidity and Mortality Weekly Report* 36, suppl. 1 (14 August 1987): 3S–15S.

105. Ibid., 288.

106. Duesberg and Ellison, "Is the AIDS Virus a Science Fiction?" 46.

107. Robert S. Root-Bernstein, "AIDS and Kaposi Sarcoma Pre-1979," *Lancet* 335 (21 April 1990): 969 (letter to the editor).

108. Duesberg and Ellison, "Is the AIDS Virus a Science Fiction?" 48.

109. Both Duesberg and Ellison agreed in retrospect that it was Ellison who advocated inclusion of the immune overload argument, while Duesberg at this point became suspicious of the linkage between sexual practices and AIDS. See the discussion of the evolution of Duesberg's causal argument after this point, in chapter 4.

110. Duesberg and Ellison, "Is the AIDS Virus a Science Fiction?" 49.

111. This decidedly odd reference to malnourished homosexuals is perhaps an allusion to the "gay bowel syndrome," which was often mentioned in the early medical literature on AIDS during the heyday of the immune overload hypothesis (see chapter 1).

112. Duesberg and Ellison, "Is the AIDS Virus a Science Fiction?" 48.

113. John Lauritsen, letter to Peter Duesberg, 27 March 1990.

114. Duesberg and Ellison, "Is the AIDS Virus a Science Fiction?" 49.

115. Ibid., 50–51.

116. Ibid.

117. Howard M. Temin, "Proof in the Pudding," *Heritage Foundation Policy Review,* fall 1990, 71–72 (letter to the editor).

118. Warren Winkelstein Jr., "Evidence for HIV," *Heritage Foundation Policy Review,* fall 1990, 71 (letter to the editor).

119. Michael Fumento, "Duesberg Injected," *Heritage Foundation Policy Review,* fall 1990, 80–81 (letter to the editor).

120. Peter H. Duesberg and Bryan J. Ellison, "Peter H. Duesberg and

Bryan J. Ellison Respond," *Heritage Foundation Policy Review,* fall 1990, 81–83 (letter to the editor).

121. Ibid.

122. Alfred S. Evans, "Does HIV Cause AIDS? An Historical Perspective," *Journal of Acquired Immune Deficiency Syndromes* 2 (April 1989): 107–113; Peter Duesberg, "Does HIV Cause AIDS?" *Journal of Acquired Immune Deficiency Syndromes* 2 (October 1989): 514–515 (letter to the editor); Alfred S. Evans, "Author's Reply," *Journal of Acquired Immune Deficiency Syndromes* 2 (October 1989): 515–517 (letter to the editor).

123. Evans, "Does HIV Cause AIDS?" 107, 112.

124. Duesberg cited a *New York Native* article by Joseph Sonnabend in his "HIV Is Not the Cause of AIDS"; he cited Celia Farber, Katie Leishman, and John Lauritsen in Duesberg, "Human Immunodeficiency Virus and Acquired Immunodeficiency Syndrome"; he cited Jad Adams, Farber, and Lauritsen in P. H. Duesberg, "AIDS: Non-Infectious Deficiencies Acquired by Drug Consumption and Other Risk Factors," *Research in Immunology* 141 (January 1990): 5–11; and so on.

125. Robert Root-Bernstein, "Do We Know the Cause(s) of AIDS?" *Perspectives in Biology and Medicine* 33 (summer 1990): 480–500.

126. Robert Gallo, *Virus Hunting* (New York: Basic Books, 1991).

127. Ibid., 276, 277.

128. Gallo, interview.

129. Gallo, *Virus Hunting,* 286, 296.

130. Ibid., 285, 289.

131. Garry Abrams, "Hero or Heretic? Peter Duesberg, One of the Country's Top Virus Specialists, Risks Reputation with Theory That HIV Doesn't Cause AIDS," *Los Angeles Times,* 21 May 1991, E-1.

132. Kim Painter, "A Controversial 'Spin' on AIDS," *USA Today,* 21 March 1989, D-5.

133. Charles Trueheart, "Down at the Healers," *Washington Post,* 24 July 1990, E-7.

134. Nathaniel S. Lehrman, "AIDS Controversy and the Media," *Lies of Our Times,* July-August 1991, 20.

135. John Lauritsen, "Science by Press Release," *New York Native,* 21 August 1989, 20–22; John Lauritsen, "The 'AIDS' War: Censorship and Propaganda Dominate Media Coverage of the Epidemic," *New York Native,* 12 August 1991, 14–18.

136. Michael C. Botkin, "The Great KS Debate," *Bay Area Reporter,* 29 August 1991, 19, 24.

137. Ralph Garrett, "Blind Trust," *San Diego Gay Times,* 20 June 1991, 16 (letter to the editor).

138. Stephen Hilgartner, "The Dominant View of Popularization: Conceptual Problems, Political Uses," *Social Studies of Science* 20 (August 1990): 519–539, quote from 522.

139. See note 124 above.

140. Hilgartner, "Dominant View of Popularization," 524.

Chapter 4

1. Charles A. Thomas Jr., telephone interview by author, 27 October 1992.

2. Charles A. Thomas Jr., form letter, 18 June 1991.

3. Group for the Scientific Reappraisal of the HIV/AIDS Hypothesis, unpublished letter, n.d. (ca. June 1991).

4. A different, and longer, version of the letter ultimately was published in *Science,* more than two and a half years later: Eleen Baumann et al., "AIDS Proposal," *Science* 267 (17 February 1995): 945–946 (letter to the editor).

5. Tony Perry, "San Diego at Large: Is It Politically Incorrect to Challenge AIDS-HIV Link?" *Los Angeles Times,* 9 September 1991, B-1, San Diego County edition.

6. Thomas J. DeLoughry, "40 Scientists Call on Colleagues to Re-evaluate AIDS Theory," *Chronicle of Higher Education,* 4 December 1991, A-9.

7. John Maddox, "AIDS Research Turned Upside Down," *Nature* 353 (26 September 1991): 297.

8. Roger Highfield, "Pilloried Professor May Be Right about Aids," *Daily Telegraph,* 26 September 1991, 6. (In Britain, the syndrome has generally been spelled with a combination of upper- and lowercase letters, as "Aids.")

9. Randy Peters, "New Study Vindicates Duesberg, Calls AIDS an Autoimmune Disease," *Bay Area Reporter,* 14 November 1991, 24.

10. Joseph Palca, "Duesberg Vindicated? Not Yet," *Science* 254 (18 October 1991): 376.

11. Ibid.

12. Joseph Sonnabend, "AIDS Research: All Sound and No Fury," *NYQ,* 1 December 1991, 50–51.

13. Anonymous reviews accompanying letter from Igor B. Dawid to Peter Duesberg, 12 February 1991.

14. Peter Duesberg, interview by author, tape recording, Berkeley, Calif., 28 September 1992.

15. My account here is based on a follow-up interview with Bryan Ellison, 23 October 1992.

16. P. H. Duesberg, "The Role of Drugs in the Origin of AIDS," *Biomedicine & Pharmacotherapy* 46 (January 1992): 3–15, quotes from 5, 8, 10.

17. Ibid., 5–6.

18. Margaret A. Fischl et al., "The Efficacy of Azidothymidine (AZT) in the Treatment of Patients with AIDS and AIDS-Related Complex," *New England Journal of Medicine* 317 (23 July 1987): 185–191. For debates, see Ezra Bowen, "Fateful Decisions on Treating AIDS," *Time,* 2 February 1987, 62; and John Lauritsen, *Poison by Prescription: The AZT Story* (New York: Asklepios, 1990), 19.

19. See the extended discussion of AZT studies in part two of this book.

20. In 1989, an open letter in the *New York Native* describing the use of AZT as "genocide" was signed by a range of community representatives, including Ortleb and Neenyah Ostrom from the *Native* staff; Lauritsen; James

D'Eramo; and ACT UP member Michael Petrelis ("An Open Letter to Mayor Koch," *New York Native,* 21 August 1989, 23).

21. See, for example, Michael Callen, "A Dinosaur's Diary," *NYQ,* 12 April 1992, 49–78.

22. Duesberg, "The Role of Drugs," 7, 9, 11.

23. Alfred S. Evans, "Author's Reply," *Journal of Acquired Immune Deficiency Syndromes* 2 (October 1989): 515–517 (letter to the editor).

24. Neville Hodgkinson, "Experts Mount Startling Challenge to Aids Orthodoxy," *Sunday Times* (London), 26 April 1992, 1; Neville Hodgkinson, "Aids: Can We Be Positive?" *Sunday Times* (London), 26 April 1992, 12–13; Neville Hodgkinson, "Time to Think Again on Aids Link, Claims HIV Pioneer," *Sunday Times* (London), 26 April 1992, 13.

25. Hodgkinson, "Aids: Can We Be Positive?" 12. In conversation, Duesberg identified himself to me as the observer quoted.

26. Clive Cooksun and Jenny Lynch, "A Chain Reaction—A Simple Method of Analysing Genetic Material Could Be Worth Billions of Dollars," *Financial Times,* 2 October 1992, 19.

27. Hodgkinson, "Aids: Can We Be Positive?" 12.

28. Nigel Hawkes, "Scientists Challenge Aids Link to HIV," *Times* (London), 27 April 1992.

29. "Wellcome Defends AZT Against Aids Report," *Reuters,* 27 April 1992.

30. Steve Connor, "Government Fears Complacency over Aids Prevention," *The Independent,* 2 May 1992.

31. William Leith, "New Theories, Old Prejudices," *The Independent,* 10 May 1992, 22 (op-ed).

32. Steve Connor, "The Spreading of a Terrible Myth," *The Independent,* 14 May 1992, 25 (op-ed).

33. Malcolm Dean, "London Perspective: AIDS and the Murdoch Press," *Lancet* 339 (23 May 1992): 1286 (News & Comment section).

34. Pierre Bourdieu, "The Specificity of the Scientific Field and the Social Conditions of the Progress of Reason," *Social Science Information* 14 (December 1975): 19–47, esp. 30.

35. Duesberg, interview.

36. Peter Gorner, "A Lively Cocktail Party of Scientists," *Chicago Tribune,* 15 November 1989, C-3.

37. "Last of the Great Tinkerers," *Time,* 12 August 1991, 55.

38. Tony Perry, "San Diego at Large: When You're a Flaky Genius, Problems Can Cease to Exist," *Los Angeles Times,* 1 September 1991, B-1, San Diego County edition.

39. Kary B. Mullis, "The Unusual Origins of the Polymerase Chain Reaction," *Scientific American* 262 (April 1990): 56.

40. Perry, "San Diego at Large."

41. Scott LaFee, "San Diegan Wins Chemistry Nobel," *San Diego Union-Tribune,* 14 October 1993, A-1.

42. Peter H. Duesberg, "Can Alternative Hypotheses Survive in This Era of Megaprojects?" *The Scientist,* 8 July 1991, 12 (commentary).

43. Ian Geogheagn, "U.K. Health Body Attacks Alternative Aids Claims," *Reuters,* 15 May 1992.

44. Nigel Hawkes, "Scientists Reject Role of HIV in Aids Cases," *Times* (London), 15 May 1992.

45. Tom Fennell, "What Causes AIDS," *Macleans,* 1 June 1992, 32.

46. "The New AIDS Controversy: Research World Torn by Theory That Says HIV May Not Trigger Deadly Disease," *Toronto Star,* 7 June 1992, B-1.

47. National Public Radio (segment reported by Mike Hornwick, Canadian Broadcasting Corporation), *NPR Weekend Edition,* 16 May 1992.

48. Avril McDonald, "HIV Does Not Cause AIDS, Virus Discoverer Claims," *QW,* 10 May 1992, 63.

49. Neenyah Ostrom, "Montagnier: HIV Is Not the Cause," *New York Native,* 11 May 1992, 7.

50. Arturo Jackson III, "Is the HIV Virus Really the True Cause of AIDS?" *San Francisco Sentinel,* 7 May 1992, 1.

51. On Delaney's relationship with Gallo and perceptions of him, see Jonathan Kwitny, *Acceptable Risks* (New York: Poseidon Press, 1992), 337, 343–344, 413, 460–461.

52. Reporter Lisa Krieger printed excerpts from the letter in her "AIDS-WEEK" column in the *San Francisco Examiner,* 20 May 1992, A-2.

53. Luc Montagnier, letter to Martin Delaney, Paris, 12 May 1992.

54. "Discussion Paper #5" (Project Inform, San Francisco, 3 June 1992, photocopy), 1 (boldface in the original).

55. Ibid., 5.

56. Ibid.

57. Ibid., 2.

58. Ibid.

59. Ibid., 5–6.

60. Ibid., 3.

61. Duesberg, interview.

62. Bruce Livesey and Ellen Lipsius, "AIDS: Modern Medicine's Achilles' Heel," *Canadian Dimension,* October 1989, 27–30, quote from 28.

63. Thomas, interview.

64. The quotes are from an article describing the magazine: Paul Ciotti, "John Kurzweil of Sherman Oaks Publishes a Conservative Political Magazine," *Los Angeles Times,* 14 August 1992, 20.

65. Tom Bethell, "The Case for Buchanan," *National Review,* 2 March 1992: 34–37 (cover story).

66. Tom Bethell, "Column Right: We May Regret Going Along with This: The Gay-Rights Agenda Precludes Any Public Doubts," *Los Angeles Times,* 8 July 1991, B-5 (op-ed).

67. Tom Bethell, "Conversations in the Tenderloin," *California Political Review,* fall 1991: 20–23.

68. "Discussion Paper #5," 4.

69. Ellison, interview.

70. Thomas Ryan, "AIDS as Career," *Christopher Street,* May 1988, 28–35, quote from 31.

71. Drew Hopkins, "Peter Duesberg and the Media," *Christopher Street,* April 1988, 52–59.

72. Geoffrey Cowley, "Is a New AIDS Virus Emerging?" *Newsweek,* 27 July 1992, 41.

73. Lawrence K. Altman, "New Virus Said to Cause a Condition Like AIDS," *New York Times,* 23 July 1992, B-8.

74. Cowley, "Is a New AIDS Virus Emerging?" 41.

75. See Martin Delaney's report: "Does a New Virus Stalk the Land?" *Advocate,* 25 August 1992, 33.

76. Peter Duesberg, "HIV-Free AIDS Reports," *Science* 257 (21 September 1992): 1848 (letter to the editor).

77. Steve Heimoff, "Test Ideas with Science, Not Scorn: Critics Who Insist That HIV Doesn't Cause AIDS May Be Wrong, but Their Argument Deserves Checking," *Los Angeles Times,* 28 July 1992, B-7 (op-ed).

78. Michael Fumento, "A Complicated Disease Won't Have Simple Answers: The AIDS Establishment Needs Critics, but Arguing That HIV Doesn't Cause the Disease Is Murderously Wrong," *Los Angeles Times,* 28 July 1992, B-7 (op-ed).

79. Peter H. Duesberg and Bryan J. Ellison, letter to the editor, *Los Angeles Times,* 7 August 1992, B-6.

80. Bruce Mirken, "The Twilight Zone," *QW,* 9 August 1992, 44, 67, 68; John S. James, "AIDS Treatment News," *San Francisco Bay Times,* 13 August 1992, 12–14.

81. Delaney, "Does a New Virus Stalk the Land?" 33.

82. Charles E. Ortleb, "Honey, I Blew Up the HIV Paradigm," *New York Native,* 3 August 1992, 4 (editorial).

83. Geoffrey Cowley, "AIDS or Chronic Fatigue?" *Newsweek,* 7 September 1992, 66.

84. Christine Gorman, "Invincible AIDS," *Time,* 3 August 1992, 28–37. The magazine's cover read: "Losing the Battle."

85. Daniel J. DeNoon, "Jury Still Out on Etiology of HIV-Negative CD4 Deficiency," *CDC AIDS Weekly,* 24 August 1992, 2–6 (news report).

86. "Unexplained CD4+ T-Lymphocyte Depletion in Persons without Evident HIV Infection—United States," *Morbidity and Mortality Weekly Report* 41 (31 July 1992): 541–545; "Update: CD4+ T-Lymphocytopenia in Persons without Evident HIV Infection—United States," *Morbidity and Mortality Weekly Report* 41 (7 August 1992): 578–579.

87. DeNoon, "Jury Still Out," 3.

88. World Health Organization Global Programme on AIDS, *Report of a Scientific Meeting on Unexplained Severe Immunodeficiency without Evidence of HIV Infection* (Geneva, 28–29 September 1992).

89. One report was: Omar Bagasra et al., "Detection of Human Immunodeficiency Virus Type-1 Provirus in Mononuclear Cells by In Situ Polymerase Chain Reaction," *New England Journal of Medicine* 326 (21 May 1992): 1385–1391. The other report was made by Dr. David Ho at a Burroughs Wellcome symposium in Amsterdam (described in: Ronald A. Baker, "Treatment Updates from the Harvard-Amsterdam AIDS Conference," *BETA,* August 1992, 1–11).

90. Janet Embretson et al., "Analysis of Human Immunodeficiency Virus–Infected Tissues by Amplification and *In Situ* Hybridization Reveals Latent and Permissive Infections at Single-Cell Resolution," *Proceedings of the National Academy of Sciences* 90 (January 1993): 357.

91. David Perlman, "HIV Is Never Truly Latent, Lymphoid Cell Studies Show," *San Francisco Chronicle*, 25 March 1993, A-2.

92. John Maddox, "Facing the Cruel Truth about HIV," *Times* (London), 25 March 1993 (features section).

93. Lawrence K. Altman, "Cost of Treating AIDS Patients Is Soaring," *New York Times*, 23 July 1992, B-8.

94. Kevin J. P. Craib et al., "HIV Causes AIDS: A Controlled Study" (Abstract #WeC 1027), VIII International Conference on AIDS, Amsterdam, 22 July 1992.

95. This exchange occurred in a UC Berkeley classroom debate: "IDS Seminar Series" (forum on causes of AIDS, with Peter Duesberg, Warren Winkelstein, and Chip Shepard), University of California at Berkeley, 28 September 1992 (author's field notes).

96. M. S. Ascher et al., "Does Drug Use Cause AIDS?" *Nature* 362 (11 March 1993): 103–104.

97. Sheryl Stolberg, "Studies Rebut Controversial AIDS Theory," *Los Angeles Times*, 11 March 1993, A-18; Gina Kolata, "Debunking Doubts That H.I.V. Causes AIDS," *New York Times*, 11 March 1993, B-13.

98. Ascher et al., "Does Drug Use Cause AIDS?" 103.

99. H. Tristram Engelhardt Jr. and Arthur L. Caplan, "Patterns of Controversy and Closure: The Interplay of Knowledge, Values, and Political Forces," in *Scientific Controversies: Case Studies in the Resolution and Closure of Disputes in Science and Technology,* ed. H. Tristram Engelhardt Jr. and Arthur L. Caplan (Cambridge, England: Cambridge Univ. Press, 1987), 6, 11.

100. Fujimura and Chou have contended that Duesberg relied on a "laboratory style of practice" and his adversaries employed an "epidemiological style of practice." While that may be correct, over time both sides came to emphasize epidemiology as the science that could conceivably provide the most definitive evidence. See Joan H. Fujimura and Danny Y. Chou, "Dissent in Science: Styles of Scientific Practice and the Controversy over the Cause of AIDS," *Social Science and Medicine* 38 (April 1994): 1017–1036.

101. Bryan Ellison, interview by author, Berkeley, 23 October 1992. See also the critique of the Craib et al. study in Benjamin A. Goldman and Michael Chappelle, "Is HIV = AIDS Wrong?" *In These Times,* 5 August 1992, 8–10.

102. Harry Collins and Trevor Pinch, *The Golem: What Everyone Should Know about Science* (Cambridge: Cambridge Univ. Press, 1993), 3.

103. Steven Shapin, "Cordelia's Love: Credibility and the Social Studies of Studies," *Perspectives on Science* 3, no. 3 (1995): 255–275.

104. Martin Delaney, "Evidence Does Not Back Duesberg's Views," *San Francisco Chronicle*, 4 September 1992, A-29 (op-ed).

105. See Fujimura and Chou, "Dissent in Science."

106. René Dubos, *Mirage of Health: Utopias, Progress, and Biological Change* (New York: Harper & Brothers, 1959), 86.

107. "What Causes AIDS? A Second Look" (reported by Colman Jones,

Canadian Broadcasting Corporation, Toronto), *Ideas,* 6–7 November 1991. Transcript published in 1992.

108. Robert Gallo, interview by author, tape recording, Bethesda, Md., 3 November 1994.

109. Robert S. Root-Bernstein, *Rethinking AIDS: The Tragic Cost of Premature Consensus* (New York: Free Press, 1993). For a more recent update, see Robert S. Root-Bernstein, "Five Myths about AIDS That Have Misdirected Research and Treatment," *Genetica* 95, no. 1–3 (1995): 111–132.

110. John Lauritsen, *The AIDS War: Propaganda, Profiteering and Genocide from the Medical-Industrial Complex* (New York: Asklepios, 1993).

111. Peter H. Duesberg, *Inventing the AIDS Virus* (Washington, D.C.: Regnery, 1996).

112. David W. Dunlap, "Michael Callen, Singer and Expert on Coping with AIDS, Dies at 38," *New York Times,* 29 December 1993.

113. Colin Macilwain, "AAAS Criticized over AIDS Sceptics' Meeting," *Nature* 369 (May 1994): 265; Rick Weiss, "And Now for Something Completely Different: Florida Physician Throws a Dramatic Jab at the Experts' View of AIDS," *Washington Post,* 1 November 1994, 7; Richard Stone, "Congressman Uncovers the HIV Conspiracy," *Science* 268 (14 April 1995): 191.

114. Jon Cohen, "The Duesberg Phenomenon," *Science* 266 (9 December 1994): 1642–1649 (special news report). The article prompted eight pages of letters, published in the January 13 and January 20 issues. This article marked my own entry as an actor in the controversy: I was interviewed by Cohen about the sociological bases of the controversy and quoted in the text. For a critique of Cohen's article that also takes me to task, see Tom Bethell, "The Cohen Phenomenon," *Reappraising AIDS* 3 (April 1995).

115. Cohen, "Duesberg Phenomenon," 1645, 1647, 1649.

116. Billy Goodman, "A Controversy That Will Not Die: The Role of HIV in Causing AIDS," *The Scientist,* 20 March 1995, 1, 6, 7. Goodman had read my doctoral dissertation; the title of his article was borrowed from the title of this chapter in its earlier incarnation.

117. Anthony Fauci, "Writing for My Sister Denise," *AAAS Observer,* 1 September 1989, 4.

118. Harry M. Collins and Trevor J. Pinch, "The Construction of the Paranormal: Nothing Unscientific Is Happening," in *On the Margins of Science: The Social Construction of Rejected Knowledge,* ed. Roy Wallis (Keele, England: Univ. of Keele Press, 1979), 237–270.

119. Susan Leigh Star, *Regions of the Mind: Brain Research and the Quest for Scientific Certainty* (Stanford: Stanford Univ. Press, 1989), 140.

120. See Brian Martin, *Scientific Knowledge in Controversy: The Social Dynamics of the Fluoridation Debate* (Albany: State Univ. of New York Press, 1991), esp. chapter 4 ("The Struggle over Credibility"). For similar credibility strategies, see Star, *Regions of the Mind,* 138–144.

121. Martin, *Scientific Knowledge in Controversy,* 61, 62.

122. Ibid., 89.

123. Fumento, quoted in Tom Bethell, "Heretic," *American Spectator,* May 1992, 18.

124. Martin, *Scientific Knowledge in Controversy,* 90.

125. Michael C. Botkin, "The Great KS Debate," *Bay Area Reporter*, 29 August 1991, 19.

126. These anecdotes were reported in Martin, *Scientific Knowledge in Controversy*, 93–98.

127. Ibid., 101.

128. Ibid.

129. Celia Farber, "Fatal Distraction," *Spin*, June 1992, 84.

130. Delaney, "Evidence Does Not Back Duesberg's Views," A-29.

131. Anthony Fauci, "Writing for My Sister Denise."

132. On scientists' difficulties in signaling degrees of consensus to the lay public, see Yaron Ezrahi, "The Authority of Science in Politics," in *Science and Values: Patterns of Tradition and Change,* ed. Arnold Thackray and Everett Mendelsohn (New York: Humanities Press, 1974), 215–251, esp. 222. On the media's tendency to portray scientific controversies as having "two sides, of somewhat comparable merit," see Rae Goodell, "The Role of the Mass Media in Scientific Controversies," in *Scientific Controversies: Case Studies in the Resolution and Closure of Disputes in Science and Technology,* ed. H. Tristram Engelhardt Jr. and Arthur L. Caplan (Cambridge, England: Cambridge Univ. Press, 1987), 585–597, quote from 589.

133. Duesberg, interview.

134. Ibid.

135. Anne Karpf, *Doctoring the Media: The Reporting of Health and Medicine* (London: Routledge, 1988), 111.

136. Goodell, "Role of the Mass Media in Scientific Controversies," 590.

137. Karpf, *Doctoring the Media,* 111, describing David M. Rubin and Val Hendy, "Swine Influenza and the News Media," *Annals of Internal Medicine* 87 (December 1977): 769–774.

138. Duesberg, interview.

139. For Gallo's critiques of the press, see Robert Gallo, *Virus Hunting* (New York: Basic Books, 1991).

140. Russell Schoch, "A Conversation with Peter Duesberg," *California Monthly,* April 1990, 8–11, quote from 9.

141. "An AIDS Theory That Can Kill," *San Francisco Examiner,* 11 September 1992, A-26 (editorial).

142. Celia Farber, "AIDS: Words from the Front," *Spin*, August 1992, 65–67.

143. Duesberg, interview.

Chapter 5

1. Randy Shilts, *And the Band Played On: Politics, People, and the AIDS Epidemic* (New York: St. Martin's, 1987), 451.

2. Philip M. Boffey, "A Likely AIDS Cause, but Still No Cure," *New York Times,* 29 April 1984, sec. 4, p. 22.

3. Margaret I. Johnston and Daniel F. Hoth, "Present Status and Future Prospects for HIV Therapies," *Science* 260 (28 May 1993): 1286–1293.

4. See John M. Coffin, "Introduction to Retroviruses," in *AIDS and Other*

Manifestations of HIV Infection, 2d ed., ed. Gary P. Wormser (New York: Raven Press, 1992), 37–56.

5. For an example of an argument linking this conception of pathogenesis with the search for a reverse transcriptase inhibitor, see Dani P. Bolognesi and Peter J. Fischinger, "Prospects for Treatment of Human Retrovirus-Associated Diseases," *Cancer Research* 45, Suppl. (September 1985): 4700s–4705s.

6. H. Mitsuya et al., "Suramin Protection of T Cells in Vitro Against Infectivity and Cytopathic Effect of HTLV-III," *Science* 226 (12 October 1984): 172–174.

7. W. Rozenbaum et al., "Antimoniotungstate (HPA 23) Treatment of Three Patients with AIDS and One with Prodrome," *Lancet,* 23 February 1985, 450–451.

8. Ibid., 450.

9. Matt Clark and Vincent Coppola, "AIDS: A Growing 'Pandemic'?" *Newsweek,* 29 April 1985, 71.

10. Lawrence K. Altman, "The Doctor's World: AIDS Data Pour In, Studies Proliferate," *New York Times,* 23 April 1985, C-3.

11. The following history of drug regulation in the United States draws from Harry Milton Marks, "Ideas as Reforms: Therapeutic Experiments and Medical Practice, 1900–1980" (Ph.D. diss., Massachusetts Institute of Technology, 1987); and Albert R. Jonsen and Jeff Stryker, eds., *The Social Impact of AIDS in the United States* (Washington, D.C.: National Academy Press, 1993), 84–87.

12. Marks has refuted the commonly told story that, before Kefauver-Harris, the FDA *never* looked at efficacy; see "Ideas as Reforms," 53. Ironically, thalidomide has recently resurfaced, as a potential AIDS drug.

13. Marks, "Ideas as Reforms," 85–86.

14. Harold M. Schmeck Jr., "Scientists Say Genes in AIDS May Hamper Vaccine Work," *New York Times,* 11 October 1984, A-24.

15. Altman, "Doctor's World: AIDS Data Pour In."

16. "International Conference," *BAPHRON* 7 (May-June 1985): 306.

17. William F. Buckley Jr., "Steps in Combating the AIDS Epidemic," *New York Times,* 18 March 1985 (op-ed).

18. Cindy Patton has criticized the common tendency to imagine that AIDS activism originated with the birth of ACT UP in 1987; see *Inventing AIDS* (New York: Routledge, 1990), 19.

19. Michael Specter, "The New Politics of AIDS," *Washington Post Weekly,* 19 August 1985, 9.

20. See Jackie Winnow, "Lesbians Evolving Health Care: Cancer and AIDS," *Feminist Review,* summer 1992, 68–77; Gena Corea, *The Invisible Epidemic: The Story of Women and AIDS* (New York: HarperCollins, 1992); Amber Hollibaugh, "Lesbian Denial and Lesbian Leadership in the AIDS Epidemic: Bravery and Fear in the Construction of a Lesbian Geography of Risk," in *Women Resisting AIDS: Feminist Strategies of Empowerment,* ed. Beth E. Schneider and Nancy E. Stoller (Philadelphia: Temple Univ. Press, 1995), 219–230; Nancy Stoller, "Lesbian Involvement in the AIDS Epidemic: Changing

Roles and Generational Differences," in *Women Resisting AIDS* (above), 270–285.

21. Jonathan Kwitny, *Acceptable Risks* (New York: Poseidon Press, 1992), 20–73.

22. Mark Clark et al., "AIDS Exiles in Paris," *Newsweek,* 5 August 1985, 71.

23. Irvin Molotsky, "French AIDS Drug Due for U.S. Tests," *New York Times,* 31 July 1985, A-10.

24. Lawrence K. Altman, "The Doctor's World: Search for an AIDS Drug Is Case History in Frustration," *New York Times,* 30 July 1985, C-1.

25. Kwitny, *Acceptable Risks,* 49–50, 82–83.

26. Ibid., 29–31.

27. See, for example, Robert J. Levine, *Ethics and Regulation of Clinical Research* (Baltimore: Urban & Schwarzenberg, 1986).

28. Jonsen and Stryker, *Social Impact of AIDS,* 81.

29. David J. Rothman, *Strangers at the Bedside* (New York: Basic Books, 1991), 15–18, 70–84.

30. James H. Jones, *Bad Blood: The Tuskegee Syphilis Experiment* (New York: Free Press, 1981).

31. Jonsen and Stryker, *Social Impact of AIDS,* 87–88.

32. David J. Rothman and Harold Edgar, "AIDS, Activism, and Ethics," *Hospital Practice* 26 (15 July 1991): 135–142, quote from 136.

33. Robert Yarchoan et al., "Implications of the Discovery of HTLV-III for the Treatment of AIDS," *Cancer Research* 45, Suppl. (September 1985): 4685s–4688s.

34. Samuel Broder et al., "Effects of Suramin on HTLV-III/LAV Infection Presenting as Kaposi's Sarcoma or AIDS-Related Complex: Clinical Pharmacology and Suppression of Virus Replication in Vivo," *Lancet,* 21 September 1985, 627–630.

35. Bruce Nussbaum, *Good Intentions: How Big Business and the Medical Establishment Are Corrupting the Fight against AIDS* (New York: Atlantic Monthly Press, 1990), 23.

36. See Kwitny, *Acceptable Risks,* 84–93 and the accompanying endnotes.

37. Paul Volberding and Donald Abrams, quoted in Kwitny, *Acceptable Risks,* 437.

38. Barry Adkins, "Looking at AIDS in Totality: A Conversation with Joseph Sonnabend," *New York Native,* 7 October 1985, 21–25.

39. See the account in Nussbaum, *Good Intentions,* chapter 1.

40. "A Failure Led to Drug against AIDS," *New York Times,* 20 September 1986, A-7.

41. "New Drug Shows Gain in Fight against AIDS," *New York Times,* 26 January 1986, A-17.

42. Robert Yarchoan et al., "Administration of 3'-Azido-3'-Deoxythymidine, an Inhibitor of HTLV-III/LAV Replication, to Patients with AIDS or AIDS-Related Complex," *Lancet,* 15 March 1986, 575–580.

43. Jean L. Marx, "AIDS Drug Shows Promise in Preliminary Clinical Trial," *Science* 231 (28 March 1986): 1504–1505.

44. Yarchoan et al., "Administration of 3'-Azido-3'-Deoxythymidine," 580.

45. John S. James, "What's Wrong with AIDS Treatment Research?" *AIDS Treatment News,* 9 May 1986.

46. John James, interview by author, tape recording, San Francisco, 10 December 1993; Peter S. Arno and Karyn L. Feiden, *Against the Odds: The Story of AIDS Drug Development, Politics and Profits* (New York: HarperCollins, 1992), 64; Katherine Bishop, "Underground Press Leads Way on AIDS Advice," *New York Times,* 16 December 1991, A-16.

47. This figure is given by John James in "A Wish List, Some Problems, and Recommendations: Testimony of John S. James before the Presidential Commission on the HIV Epidemic, New York City, New York, February 20, 1988," *AIDS Treatment News,* 26 February 1988.

48. Debbie Indyk and David Rier, "Grassroots AIDS Knowledge: Implications for the Boundaries of Science and Collective Action," *Knowledge: Creation, Diffusion, Utilization* 15 (September 1993): 3–43, quote from 9.

49. James, "What's Wrong with AIDS Treatment Research?"

50. John S. James, "AIDS Conspiracy—Just a Theory?" *AIDS Treatment News* (September 1986).

51. Erik Eckholm, "$100 Million for AIDS Drug Testing," *New York Times,* 1 July 1986, C-3.

52. Nussbaum, *Good Intentions,* 127–130.

53. See Marks, "Ideas as Reforms"; Theodore M. Porter, *Trust in Numbers: The Pursuit of Objectivity in Science and Public Life* (Princeton, N.J.: Princeton Univ. Press, 1995), 203–216; and the citations I provide in note 147 of the introduction.

54. Marks, "Ideas as Reforms," 173, 239, 242.

55. This estimate was offered by Dr. Curtis Meinert, editor of the specialty journal *Controlled Clinical Trials,* in Philip M. Boffey, "Thousands in U.S. Receive Treatments in Experiments," *New York Times,* 7 January 1986, C-1.

56. Boffey, "Thousands in U.S. Receive Treatments."

57. Ibid.

58. See Susan Ellenberg et al., "The Use of External Monitoring Committees in Clinical Trials of the National Institute of Allergy and Infectious Diseases," *Statistics in Medicine* 12 (March 1993): 461–467.

59. Erik Eckholm, "AIDS Drug Prolongs Lives in Some Cases," *New York Times,* 20 September 1986, A-1.

60. Deborah M. Barnes, "Promising Results Halt Trial of Anti-AIDS Drug," *Science* 234 (3 October 1986): 15–16.

61. Margaret A. Fischl et al., "The Efficacy of Azidothymidine (AZT) in the Treatment of Patients with AIDS and AIDS-Related Complex," *New England Journal of Medicine* 317 (23 July 1987): 185–191.

62. Douglas D. Richman et al., "The Toxicity of Azidothymidine (AZT) in the Treatment of Patients with AIDS and AIDS-Related Complex," *New England Journal of Medicine* 317 (23 July 1987): 192–197.

63. Erik Eckholm, "Test Group for AIDS Drug Is Broadened to Include 7,000," *New York Times,* 1 October 1986, B-6.

64. Irvin Molotsky, "U.S. Approves Drug to Prolong Lives of AIDS Patients," *New York Times,* 21 March 1987, A-1.

65. Barnaby J. Feder, "Drug Expected to Spur Growth and Profit of Its Maker," *New York Times,* 21 March 1987, A-32.

66. Gina Kolata, "Imminent Marketing of AZT Raises Problems," *Science* 235 (20 March 1987): 1462–1463 ("Research News").

67. Ezra Bowen, "Fateful Decisions on Treating AIDS," *Time,* 2 February 1987, 62.

68. Itzak Brook, "Approval of Zidovudine (AZT) for Acquired Immunodeficiency Syndrome," *Journal of the American Medical Association* 258 (18 September 1987): 1517 (commentary).

69. Bowen, "Fateful Decisions on Treating AIDS."

70. Philip J. Hilts, "Results of AIDS Drug Test Raising Ethical Questions," *Washington Post,* 14 September 1986, A-1.

71. Bowen, "Fateful Decisions on Treating AIDS."

72. Benjamin Freedman, "Equipoise and the Ethics of Clinical Research," *New England Journal of Medicine* 317 (16 July 1987): 141–145.

73. Jonsen and Stryker, *Social Impact of AIDS,* 83–84.

74. See François Blanchard and Ruth Murbach, "AIDS and Clinical Research: Ethical Controversy and Equipoise" (paper presented at the annual meeting of the Society for Social Studies of Science, Minneapolis, 19 October, 1990).

75. Robert M. Veatch, *The Patient as Partner: A Theory of Human-Experimentation Ethics* (Bloomington: Indiana Univ. Press, 1987), 7, 211.

76. Dominique Lapierre, *Beyond Love* (New York: Warner Books, 1991), 369.

77. From a conference presentation published as: Douglas D. Richman, "Public Access to Experimental Drug Therapy: AIDS Raises Yet Another Conflict between Freedom of the Individual and Welfare of the Individual and Public," *Journal of Infectious Diseases* 159 (March 1989): 412–415.

78. Ibid.

79. See Ruth Macklin and Gerald Friedland, "AIDS Research: The Ethics of Clinical Trials," *Law, Medicine & Health Care* 14 (December 1986): 273–280; David J. Rothman and Harold Edgar, "Scientific Rigor and Medical Realities: Placebo Trials in Cancer and AIDS Research," in *AIDS: The Making of a Chronic Disease,* ed. Elizabeth Fee and Daniel M. Fox (Berkeley: Univ. of California Press, 1992), 194–206.

80. These anecdotes are reported in Lapierre, *Beyond Love,* 366–367.

81. See Gary B. Melton et al., "Community Consultation in Socially Sensitive Research: Lessons from Clinical Trials of Treatments for AIDS," *American Psychologist* 43 (July 1988): 573–581, esp. 574.

82. Harry Collins has emphasized that perceptions of certainty in science typically depend on one's "distance from the research front": the closer one gets to the center, the messier things appear (H. M. Collins, "Certainty and the Public Understanding of Science: Science on Television," *Social Studies of Science* 17 [1987]: 692).

83. Ivan Emke, "Medical Authority and Its Discontents: The Case of Organized Non-Compliance," *Critical Sociology* 19 (Fall 1993): 57–80.

84. Norman Fineman, "The Social Construction of Noncompliance: A Study of Health Care and Social Service Providers in Everyday Practice," *Sociology of Health & Illness* 13 (September 1991): 354–374.

85. Emke, "Questioning Medical Authority."

86. Eliot Freidson, "The Impurity of Professional Authority," in *Institutions and the Person*, ed. Howard S. Becker, Blanche Geer, et al. (Chicago: Aldine, 1968), 25–34, esp. 29–30.

87. On models of the doctor-patient relationship, see Thomas S. Szasz and Marc H. Hollender, "A Contribution to the Philosophy of Medicine: The Basic Models of the Doctor-Patient Relationship," *Archives of Internal Medicine* 97 (May 1956): 585–592. On the transformation of the patient into a surgical "object," see Stefan Hirschauer, "The Manufacture of Bodies in Surgery," *Social Studies of Science* 21 (May 1991): 279–319.

88. Indyk and Rier, "Grassroots AIDS Knowledge," 6.

89. PWA Coalition, "Founding Statement of People with AIDS/ARC," in *AIDS: Cultural Analysis, Cultural Activism*, ed. Douglas Crimp (Cambridge, Mass.: Massachusetts Institute of Technology Press, 1988), 148–149.

90. PWA Coalition, "A Patient's Bill of Rights," in *AIDS: Cultural Analysis, Cultural Activism*, ed. Douglas Crimp (Cambridge, Mass.: Massachusetts Institute of Technology Press, 1988), 160.

91. Tim Kingston, "The AIDS Industry vs. the Healing Workers," *Coming Up!* April 1988, 10–13. The anthropologist cited was Ronald Frankenberg of the University of Keele in England.

92. Michelle Roland, "Managing Your Doctor," *AIDS Treatment News*, 21 September 1990, 4.

93. John D. Arras, "Noncompliance in AIDS Research," *Hastings Center Report*, September-October 1990, 24–32.

94. Barrie R. Cassileth and Helene Brown, "Unorthodox Cancer Medicine," *Ca—A Cancer Journal for Clinicians* 38 (May-June 1988): 176–186.

95. Paul Monette, *Borrowed Time: An AIDS Memoir* (San Diego: Harcourt Brace Jovanovich, 1987), 92.

96. Lapierre, *Beyond Love*, 214.

97. Charles L. Bosk and Joel E. Frader, "AIDS and Its Impact on Medical Work: The Culture and Politics of the Shop Floor," *Milbank Quarterly* 68, suppl. 2 (1990): 257–279, esp. 271.

Chapter 6

1. Robert C. Gallo et al., "HTLV-III/LAV and the Origin and Pathogenesis of AIDS," *International Archives of Allergy and Applied Immunology* 82 (March-April 1987): 471–475.

2. Gina Kolata, "The Evolving Biology of AIDS: Scavenger Cell Looms Large," *New York Times*, 7 June 1988, C-1.

3. See Wendy K. Mariner and Robert C. Gallo, "Getting to Market: The Scientific and Legal Climate for Developing an AIDS Vaccine," *Law, Medi-*

cine & Health Care 15 (summer 1987): 17–26; Jay A. Levy, "Can an AIDS Vaccine Be Developed?" *Transfusion Medicine Reviews* 2 (December 1988): 264–271.

4. Lawrence K. Altman, "The Doctor's World: Who Will Volunteer for an AIDS Vaccine?" *New York Times,* 15 April 1986, C-1. The official was not identified.

5. Ibid. From a statistical standpoint, the only solution is to do a larger trial or have it run for a longer period of time, so as to generate more "events" of HIV infection—or simply to assume that AIDS education is never going to be entirely effective in preventing new infections.

6. Philip M. Boffey, "Experts Find Lag on Testing Drugs in AIDS Patients," *New York Times,* 12 April 1987, A-1.

7. Ibid.

8. Bruce Nussbaum, *Good Intentions: How Big Business and the Medical Establishment Are Corrupting the Fight against AIDS* (New York: Atlantic Monthly Press, 1990), 143 ff.

9. Daniel Hoth, interview by author, tape recording, Foster City, Calif., 11 July and 19 October, 1994.

10. Ibid.

11. Philip M. Boffey, "Campaign to Find Drugs for Fighting AIDS Is Intensified," *New York Times,* 14 February 1988, A-1.

12. Ibid.

13. Dick Thompson, "A Decoy for the Deadly AIDS Virus: Human Tests Begin for a New Genetically Engineered Drug," *Time,* 22 August 1988, 69.

14. Ellen Cooper, interview by author, tape recording, Rockville, Md., 25 April 1994.

15. Gina Kolata, "Doctors Stretch Rules on AIDS Drug," *New York Times,* 21 December 1987, A-1.

16. Mathilde Krim, "Making Experimental Drugs Available for AIDS Treatment," *AIDS & Public Policy* 2 (spring-summer 1987): 1–5.

17. Tim Kingston, "Death by Placebo: The Sacrificial Lambs of Protocol 019," *Coming Up!* September 1988, 10–11.

18. Thomas C. Chalmers, "The Need for Early Randomization in the Development of New Drugs for AIDS," *Journal of Acquired Immune Deficiency Syndromes* 3, suppl. 2 (1990): S11.

19. Kingston, "Death by Placebo," 10.

20. Robert J. Levine, "Clinical Trials and Physicians as Double Agents," *Yale Journal of Biology and Medicine* 65 (March-April 1992): 65–74.

21. David J. Rothman and Harold Edgar, "Scientific Rigor and Medical Realities: Placebo Trials in Cancer and AIDS Research," in *AIDS: The Making of a Chronic Disease,* ed. Elizabeth Fee and Daniel M. Fox (Berkeley: Univ. of California Press, 1992), 194–206, quote from 205.

22. Andrew Abbott, *The System of Professions: An Essay on the Division of Expert Labor* (Chicago: Univ. of Chicago Press, 1988), 188 ff; Andrew Abbott, "Status and Status Strain in the Professions," *American Journal of Sociology* 86 (January 1981): 819–835.

23. See Mary-Rose Mueller, "Science in the Community: The Redistribution of Medical Authority in Federally Sponsored Treatment Research for AIDS" (Ph.D. diss., University of California at San Diego, 1995).

24. John S. James, "Treatment Research Ideas for Community-Based Trials," *AIDS Treatment News*, 7 October 1988.

25. Mueller, "Science in the Community," quote from 276n.

26. Bruno Latour, "Give Me a Laboratory and I Will Raise the World," in *Science Observed: Perspectives on the Social Study of Science*, ed. Karin D. Knorr-Cetina and Michael Mulkay (London: Sage, 1983), 141-170.

27. John S. James, "Community Research Alliance: New San Francisco Effort for Community-Based Trials," *AIDS Treatment News*, 2 December 1988.

28. Albert R. Jonsen and Jeff Stryker, eds., *The Social Impact of AIDS in the United States* (Washington, D.C.: National Academy Press, 1993), 100.

29. Donald Abrams, interview by author, tape recording, San Francisco, 16 December 1993.

30. James, "Community Research Alliance."

31. "Decisions for Community-Based Trials," *AIDS Treatment News*, 7 October 1988; Gina Kolata, "Doctors and Patients Take AIDS Drug Trials into Their Own Hands," *New York Times*, 15 March 1988, C-3.

32. Peter S. Arno and Karyn L. Feiden in *Against the Odds: The Story of AIDS Drug Development, Politics, and Profits* (New York: HarperCollins, 1992) 111.

33. Ibid., 93-95, 116.

34. Ibid., 118; Nussbaum, *Good Intentions*, 233.

35. Nussbaum, *Good Intentions*, 234.

36. Presidential Commission on the Human Immunodeficiency Virus Epidemic, *Report of the Presidential Commission on the Human Immunodeficiency Virus Epidemic, Submitted to the President of the United States, June 24, 1988* (Washington, D.C., 1988), 56.

37. Dr. Burton J. Lee Jr., quoted in Kolata, "Doctors and Patients Take AIDS Drug Trials into Their Own Hands."

38. Gina Kolata, "Private Doctors Testing AIDS Drugs in Novel Approach," *New York Times*, 9 July 1989, A-1.

39. Charles Linebarger, "CMJ Zaps Drug Maker for AIDS Profiteering," *Bay Area Reporter*, 4 June 1987, 14.

40. "AIDS Action Pledge Holds First Meeting," *Bay Area Reporter*, 27 August 1987, 14.

41. On ACT UP, see "ACT UP/New York Capsule History" (AIDS Coalition to Unleash Power, New York, 1991, photocopy); ACT UP/New York Women and AIDS Book Group, *Women, AIDS, and Activism* (Boston: South End Press, 1990); Cathy Jean Cohen, "Power, Resistance and the Construction of Crisis: Marginalized Communities Respond to AIDS" (Ph.D. diss., University of Michigan, 1993); Douglas Crimp and Adam Rolston, *AIDS Demographics* (Seattle: Bay Press, 1990); Gilbert Elbaz, "The Sociology of AIDS Activism, the Case of ACT UP/New York, 1987-1992" (Ph.D. diss., City University of New York, 1992); Josh Gamson, "Silence, Death, and the Invisible Enemy: AIDS Activism and Social Movement 'Newness,'" *Social Problems* 36 (October 1989): 351-365; Maxine Wolfe, "The AIDS Coalition to Unleash

Power, New York (ACT UP NY): A Direct Action Political Model of Community Research for AIDS Prevention," in *AIDS Prevention and Services: Community Based Research,* ed. J. Van Vugt (Westport, Conn.: Bergin Garvey, forthcoming).

42. On the cultural sources of ACT UP's representational politics, see also Stephen O. Murray, *American Gay* (Chicago: Univ. of Chicago Press, 1996), chapter 5.

43. Gamson, "Silence, Death, and the Invisible Enemy," 354–355. For the literature on "new social movements," see the sources cited in the introduction of my book, note 87.

44. On ACT UP's demonstrations as "performances," see Cindy J. Kistenberg, "Theatrical Intervention in the AIDS Crisis: Performance, Politics, and Social Change" (Ph.D. diss., Louisiana State University, 1992).

45. David Firestone, "A Monument to AIDS: GMHC's New Six-Story Home Is a Symbol of 'Success' for Service Organizations That Would Rather Go Out of Business," *Newsday,* 29 December 1988, II-4.

46. Elbaz, "Sociology of AIDS Activism," 65–66, 71–77.

47. David Barr, interview by author, tape recording, New York City, 28 April 1994.

48. Michelle Roland, interview by author, tape recording, San Francisco, 18 December 1993.

49. Roland, interview; Mark Harrington, interview by author, tape recording, New York City, 29 April 1994; Brenda Lein, interview by author, tape recording, San Francisco, 18–19 December 1993.

50. Larry Kramer, *Reports from the Holocaust: The Making of an AIDS Activist* (New York: St. Martin's, 1989), 265, 270 (emphasis in the original).

51. Early debates involving AIDS, drug regulation, and access to experimental medications have been well described by Arno and Feiden in *Against the Odds* and Jonathan Kwitny in *Acceptable Risks* (New York: Poseidon Press, 1992).

52. Frank E. Young et al., "The FDA's New Procedures for the Use of Investigational Drugs in Treatment," *Journal of the American Medical Association* 259 (April 15, 1988): 2267–2270.

53. Larry Kramer, "The F.D.A.'s Callous Response to AIDS," *New York Times,* 23 March 1987, A-19 (op-ed).

54. Martin Delaney, "The Case for Patient Access to Experimental Therapy," *Journal of Infectious Diseases* 159 (March 1989): 416–419.

55. Barr, interview.

56. James C. Petersen and Gerald E. Markle, "The Laetrile Phenomenon: An Overview," in *Politics, Science, and Cancer: The Laetrile Phenomenon,* ed. Gerald E. Markle and James C. Petersen (Boulder, Colo.: Westview Press, 1980), 1–10.

57. John S. James, "FDA Reform: Major New Position Paper," *AIDS Treatment News,* 3 June 1988.

58. Gina Kolata, "Odd Alliance Would Speed New Drugs," *New York Times,* 26 November 1988, A-9.

59. "A New Era for New Drugs," *Wall Street Journal,* 13 March 1987, 18 (editorial).

60. Jonathan Kwitny has extensively profiled the most famous such courier, a Los Angeles nurse named Jim Corti, nicknamed "Dextran Man," in *Acceptable Risks.*

61. Miranda Kolbe, "A PWA Movement of Guerrilla Clinics," *Gay Community News,* 7 August 1988, 8.

62. "Clinic Update," *PI Perspectives,* October 1987.

63. Gina Kolata, "AIDS Patients and Their Above-Ground Underground," *New York Times,* 10 July 1988, 32 (section 4).

64. "FDA Allows AIDS Patients to Import Banned Drugs," *Los Angeles Times,* 24 July 1988, 18.

65. Philip M. Boffey, "F.D.A. Will Allow AIDS Patients to Import Unapproved Medicines," *New York Times,* 24 July 1988, A-1; Philip M. Boffey, "Importing AIDS Drugs: Analysis of F.D.A. Policy," *New York Times,* 26 July 1988, C-1.

66. William Booth, "An Underground Drug for AIDS," *Science* 241 (9 September 1988): 1279.

67. Jim Eigo et al., "FDA Action Handbook" (ACT UP/New York, New York, 21 September, 1988, photocopy), 1.

68. See Scott A. Hunt and Robert D. Benford, "Identity Talk in the Peace and Justice Movement," *Journal of Contemporary Ethnography* 22 (January 1994): 488–517; Scott A. Hunt, Robert D. Benford, and David A. Snow, "Identity Fields: Framing Processes and the Social Construction of Movement Identities," in *New Social Movements: From Ideology to Identity,* ed. Enrique Laraña, Hank Johnston, and Joseph R. Gusfield (Philadelphia: Temple Univ. Press, 1994), 185–208.

69. Eigo et al., "FDA Action Handbook," 17.

70. Chris Bull, "Seizing Control of the FDA," *Gay Community News,* 16 October 1988, 1, 3.

71. Crimp and Rolston, *AIDS Demographics,* 76.

72. Ibid., 78–81.

73. Barr, interview.

74. James M. Jasper and Dorothy Nelkin, *The Animal Rights Crusade: The Growth of a Moral Protest* (New York: Free Press, 1992).

75. Harrington, interview.

76. "The FDA for Itself," *Wall Street Journal,* 13 October 1988 (editorial).

77. "FDA Relaxes Drug Access Policy," *AIDS Treatment News,* 29 July 1988.

78. Ellen C. Cooper, "Controlled Clinical Trials of AIDS Drugs: The Best Hope," *Journal of the American Medical Association* 261 (28 April 1989): 2445.

79. Cooper, interview.

80. See Cooper's comments in Philip M. Boffey, "Washington Talk: Food and Drug Administration: At Fulcrum of Conflict, Regulator of AIDS Drugs," *New York Times,* 19 August 1988, A-13.

81. Martin Delaney, "Patient Access to Experimental Therapy," *Journal of the American Medical Association* 261 (28 April 1989): 2444, 2447.

82. The text from this presentation was published as: Martin Delaney, "The Case for Patient Access to Experimental Therapy," *Journal of Infectious Diseases* 159 (March 1989): 416–419.

83. On "community" as a "micro-mobilization context" for social movement formation, see Clarence Y. H. Lo, "Communities of Challengers in Social Movement Theory," in *Frontiers in Social Movement Theory,* ed. Aldon D. Morris and Carol McClurg Mueller (New Haven: Yale Univ. Press, 1992), 224–247.

84. Kolbe, "PWA Movement of Guerrilla Clinics," 8.

85. Nussbaum, *Good Intentions,* 189–192.

86. The quote is from an obituary following Zysman's death from HIV-related causes in 1993 at the age of 38: Obituaries, *AAPHR Reporter,* fall 1993, 28.

87. Antiviral Advisory Committee, meeting transcript (Food and Drug Administration, Bethesda, Md., 13–14 February 1991, photocopy), 50.

88. See Pierre Bourdieu and Loïc J. D. Wacquant, *An Invitation to Reflexive Sociology* (Chicago: Univ. of Chicago Press, 1992), 98–99.

89. David Handelman, "Act Up in Anger," *Rolling Stone,* 8 March 1990, 80–90, 116.

90. Harrington, interview.

91. Harrington, interview; Handelman, "Act Up in Anger."

92. On the struggles and tensions between the humanistic and the technical intelligentsia, see Alvin W. Gouldner, *The Future of Intellectuals and the Rise of the New Class* (New York: Oxford Univ. Press, 1979).

93. Quoted in Arno and Feiden, *Against the Odds,* 10.

94. Steven Shapin, "Science and the Public," in *Companion to the History of Modern Science,* ed. R. C. Olby et al. (London: Routledge, 1990), 990–1007, quote from 993.

95. G'dali Braverman, interview by author, tape recording, San Francisco, 17 December 1993.

96. Brenda Lein, interview by author, tape recording, San Francisco, 18–19 December 1993.

97. See Jasper and Nelkin, *Animal Rights Crusade, 7.*

98. Louis Lasagna, interview by author, tape recording, Boston, 26 October 1994.

99. Harrington, interview.

100. See Barbara Epstein, *Political Protest and Cultural Revolution: Nonviolent Direct Action in the 1970s and 1980s* (Berkeley: Univ. of California Press, 1991), 122.

101. "Evaluating New Treatment Alternatives," *PI Perspectives,* October 1987.

102. Ibid.

Chapter 7

1. Michael Specter, "Pressure from AIDS Activists has Transformed Drug Testing," *Washington Post,* 2 July 1989, A-1.

2. See Peter S. Arno and Karyn L. Feiden, *Against the Odds: The Story of AIDS Drug Development, Politics and Profits* (New York: HarperCollins, 1992), chapter 13.

3. Anthony S. Fauci, "AIDS—Challenges to Basic and Clinical Biomedical Research," *Academic Medicine* 64 (March 1989): 117.

4. J. Eigo and M. Harrington, "AIDS Drugs and the Politics of Biomedicine" (abstract of presentation at the Fifth International Conference on AIDS), Montreal, 4–9 June 1989; J. Eigo et al., "Drug Regulation Gone Wrong: The Saga of Ganciclovir" (abstract of presentation at the Fifth International Conference on AIDS), Montreal, 4–9 June 1989.

5. Arno and Feiden, *Against the Odds,* 173–174.

6. Gina Kolata, "AIDS Researcher Seeks Wide Access to Drugs in Tests," *New York Times,* 26 June 1989, A-1.

7. Ibid.

8. On parallel track and the approval of ddI, see Jeffrey Levi, "Unproven AIDS Therapies: The Food and Drug Administration and ddI," in *Biomedical Politics,* ed. Kathi E. Hanna (Washington, D.C.: National Academy Press, 1991), 9–37.

9. Anthony Fauci, interview by author, tape recording, Bethesda, Md., 31 October 1994.

10. For a formal expression of the idea, see Samuel Broder, "Controlled Trial Methodology and Progress in Treatment of the Acquired Immunodeficiency Syndrome (AIDS): A Quid Pro Quo," *Annals of Internal Medicine* 110 (15 March 1989): 417–418.

11. Philip J. Hilts, "Drug Said to Help AIDS Cases with Virus but No Symptoms," *New York Times,* 18 August 1989, A-1.

12. Gina Kolata, "Strong Evidence Discovered That AZT Holds Off AIDS," *New York Times,* 4 August 1989, A-1.

13. Hilts, "Drug Said to Help AIDS Cases."

14. Paul A. Volberding et al., "Zidovudine in Asymptomatic Human Immunodeficiency Virus Infection," *New England Journal of Medicine* 322 (5 April 1990): 941–949.

15. Paul Volberding, interview by author, tape recording, San Francisco, 7 July 1994.

16. Volberding et al., "Zidovudine in Asymptomatic Human Immunodeficiency Virus Infection," 948.

Zidovudine is the name that tends to get used in the medical journals and at conferences. It is a testament to the drug's construction as a "boundary object," existing simultaneously in multiple social worlds, that it bears different names in different places (azidothymidine, AZT, zidovudine, and Retrovir). (On "boundary objects" in science, see Susan Leigh Star and James R. Griesemer, "Institutional Ecology, 'Translations' and Boundary Objects: Amateurs and Professionals in Berkeley's Museum of Vertebrate Zoology, 1907–39," *Social Studies of Science* 19 [August 1989]: 387–420.)

17. Volberding et al., "Zidovudine in Asymptomatic Human Immunodeficiency Virus Infection," 948.

18. See Donald I. Abrams, "On the Matter of Survival," *BETA,* November 1992.

19. Gerald H. Friedland, "Early Treatment for HIV: The Time Has Come," *New England Journal of Medicine* 322 (5 April 1990): 1001 (editorial).

20. On the relation between diagnostic conditions and identity in AIDS, see the discussion of "becoming a person with HIV" in Rose Weitz, *Life with AIDS* (New Brunswick, N.J.: Rutgers Univ. Press, 1991), chapter 4.

21. Friedland, "Early Treatment for HIV," 1001.

22. "Incorporation of Trial Results into Clinical Practice: Open Discussion," *Journal of Acquired Immune Deficiency Syndromes* 3, suppl. 2 (1990): S145–S147.

23. "Recommendations for Zidovudine: Early Infection," *Journal of the American Medical Association* 263 (23–30 March 1990): 1606, 1609. This is a summary of the "State-of-the-Art Conference on AZT Therapy for Early HIV Infection" sponsored by NIAID, 3–4 March 1990.

24. "U.S. Urges Wider Use of AZT for Adults with AIDS Virus," *New York Times,* 3 March 1990, A-10.

25. Neville Hodgkinson, "The Cure That Failed," *Sunday Times* (London), 4 April 1993, Features section.

26. "AZT News: The Final Chapter?" *PI Perspectives,* November 1989.

27. Gina Kolata, "Medical Data: Who Should Hear It First?" *New York Times,* 22 May 1990, C-1.

28. John Lauritsen, "Science by Press Release," *New York Native,* 21 August 1989, 20–22; Kolata, "Medical Data: Who Should Hear It First?"

29. Kolata, "Medical Data: Who Should Hear It First?"

30. "An Open Letter to Mayor Koch," *New York Native,* 21 August 1989, 23.

31. John Lauritsen, "First Things First: Some Thoughts on the 'AIDS Virus' and AZT," *New York Native,* 1 June 1987, 1, 14–16 (cover story).

32. John Lauritsen, *Poison by Prescription: The AZT Story* (New York: Asklepios, 1990), 19.

33. Susan Leigh Star, "Scientific Work and Uncertainty," *Social Studies of Science* 15 (August 1985): 391–427, quote from 392.

34. H. M. Collins, "Certainty and the Public Understanding of Science: Science on Television," *Social Studies of Science* 17 (November 1987): 692.

35. Harry Collins, *Changing Order: Replication and Induction in Scientific Practice,* 2d ed. (Chicago: Univ. of Chicago Press, 1992), 162.

36. Gina Kolata, "Recruiting Problems in New York Slowing U.S. Trials of AIDS Drug," *New York Times,* 18 December 1988, A-1.

37. Randy Shilts, *And the Band Played On: Politics, People, and the AIDS Epidemic* (New York: St. Martin's, 1987), 539–543.

38. See Michael Wright, "East West Gulf, Project Inform's Consensus Statement on ddI and ddC and Ellen Cooper Resignation Fallout?" *ACT UP/ Golden Gate Treatment Issues Report* 2, no. 3 (1991).

39. Paul Harding Douglas, ed., *Improving the Odds: 1988* (New York: Columbia Gay Health Advocacy Project, 1989), 28 (proceedings of conference held at Columbia University, November 19, 1988). For analytical commentary see also Paula A. Treichler, "How to Have Theory in an Epidemic:

The Evolution of AIDS Treatment Activism," in *Technoculture*, ed. Constance Penley and Andrew Ross (Minneapolis and Oxford: Univ. of Minnesota Press, 1991), 83–93.

40. "AZT-Resistant Strains of HIV Appear," *PI Perspectives*, March 1989.

41. On obligatory passage points in science, see Bruno Latour, *Science in Action* (Cambridge, Mass.: Harvard Univ. Press, 1987). For a similar analysis of Delaney's reliance on AZT, see Treichler, "How to Have Theory in an Epidemic," 93.

42. "AZT News: The Final Chapter?"

43. "Zidovudine for Symptomless HIV Infection," *Lancet* 335 (7 April 1990): 821–822 (editorial).

44. Anthony J. Pinching, "Zidovudine in Asymptomatic HIV Infection: Knowledge and Uncertainty," *International Journal of STD & AIDS* 2 (May-June 1991): 157–161 (editorial review).

45. See Meurig Horton, "Bugs, Drugs and Placebos: The Opulence of Truth, or How to Make a Treatment Decision in an Epidemic," in *Taking Liberties: AIDS and Cultural Politics,* ed. Erica Carter and Simon Watney (London: Serpent's Tail, 1989), 161–181.

46. Jeremy Cherfas, "AZT Still on Trial," *Science* 246 (17 November 1989): 882.

47. Ibid.

48. Susan Ellenberg, interview by author, tape recording, Rockville, Md., 25 April 1994.

49. Martin Hirsch, interview by author, tape recording, Boston, 25 October 1994.

50. Cherfas, "AZT Still on Trial."

51. Ellenberg, interview.

52. David Byar, "Design Considerations for AIDS Trials," *Journal of Acquired Immune Deficiency Syndromes* 3, suppl. 2 (1990): S16–S19.

53. See William Francis Patrick Crowley III, *Gaining Access: The Politics of AIDS Clinical Drug Trials in Boston* (undergraduate thesis, Harvard College, 1991), 40.

54. Rebecca Smith, "AIDS Drug Trials," *Science* 246 (22 December 1989): 1547 (letter to the editor).

55. From the public forum "Clinical Trials," Davies Hospital, San Francisco, 6 October 1990 (author's field notes).

56. David Byar, quoted in Joseph Palca, "AIDS Drug Trials Enter New Age," *Science* 246 (6 October 1989): 20. For other criticisms of researchers' assumptions, see, for example, Byar, "Design Considerations for AIDS Trials." For an example of the role of biostatisticians in rethinking AIDS trials in the Boston area, see also Crowley, *Gaining Access,* 51.

57. Rebecca Smith, interview by author, tape recording, Providence, R.I., 26 October 1994.

58. Ellenberg, interview.

59. Susan S. Ellenberg et al., "Studying Treatments for AIDS: New Challenges for Clinical Trials—A Panel Discussion at the 1990 Annual Meeting of

the Society for Clinical Trials," *Controlled Clinical Trials* 13 (August 1992): 272–292.

60. Douglas Richman, interview by author, tape recording, San Diego, 1 June 1994.

61. Smith, interview.

62. Fauci, interview. On "situated knowledges," see Donna J. Haraway, *Simians, Cyborgs, and Women: The Reinvention of Nature* (New York: Routledge, 1991), chapter 9.

63. Smith, interview.

64. *Deciding to Enter an AIDS/HIV Drug Trial* (New York: AIDS Treatment Registry, 1989).

65. Ellenberg, interview; Mark Harrington, interview by author, tape recording, New York City, 29 April 1994.

66. David Byar, "Design Options for AIDS Trials" (paper presented at the annual conference of the American Academy for the Advancement of Science, Washington, D.C., 17 February 1991), tape recorded proceedings.

67. D. Bruce Burlington, "Statutory and Regulatory Framework for Drug Approval," *Journal of Acquired Immune Deficiency Syndromes* 3, suppl. 2 (1990): S4–S9.

68. Jim Eigo, "How AIDS Will Change the Way We Test Drugs" (paper presented at the annual conference of the American Academy for the Advancement of Science, Washington, D.C., 17 February 1991), tape recorded proceedings.

69. Douglas Richman et al., "Design of Clinical Trials—Active Control (Equivalence) Trials," *Journal of Acquired Immune Deficiency Syndromes* 3, suppl. 2 (1990): S88–S91. This issue of the journal contains the transcript of the conference, which was held in the Washington, D.C., area in November 1989.

70. Paul Lietman et al., "Design of Clinical Trials—Approaches to Clinical Trials Design: Discussion," *Journal of Acquired Immune Deficiency Syndromes* 3, suppl. 2 (1990): S27–S36.

71. Paul A. Volberding, "Rationale for Variations in Clinical Trial Design in Different HIV Disease Stages," *Journal of Acquired Immune Deficiency Syndromes* 3, suppl. 2 (1990): S40–S44.

72. Donald Abrams, interview by author, tape recording, San Francisco, 16 December 1993.

73. Michelle Roland, interview by author, tape recording, Davis, Calif., 18 December 1993.

74. On this point, see also Crowley, *Gaining Access*.

75. Lietman et al., "Design of Clinical Trials—Approaches to Clinical Trial Design," S31.

76. Quoted in Tim Kingston, "Justice Gone Blind: CMV Patients Fight for Their Sight," *Coming Up!* February 1989, 4. Sutton died of AIDS-related causes on April 11, 1989.

77. "Alternative Approaches to Clinical Trials"; Smith, interview.

78. See Palca, "AIDS Drug Trials Enter New Age," S20.

79. Byar, "Design Considerations for AIDS Trials," S18.

80. Alvan R. Feinstein, "An Additional Basic Science for Clinical Medicine: II. The Limitations of Randomized Trials," *Annals of Internal Medicine* 99 (October 1983): 545.

81. Harry Milton Marks, "Ideas as Reforms: Therapeutic Experiments and Medical Practice, 1900–1980" (Ph.D. diss., Massachusetts Institute of Technology, 1987).

82. Robert J. Levine, *Ethics and Regulation of Clinical Research* (Baltimore: Urban & Schwarzenberg, 1986), 208; "Scientific Justification for Community-Based Trials," *AIDS Treatment News,* 23 September 1988.

83. Volberding, "Rationale for Variations in Clinical Trial Design," S41.

84. See Steven Shapin, "Cordelia's Love: Credibility and the Social Studies of Studies," *Perspectives on Science* 3, no. 3 (1995): 255–275, esp. 261–266.

85. Ellenberg, interview.

86. I am grateful to Evelleen Richards for discussion of similarities and differences between AIDS trials and cancer trials.

87. Eliot Marshall, "Quick Release of AIDS Drugs," *Science* 245 (28 July 1989): 345–347, quote from 345.

88. John S. James, "The Drug-Trials Debacle—And What to Do about It (Part I)," *AIDS Treatment News,* 21 April 1989.

89. "AIDS Treatment Research and Care Issues: The Need for Advocacy," *AIDS Treatment News,* 26 February 1988.

90. Cf. Pierre Bourdieu, "The Specificity of the Scientific Field and the Social Conditions of the Progress of Reason," *Social Science Information* 14 (December 1975): 19–47.

91. On the cultural significance of metaphors of purity and contamination, see Mary Douglas, *Purity and Danger* (New York: Routledge & Kegan Paul, 1979). On the "sacred" character of "pure science," see Sal Restivo, "The Social Roots of Pure Mathematics," in *Theories of Science in Society,* ed. Susan E. Cozzens and Thomas F. Gieryn (Bloomington: Indiana Univ. Press, 1990), 120–143.

92. Roland, interview.

93. See Jonathan Kwitny, *Acceptable Risks* (New York: Poseidon Press, 1992).

94. From the session "Clinical Trials and Drug Development" at the VI International Conference on AIDS, San Francisco, 22 June 1990 (author's field notes).

95. Scott Brookie, "Unofficial Compound Q Trial Continues," *Gay Community News,* 30 July 1989, 3.

96. "Clinical Trials and Drug Development."

97. From the public forum "Community Outreach Session," held in conjunction with the VI International AIDS Conference, San Francisco, 22 June 1990 (author's field notes).

98. Robert Steinbrook, "AIDS Trials Shortchange Minorities and Drug Users," *Los Angeles Times,* 25 September 1989, 1.

99. J. E. D'Eramo et al., "Women and Minorities Have Less Access to AIDS Drug Trials" (abstract of presentation at the VII International Conference on AIDS, Florence, 16–21 June 1991).

100. Gina Kolata, "AIDS Research on New Drugs Bypasses Addicts and Women," *New York Times,* 5 January 1988, C-1.

101. Donald E. Craven et al., "AIDS in Intravenous Drug Users: Issues Related to Enrollment in Clinical Trials," *Journal of Acquired Immune Deficiency Syndromes* 3, suppl. 2 (1990): S48.

102. Quoted in Stephen B. Thomas and Sandra Crouse Quinn, "The Tuskegee Syphilis Study, 1932 to 1972: Implications for HIV Education and AIDS Risk Education Programs in the Black Community," *American Journal of Public Health* 81 (November 1991): 1498–1505.

103. The survey was reported in the editorial "The AIDS 'Plot' against Blacks," *New York Times,* 12 May 1992, A-22.

104. The delay was due, in part, to Burroughs Wellcome's slowness in filing with the FDA; see Gina Kolata, "Hundreds of Children with AIDS Are Unable to Obtain AZT," *New York Times,* 23 September 1989, A-8.

105. Lisa Auer, "Developing a Clinical Research Agenda for Women," *PI Perspectives,* 9 October 1990.

106. Gina Kolata, "N.I.H. Neglects Women, Study Says," *New York Times,* 19 June 1990, C-6.

107. Scott Jaschik, "Report Says NIH Ignores Own Rules on Including Women in Its Research," *Chronicle of Higher Education,* 27 June 1990, A27.

108. Paul Cotton, "Examples Abound of Gaps in Medical Knowledge Because of Groups Excluded from Scientific Study," *Journal of the American Medical Association* 263 (23 February 1990): 1051, 1055.

109. Fauci, interview.

110. On recent trends toward the understanding of racial differences in genetic and biological terms, see Troy Duster, *Backdoor to Eugenics* (New York and London: Routledge, 1990).

111. Malcolm Gladwell, "AIDS Study Suggests Drug May Have Racial Limits," *Washington Post,* 15 February 1991, A-4.

112. Gina Kolata, "Federal Study Questions Ability of AZT to Delay AIDS," *New York Times,* 15 February 1991, A-1; see also Gina Kolata, "In Medical Research Equal Opportunity Doesn't Always Apply," *New York Times,* 10 March 1991, 16 (Section 4).

113. Quoted in Paul Rykoff Coleman, "AZT Efficacy Study Angers Blacks and Latinos," *Outweek,* 6 March 1991, 28, 29, 102. For more on the issue of AZT's efficacy in different racial groups, see Gina Kolata, "AIDS Drug Unaffected by Race or Sex," *New York Times,* 20 November 1991, A-25.

114. Paul Cotton, "Is There Still Too Much Extrapolation from Data on Middle-Aged White Men?" *Journal of the American Medical Association* 263 (23 February 1990): 1049–1050.

115. "Incorporation of Trial Results into Clinical Practice," S146.

116. David P. Byar et al., "Sounding Board: Design Considerations for AIDS Trials," *New England Journal of Medicine* 323 (8 November 1990): 1343–1347.

117. Thomas C. Merigan, "Sounding Board: You *Can* Teach an Old Dog New Tricks: How AIDS Trials Are Pioneering New Strategies," *New England Journal of Medicine* 323 (8 November 1990): 1341–1343.

118. Carol Levine, Nancy Neveloff Dubler, and Robert J. Levine, "Building a New Consensus: Ethical Principles and Policies for Clinical Research on HIV/AIDS," *AIDS Patient Care,* April 1992, 67–85.

119. Robert J. Levine, "Community Consultation in Clinical Trials" (paper presented at the annual conference of the American Academy for the Advancement of Science, Washington, D.C., 17 February 1991), tape recorded proceedings.

120. Byar, "Design Options for AIDS Trials."

121. Eigo, "How AIDS Will Change the Way We Test Drugs."

Chapter 8

1. See, for example, Samuel Broder, "Controlled Trial Methodology and Progress in Treatment of the Acquired Immunodeficiency Syndrome (AIDS): A Quid Pro Quo," *Annals of Internal Medicine* 110 (15 March 1989): 417–418.

2. See the published report of the study in Tze-Chiang Meng et al., "Combination Therapy with Zidovudine and Dideoxycytidine in Patients with Advanced Human Immunodeficiency Virus Infection: A Phase I/II Study," *Annals of Internal Medicine* 116 (1 January 1992): 13–20.

3. John S. James, "ddC Background," *AIDS Treatment News,* 21 February 1992.

4. Meng et al., "Combination Therapy with Zidovudine and Dideoxycytidine," 18–19.

5. G'dali Braverman, interview by author, tape recording, San Francisco, 17 December 1993.

6. James, "ddC Background."

7. Warren J. Blumenfeld, "FDA, Buyers Clubs Negotiate New Relationship," *Advocate,* 19 November 1991, 62–63.

8. Gina Kolata, "Patients Going Underground to Buy Experimental Drugs," *New York Times,* 4 November 1991, A-1.

9. Ibid.

10. Rachel Nowak, "Conditional Approval Touted," *Nature* 352 (8 August 1991): 464.

11. Blumenfeld, "FDA, Buyers Clubs Negotiate New Relationship."

12. Jonathan Kwitny, *Acceptable Risks* (New York: Poseidon Press, 1992), 97.

13. Blumenfeld, "FDA, Buyers Clubs Negotiate New Relationship."

14. Deborah R. Gordon, "Clinical Science and Clinical Expertise: Changing Boundaries between Art and Science in Medicine," in *Biomedicine Examined,* ed. M. Lock and D. R. Gordon (Dordrecht, Holland: Kluwer Academic Publishing, 1988), 257–295, quote from 257; Harry Milton Marks, "Ideas as Reforms: Therapeutic Experiments and Medical Practice, 1900–1980" (Ph.D. diss., Massachusetts Institute of Technology, 1987).

15. John S. James, "ddC: AZT Combination Approval Recommended," *AIDS Treatment News,* 1 May 1992.

16. Mark Harrington, "Gina Kolata Sings the ddI Blues (Again)," *Outweek*, 28 March 1990, 34–35, quote from 35.

17. John S. James, "ddI and ddC: The Call for Early Approval," *AIDS Treatment News*, 5 October 1990.

18. John S. James, "Montreal Conference: Overview and Comment," *AIDS Treatment News*, 29 June 1989.

19. John S. James, "Why No Antivirals: A Case History of Failed Trial Design," *AIDS Treatment News*, 29 June 1989.

20. Andrew R. Moss, "Laboratory Markers as Potential Surrogates for Clinical Outcomes in AIDS Trials," *Journal of Acquired Immune Deficiency Syndromes* 3, suppl. 2 (1990), S69–S71; David Amato and Stephen W. Lagakos, "Considerations in the Selection of End Points for AIDS Clinical Trials," *Journal of Acquired Immune Deficiency Syndromes* 3, suppl. 2 (1990), S64–S68.

21. "Surrogate Endpoints in Evaluating the Effectiveness of Drugs against HIV Infection and AIDS" (transcript of conference of the National Academy of Sciences, Washington, D.C., 11–12 September 1989, photocopy).

22. This account is from Moss, "Laboratory Markers as Potential Surrogates."

23. See the discussion in Kwitny, *Acceptable Risks*, 225, 297, 331.

24. Amato and Lagakos, "Considerations in the Selection of Endpoints," S66.

25. "Design of Clinical Trials—End Points: Open Discussion," *Journal of Acquired Immune Deficiency Syndromes* 3, suppl. 2 (1990): S75.

26. "Surrogate Endpoints in Evaluating the Effectiveness of Drugs," 100–101.

27. "A Barrier Falls at the FDA," *PI Perspectives*, April 1991.

28. Paul Cotton, "HIV Surrogate Markers Weighed," *Journal of the American Medical Association* 265 (20 March 1991): 1357, 1361, 1362.

29. See Bruce Nussbaum, *Good Intentions: How Big Business and the Medical Establishment Are Corrupting the Fight against AIDS* (New York: Atlantic Monthly Press, 1990); Kwitny, *Acceptable Risks*.

30. John S. James, "Drug Development: What's Needed Now?" *AIDS Treatment News*, 8 March 1990.

31. On the role of "standing-for" (or "metonymical") relationships in the construction of scientific credibility, see Steven Shapin, "Cordelia's Love: Credibility and the Social Studies of Studies," *Perspectives on Science* 3, no. 3 (1995): 255–275.

32. James, "Drug Development: What's Needed Now?"

33. John S. James, "The Wrong Nightmare: The Worst Delay of Clinical Trials," *AIDS Treatment News*, 21 December 1989.

34. Tim Kingston, "The Coming Storm over Expedited Drug Approval," *San Francisco Bay Times*, June 1991, 10–12.

35. John S. James, "Expanded Access to Experimental Drugs: Interview with David Feigal, M.D., of the FDA," *AIDS Treatment News*, 30 May 1993.

36. Paul Houston, "Administration Revamps Drug-Approval Policies," *Los Angeles Times*, 10 April 1992, A-1.

37. Kingston, "Coming Storm," 12.

38. Henry A. Waxman, letter to Dr. David Kessler, Washington, D.C., 10 April 1991.

39. Martin Delaney, letter to Congressman Henry Waxman, San Francisco, 2 May 1991.

40. Paul Cotton, "Surrogate Markers of Disease Studied as Means of Determining AIDS Drugs' Effectiveness," *Journal of the American Medical Association* 264 (14 November 1990): 2362, 2365.

41. John S. James, "ddI and ddC Approval Effort—Interview with Martin Delaney," *AIDS Treatment News,* 7 December 1990.

42. See Kwitny, *Acceptable Risks,* 383; Victor F. Zonana, "Top AIDS Drug Regulator to Step Down," *Los Angeles Times,* 22 December 1990, A-6.

43. "Barrier Falls at the FDA."

44. Antiviral Advisory Committee, meeting transcript (Food and Drug Administration, Bethesda, Md., 13–14 February 1991, photocopy), 162–163.

45. Cotton, "HIV Surrogate Markers Weighed," 1362.

46. Kwitny, *Acceptable Risks,* 391.

47. "ddI Approval: Today and Tomorrow," *PI Perspectives,* October 1991.

48. Ibid.

49. Paul Cotton, "FDA 'Pushing Envelope' on AIDS Drug," *Journal of the American Medical Association* 266 (14 August 1991): 757–758, quotes from 757.

50. Donald Abrams, interview by author, tape recording, San Francisco, 16 December 1993.

51. Sheila Jasanoff, *The Fifth Branch: Science Advisers as Policymakers* (Cambridge, Mass.: Harvard Univ. Press, 1990), 178, 229.

52. Cotton, "FDA 'Pushing Envelope,'" 757.

53. Ibid.

54. Gina Kolata, "U.S. Panel Backs Sale of Experimental AIDS Drug," *New York Times,* 20 July 1991, A-1.

55. Gina Kolata, "Speeded Approval of AIDS Drug Is Termed Justified by Test Data," *New York Times,* 20 April 1992, C-3.

56. See James, "ddC: AZT Combination Approval Recommended."

57. David Feigal, interview by author, tape recording, Rockville, Md., 1 November 1994.

58. Michael C. Botkin, "ddC's Bumpy Road," *Bay Area Reporter,* 7 May 1992, 20, 23.

59. Liz Hunt, "Panel Recommends Conditional Approval for New AIDS Drug," *Washington Post,* 20 July 1991, A-9.

60. Botkin, "ddC's Bumpy Road," 23.

61. Marlene Cimons, "FDA Approves AIDS Drug for Use with AZT," *Los Angeles Times,* 23 June 1992, A-1.

62. Botkin, "ddC's Bumpy Road," 20.

63. Ibid.

64. Jon Cohen, "Searching for Markers on the AIDS Trail," *Science* 258 (16 October 1992): 388–390, quote from 388 (brackets are Cohen's).

65. Deborah Cotton, interview by author, tape recording, Boston, Mass., 25 October 1994.

66. Cohen, "Searching for Markers," 389–390.

67. Ibid., 390.

68. "AIDS Treatment Research Agenda" (ACT UP/New York Treatment & Data Committee, New York, 1990, photocopy), 2.

69. Larry Kramer, "Second-Rated to Death," *Outweek*, 24 October 1990, 48–50.

70. "AIDS Treatment Research Agenda," 9, 11–13.

71. Gina Kolata, "AIDS Research Finds 13 Vulnerable Spots in Virus Life Cycle," *New York Times*, 2 October 1990, C-3; see also Hiroaki Mitsuya, Robert Yarchoan, and Samuel Broder, "Molecular Targets for AIDS Therapy," *Science* 249 (28 September 1990): 1533–1544.

72. John S. James, "AIDS Antivirals: A New Generation," *AIDS Treatment News*, 19 April 1991.

73. John S. James, "1992: Treatments to Watch," *AIDS Treatment News*, 23 December 1991.

74. David Baltimore and Mark B. Feinberg, "HIV Revealed: Toward a Natural History of the Infection," *New England Journal of Medicine* 321 (14 December 1989): 1673 (editorial).

75. See "Therapeutic Vaccines," *PI Perspectives*, April 1992.

76. Veronica T. Jennings and Malcolm Gladwell, "1,000 Rally for More Vigorous AIDS Effort," *Washington Post*, 22 May 1990, B-1.

77. John S. James, "ACT UP Calls for NIH Demonstration May 21," *AIDS Treatment News*, 28 April 1990.

78. Mark Harrington, "Eating Where They . . . ," *Outweek*, 18 February 1990, 34; Mark Harrington, "Anatomy of a Disaster: Why Is Federal AIDS Research at a Standstill?" *Village Voice*, 13 March 1990, 40–41.

79. See David Concar, "Protests Oust Science at AIDS Conference," *Nature* 345 (28 June 1990): 753.

80. Victor F. Zonana, "Did AIDS Protest Go Too Far?" *Los Angeles Times*, 2 July 1990, A-3.

81. Anthony Fauci, interview by author, tape recording, Bethesda, Md., 31 October 1994.

82. Nussbaum, *Good Intentions*, 306–307.

83. Arno and Feiden, *Against the Odds*, 227–229; David Barr, interview by author, tape recording, New York City, 28 April 1994.

84. Arno and Feiden, *Against the Odds*, 234–235.

85. Philip J. Hilts, "82 Held in Protest on Pace of AIDS Research," *New York Times*, 22 May 1990, C-2; Arno and Feiden, *Against the Odds*, 232.

86. Mark Harrington, interview by author, tape recording, New York City, 29 April 1994.

87. See the arguments in the introduction and chapter 1.

88. Gena Corea, *The Invisible Epidemic: The Story of Women and AIDS* (New York: HarperCollins, 1992), 265.

89. See Cindy Patton, "Resistance and the Erotic: Reclaiming History,

Setting Strategy as We Face AIDS," *Radical America* 20 (November-December 1986): 68–78.

90. Maxine Wolfe, "The AIDS Coalition to Unleash Power, New York (ACT UP NY): A Direct Action Political Model of Community Research for AIDS Prevention," in *AIDS Prevention and Services: Community Based Research,* ed. J. Van Vugt (Westport, Conn.: Bergin Garvey, forthcoming). On the varieties of AIDS activism by women, see also Beth E. Schneider and Nancy E. Stoller, eds., *Women Resisting AIDS: Feminist Strategies of Empowerment* (Philadelphia: Temple Univ. Press, 1995).

91. Cathy Jean Cohen, "Power, Resistance and the Construction of Crisis: Marginalized Communities Respond to AIDS" (Ph.D. diss., University of Michigan, 1993), 325.

92. Moisés Agosto, interview by author, tape recording, New York City, 26 April 1994.

93. Jonathan Wadleigh, interview by author, tape recording, Brookline, Mass., 25 October 1994.

94. Ibid.

95. Anne-Christine d'Adesky, "Empowerment or Co-Optation?" *The Nation,* 11 February 1991, 158–160.

96. See Carrie Wofford, "Sitting at the Table," *Outweek,* 3 April 1991, 22–23; Cohen, "Power, Resistance, and the Construction of Crisis," 320–324.

97. For a range of perspectives on the causes and significance of the ACT UP/San Francisco split, see: Tim Vollmer, "ACT-UP/SF Splits in Two over Consensus, Focus," *San Francisco Sentinel,* 20 September 1990, 1; Jesse Dobson, "Why ACT-UP Split in Two" (same issue), 4; Kate Raphael, "ACT-UP: Growing Apart" (same issue), 5; Michele DeRanleau, "How the 'Conscience of an Epidemic' Unraveled," *San Francisco Examiner,* 1 October 1990, A-15.

98. Risa Dennenberg, "Women, AIDS, Lesbians and Politics," *Outweek,* 20 March 1991, 27.

99. Harrington, interview.

100. Barr, interview.

101. Gilbert Elbaz, "The Sociology of AIDS Activism, the Case of ACT UP/New York, 1987–1992" (Ph.D. diss., City University of New York, 1992), 488.

102. Michelle Roland, interview by author, tape recording, Davis, Calif., 18 December 1993.

103. Barr, interview.

104. Theo Smart, "This Side of Despair," *QW,* 13 September 1992, 43–44, 69.

105. Mark Golden, "ACT UP Redux," *QW,* 11 October 1992, 22–25.

106. Jason Heyman, interview by author, tape recording, San Francisco, 12 July 1994.

107. On boundary work in science, see Thomas F. Gieryn, "Boundary Work and the Demarcation of Science from Non-Science: Strains and Interests in Professional Ideologies of Scientists," *American Sociological Review* 48 (December 1983): 781–795; Thomas F. Gieryn, "Boundaries of Science," in

Handbook of Science and Technology Studies, ed. Sheila Jasanoff et al. (Thousand Oaks, Calif.: Sage, 1995), 393–443.

108. Heyman, interview.

Chapter 9

1. Theo Smart, "This Side of Despair," *QW,* 13 September 1992, 44.

2. Jayne Garrison, "Experts Glum as New Drugs for AIDS Flop," *San Francisco Examiner,* 2 February 1992, A-1.

3. Jayne Garrison, "Activists Despondent and the Movement Is Splintering," *San Francisco Examiner,* 2 February 1992, A-10.

4. Garrison, "Experts Glum as New Drugs for AIDS Flop." Arguably, activists were *too quick* to dismiss the class of non-nucleoside reverse transcriptase inhibitors, since some of them, such as nevirapine, would later attract attention when used in higher doses or in combination with other drugs. In this sense, activist impatience risked contributing to the discrediting of some drugs, just as activist enthusiasm magnified the credibility of others. See Smart, "This Side of Despair."

5. Delaney's rebuttal took the form of a letter to the editor of the *Examiner,* reprinted in "No Room for Hope?" *PI Perspectives,* April 1992.

6. John S. James, "Tat Inhibitor Trials Canceled; Business Reasons Cited," *AIDS Treatment News,* 17 May 1991.

7. John S. James, "Tat Inhibitor Update," *AIDS Treatment News,* 3 January 1992.

8. This letter was printed in Ronald A. Baker, "Epidemic of Mistrust: Hoffman-LaRoche and the Treatment Activist Community," *BETA,* March 1993.

9. Martin Delaney, "The TAT Offensive," *Advocate,* 9 March 1993, 35.

10. John S. James, "AIDS Treatments 1992/1993: Where Are We Now?" *AIDS Treatment News,* 1 January 1993.

11. Lawrence K. Altman, "At AIDS Talks, Reality Weighs Down Hope," *New York Times,* 26 July 1992, A-1.

12. Gregg Gonsalves and Mark Harrington, "AIDS Research at the NIH: A Critical Review. Part I: Summary" (Treatment Action Group, New York, 1992, photocopy).

13. Gregg Gonsalves, interview by author, tape recording, New York City, 28 April 1994.

14. Gonsalves and Harrington, "AIDS Research at the NIH," 1, 12–13.

15. Ibid., 7.

16. Jon Cohen, "Reorganization Plan Draws Fire at NIH," *Science* 259 (5 February 1993): 753–754.

17. John Lauritsen, *Poison by Prescription: The AZT Story* (New York: Asklepios, 1990), 121; "Pimping for AZT," *New York Native,* 8 October 1990, 4.

18. Michael Broder, "Wellcome Gives $1 Mil to Community Research," *QW,* 12 July 1992, 16, 19.

19. Robert Massa, "Drug Money: Should Activists Take Donations from Pharmaceuticals?" *Village Voice*, 23 June 1992, 18.

20. From the leaflet "Time & Lives Are Running Out!!!" (San Francisco: ACT UP/Underground, 1992, photocopy); for a discussion see Michael C. Botkin, "The 1992 Scabbies," *Bay Area Reporter*, 21 January 1993, 18.

21. Gina Kolata, "After 5 Years of Use, Doubt Still Clouds Leading AIDS Drug," *New York Times*, 2 June 1992, C-3.

22. One study sometimes cited as demonstrating that AZT prolongs life, in fact—by its own account—failed to distinguish between the benefits of AZT and the benefits of "other aspects of care associated with zidovudine [AZT] therapy," such as PCP prophylaxis, in the group studied. See Richard D. Moore et al., "Zidovudine and the Natural History of the Acquired Immunodeficiency Syndrome," *New England Journal of Medicine* 324 (16 May 1991): 1412–1416.

23. See Mark D. Smith, "Zidovudine: Does It Work for Everyone?" *Journal of the American Medical Association* 266 (20 November 1991): 2750–2751 (editorial).

24. D. Cotton and D. Weinberg, "Survey Results: Treatment Decisions in HIV Care," *AIDS Clinical Care* 4 (1991): 85–91.

25. Jean-Pierre Aboulker and Ann Marie Swart, "Preliminary Analysis of the Concorde Trial," *Lancet* 341 (3 April 1993): 889–890 (letter to the editor).

26. Tim Kingston, "The Concorde AZT Trial: Does It Fly?" *San Francisco Bay Times*, 22 April 1993, 6–7.

27. J. Lange, "Antiretroviral Treatment," Session PS-03-2, IX International Conference on AIDS, Berlin, 8 June 1993.

28. John S. James, "AZT, Early Intervention, and the Concorde Controversy," *AIDS Treatment News*, 23 April 1993.

29. Kingston, "Concorde AZT Trial."

30. David Gold, "The Concorde Study," *Treatment Issues*, May 1993; Lawrence K. Altman, "New Study Questions Use of AZT in Early Treatment of AIDS Virus," *New York Times*, 1 April 1993, A-1.

31. Kingston, "Concorde AZT Trial."

32. "After Concorde," *Treatment Issues*, May 1993 (editorial).

33. Larry Kramer, "AZT Is Shit," *Advocate*, 18 May 1993, 80 (editorial).

34. Kingston, "Concorde AZT Trial."

35. Linda Marsa, "Toxic Hope: Widely Embraced, the AIDS Drug is Now Under Heavy Fire," *Los Angeles Times*, 20 June 1993, 14.

36. Charles R. Caulfield, "AZT: People or Profits?" *San Francisco Sentinel*, 8 April 1993, 1, 19–20.

37. Quoted in Caulfield, "AZT: People or Profits?" 20.

38. Neville Hodgkinson, "New Realism Puts the Brake on HIV Bandwagon," *Sunday Times* (London), 9 May 1993, Features section.

39. Neville Hodgkinson, "How Giant Drug Firm Funds the Aids Lobby," *Sunday Times* (London), 30 May 1993, Home News section; "GAG Claims Doctors Are Killing Babies," *Capital Gay*, 4 June 1993, 9.

40. See the statement by Marcus Conant in Kingston, "Concorde AZT

Trial"; and see ACT UP/Golden Gate Treatment Issues Committee, "ACT UP/ Golden Gate Responds to AZT Criticism," *San Francisco Sentinel,* 15 April 1993, 14 (op-ed).

41. Kim Painter, "Despite Questions, Experts Still Back AZT," *USA Today,* 5 April 1993, 6D.

42. Altman, "New Study Questions Use of AZT."

43. "After Concorde," *Treatment Issues,* May 1993 (editorial).

44. James, "AZT, Early Intervention, and the Concorde Controversy."

45. See Anastasios Tsiatis, "Intent-to-Treat Analysis," *Journal of Acquired Immune Deficiency Syndromes* 3, suppl. 2 (1990): S120–S123.

46. Kingston, "Concorde AZT Trial"; see also the statement by Burroughs Wellcome in David Gold, "The Concorde Study," *Treatment Issues,* May 1993.

47. James, "AZT, Early Intervention, and the Concorde Controversy."

48. Kramer, "AZT Is Shit."

49. Lawrence K. Altman, "The Doctor's World: AIDS Study Casts Doubt on Value of Hastened Drug Approval in U.S.," *New York Times,* 6 April 1993, C-3.

50. "After Concorde."

51. Jon Cohen, "AIDS Research: The Mood Is Uncertain," *Science* 260 (28 May 1993): 1254–1265, quotes from 1254.

52. A. S. Fauci, "Pathogenesis of HIV Infection" (paper presented at Plenary Session 01, IX International Conference on AIDS, Berlin, 7 June 1993); J. Levy, "Mechanisms of Pathogenesis and Long-Term Survival with HIV/AIDS" (paper presented at Plenary Session 05, IX International Conference on AIDS, Berlin, 9 June 1993). Another perspective was presented by Montagnier in back-to-back presentations on 10 June 1993: "HIV, Cofactors and AIDS," Session OP-03–1; and "Report of the EEC Group: Mechanisms of CD4+ Lymphocyte Depletion," Session OP-03–2.

53. Jay A. Levy, "Pathogenesis of Human Immunodeficiency Virus Infection," *Microbiological Reviews* 57 (March 1993): 183–289.

54. Quoted in Dave Gilden, "Groping toward a New Understanding," *San Francisco Bay Times,* 17 June 1993, 14–15. McKean died of HIV-related causes in 1994.

55. Robin A. Weiss, "How Does HIV Cause AIDS?" *Science* 260 (28 May 1993): 1273–1279.

56. R. Gallo, "Perspectives for the Future Control of AIDS," Session OP-01–1, IX International Conference on AIDS, Berlin, 8 June 1993.

57. M. Seligmann, "The Concorde Trial: First Results," Session WS-B24–5, IX International Conference on AIDS, Berlin, 10 June 1993; M. Seligmann, "Report of the Coordinating Committee of the Concorde Trial," Session OP-01–2, IX International Conference on AIDS, Berlin, 8 June 1993.

58. Delaney's comments are from a press conference and a Project Inform "Town Meeting," both held on June 9, 1993 (author's field notes).

59. M. A. Fischl, "Combination Therapy: Now and the Future" (paper presented at Harvard AIDS Institute—AIDS Clinical Research Symposium, Berlin, 8 June 1993).

60. From the press release "Effectiveness of AZT/ddC Combination Depends on Pretreatment Immune Cell Count," *News from NIAID,* 7 June 1993.

61. From the press release "The Effectiveness of AZT Alone, ddC Alone or AZT/ddC Combination Is Similar Overall for Patients with Advanced HIV Disease," *News from NIAID,* 10 June 1993. My thanks to Jon Cohen, AIDS reporter for *Science,* for this anecdote.

62. M. Fischl, "The Safety and Efficacy of Zidovudine (ZDV) and Zalcitabine (ddC) or ddC Alone versus ZDV," Session WS-B25-1, IX International Conference on AIDS, Berlin, 10 June 1993.

63. Author's field notes, Session WS-B25-1; Robert Massa, "Two Steps Back," *Village Voice,* 22 June 1993.

64. "When to Start Antiretroviral Treatment: Research Issues," Session ME-13, IX International Conference on AIDS," Berlin, 10 June 1993. Quotes that follow are from author's field notes.

65. As Montini and Slobin noted in a study of NIH Consensus Development Conferences that try to create "standards of care," practitioners and researchers confront different work environments and pressures, and their expectations are shaped accordingly. Typically, practicing physicians have a "desire for certainty," while researchers (even those who also see patients) may have a much higher "tolerance for uncertainty." See Theresa Montini and Kathleen Slobin, "Tensions Between Good Science and Good Practice: Lagging Behind and Leapfrogging Ahead Along the Cancer Continuum," *Research in the Sociology of Health Care* 9 (1991): 127–140, quote from 130. On the professional socialization that teaches doctors to manage uncertainty, see Renée C. Fox, "Training for Uncertainty," in Phil Brown, ed., *Perspectives in Medical Sociology* (Prospect Heights, Ill.: Waveland Press, 1992), 450–459. For a dissenting view arguing that doctors are trained to suppress and deny uncertainty, see Jay Katz, *The Silent World of Doctor and Patient* (New York: Free Press, 1984), chapter 7.

66. Lawrence K. Altman, "Experts Change Guides to Using Drugs for H.I.V.," *New York Times,* 27 June 1993, A-1, A-10.

67. Lawrence K. Altman, "The Doctor's World: Government Panel on H.I.V. Finds the Prospect for Treatment Bleak," *New York Times,* 29 June 1993, C-3.

68. David A. Cooper et al., "Zidovudine in Persons with Asymptomatic HIV Infection and CD4 + Cell Counts Greater than 400 Per Cubic Millimeter," *New England Journal of Medicine* 329 (29 July 1993): 297–303.

69. John B. Bartlett, "Zidovudine Now or Later?" *New England Journal of Medicine* 329 (29 July 1993): 351–352 (editorial).

70. Natalie Angier, "Australian Study Says AZT Slows Progression toward Full-Blown AIDS," *New York Times,* 29 July 1993, A-9.

71. Paul Volberding, interview by author, tape recording, San Francisco, 7 July 1994.

72. P. A. Volberding et al., "The Duration of Zidovudine Benefit in Persons with Asymptomatic HIV Infection: Prolonged Evaluation of Protocol 019 of the AIDS Clinical Trials Group," *Journal of the American Medical Association* 272 (10 August 1994): 437–442.

73. Centers for Disease Control and Prevention, "Zidovudine for the Prevention of HIV Transmission from Mother to Infant," *Journal of the American Medical Association* 271 (25 May 1994): 1567–1570.

74. Rae Trewartha, "AZT, Perinatal Transmission: Unanswered Questions," *AIDS Treatment News,* 16 September 1994.

75. Ronald Bayer, "Ethical Challenges Posed by Zidovudine Treatment to Reduce Vertical Transmission of HIV," *New England Journal of Medicine* 331 (3 November 1994): 1223–1225 (editorial).

76. Concorde Coordinating Committee, "Concorde: MRC/ANRS Randomised Double-Blind Controlled Trial of Immediate and Deferred Zidovudine in Symptom-Free HIV Infection," *Lancet* 343 (9 April 1994): 871–881.

77. Quoted in "Burroughs Wellcome Responds to Publication of Concorde Study," *New York Native,* 2 May 1994, 12.

78. Paul Cotton, "Use of Antiretroviral Drugs in HIV Disease Declines Following Preliminary Results from Concorde Trial," *Journal of the American Medical Association* 271 (16 February 1994): 487.

79. Deborah Cotton, interview by author, tape recording, Boston, 25 October 1994.

80. Douglas Richman, interview by author, tape recording, San Diego, 1 June 1994.

81. Margaret A. Fischl et al., "Combination and Monotherapy with Zidovudine and Zalcitabine in Patients with Advanced HIV Disease," *Annals of Internal Medicine* 122 (1 January 1995), 24–32, esp. 25.

82. Stephen Lagakos, interview by author, tape recording, Boston, 27 October 1994. In the published report, the authors themselves noted that "caution should be used when interpreting subgroup analysis because subgroup analyses may produce spurious results." The researchers supplemented the subgroup analysis with a "trend analysis, which used pretreatment CD4 cell counts as a continuous variable" and which, therefore, did not "suffer from the same limitations" (Fischl et al., "Combination and Monotherapy with Zidovudine and Zalcitabine," 27, 30).

83. Susan Ellenberg, interview by author, tape recording, Rockville, Md., 25 April 1994.

84. Fischl et al., "Combination and Monotherapy with Zidovudine and Zalcitabine," 30.

85. Lagakos, interview.

86. Martin Hirsch, interview by author, tape recording, Boston, 25 October 1994.

87. Ibid.

88. Fischl et al., "Combination and Monotherapy with Zidovudine and Zalcitabine," 30.

89. Richman, interview.

90. Mark Harrington, "The Crisis in Clinical AIDS Research" (Treatment Action Group, New York, 1 December 1993, photocopy), 13–14, 16.

91. See Evelleen Richards, *Vitamin C and Cancer: Medicine or Politics?* (New York: St. Martin's, 1991).

92. Edward A. Wyatt, "Rushing to Judgment," *Barron's,* 15 August 1994, 23.

93. Christine Gorman, "Let's Not Be Too Hasty: Activists Who Once Clamored for Speedier Approval of AIDS Drugs Now Favor a More Deliberate Approach," *Time*, 19 September 1994, 71.

94. John S. James, "BARRON'S: 'Do We Have Too Many Drugs for AIDS?'" *AIDS Treatment News*, 19 August 1994.

95. David Feigal, interview by author, tape recording, Rockville, Md., 1 November 1994.

96. Kessler has provided an overview of his position on rapid approval of AIDS drugs in: David A. Kessler and Karyn L. Feiden, "Faster Evaluation of Vital Drugs," *Scientific American*, March 1995, 48–54.

97. Derek Link, interview by author, tape recording, New York City, 28 April 1994.

98. Gina Kolata, "Debate Reopens on AIDS Drug Access," *New York Times*, 12 September 1994, A-16.

99. Anthony Fauci, interview by author, tape recording, Bethesda, Md., 31 October 1994.

100. David D. Ho et al., "Rapid Turnover of Plasma Virions and CD4 Lymphocytes in HIV-1 Infection," *Nature* 373 (12 January 1995): 123–126; Xiping Wei et al., "Viral Dynamics in Human Immunodeficiency Virus Type 1 Infection," *Nature* 373 (12 January 1995): 117–122.

101. Gina Kolata, "New AIDS Finding on Why Drugs Fail," *New York Times*, 12 January 1995, A-1.

102. Lagakos, interview.

103. "With Good Intentions, Overzealous Researchers May Be Setting the Stage for Yet Another Colossal Failure," *TAGline*, January 1995, 5.

104. "With Its First Protease Trial Completed, Roche Races to FDA with Lukewarm Results, Activists Cry 'Foul,'" *TAGline*, July 1994, 1.

105. Robert Trautman, "AIDS Group Urges Wider Use of Experimental Drug," *Reuters*, 27 October 1994.

106. John S. James, "'Access' and 'Answers': FDA Antiviral Advisory Meeting, September 12–13," *AIDS Treatment News*, 16 September 1994.

107. G'dali Braverman, interview by author, tape recording, San Francisco, 17 December 1993.

108. Brenda Lein, interview by author, tape recording, San Francisco, 18 December 1993.

109. Peter Staley, "The Responsibilities of Empowerment" (paper presented at "Until There Is a Cure, VI" Conference, Palmetto, Fla., 2 December 1994, photocopy). This was the keynote address, distributed by Treatment Action Group in New York.

110. Harrington, "Crisis in Clinical AIDS Research," 11–12.

111. David Barr, interview by author, tape recording, New York City, 28 April 1994.

112. Tim Kingston, "Coppola's Kids: Leading AIDS Researchers Gather at Project Inform Think Tank in Napa," *San Francisco Bay Times*, 28 January 1993, 6–7.

113. Gregg Gonsalves, "Basic Research on HIV Infection: A Report from the Front" (Treatment Action Group, New York, 1993, photocopy), 1–2.

114. Ibid., 4, 5.

115. Quoted in Simon Watney, "Dutch Dating," *QW*, 9 August 1992, 44, 45, 67.

116. Donald Abrams, interview by author, tape recording, San Francisco, 16 December 1993.

117. Gina Kolata, "Scientists Say U.S. Research on AIDS Needs Redirection," *New York Times*, 12 May 1994, A-12.

118. Bernard N. Fields, "AIDS: Time to Turn to Basic Science," *Nature* 369 (12 May 1994): 95–96.

119. Kolata, "Scientists Say U.S. Research on AIDS Needs Redirection." On William Paul's appointment, see Jon Cohen, "New AIDS Chief Takes Charge," *Science* 263 (11 March 1994): 1364–1366.

120. Andrew Pollack, "Meeting Lays Bare the Abyss between AIDS and Its Cure," *New York Times*, 12 August 1994, A-1.

121. Julio S. G. Montaner and Martin T. Schechter, "Time for Realism over HIV Infection," *Lancet* 344 (20 August 1994): 535.

122. Andrew Pollack, "U.S. Official to Shift Funds toward Basic AIDS Research," *New York Times*, 10 August 1994, A-6.

123. The transcript of this presentation was published in William E. Paul, "A Turning Point in AIDS Research: Building on Firmer Foundations," *Vital Speeches* 60 (September 1994): 709–712.

124. Martin Delaney, "The Evolution of Community-Based Research," Session PS-02–3, IX International Conference on AIDS, Berlin, 8 June 1993.

125. Fauci, interview.

126. Link, interview.

127. Lein, interview.

128. Robert Gallo, interview by author, tape recording, Bethesda, Md., 3 November 1994.

129. The term "pollination" was suggested to me by Michael Botkin, interview by author, tape recording, San Francisco, 16 December 1993.

130. Gallo, interview.

131. Link, interview.

132. Ho, Neumann et al., "Rapid Turnover of Plasma Virions"; Wei, Ghosh et al., "Viral Dynamics." On the persistence of imagery of warfare in discourses about the immune system, see Emily Martin, *Flexible Bodies: Tracking Immunity in American Culture—From the Days of Polio to the Age of AIDS* (Boston: Beacon Press, 1994).

133. David D. Ho, "Time to Hit HIV, Early and Hard," *New England Journal of Medicine* 333 (17 August 1995): 450–451.

134. Marlene Cimons, "New Strategies Fuel Optimism in AIDS Fight," *Los Angeles Times*, 20 February 1995, A-1.

135. John S. James, "3TC Plus AZT: Important Treatment Advance?" *AIDS Treatment News*, 12 December 1994.

136. "Like the Wings of Icarus, Treatment Hype Sweeps Its Prey Upward to the Heavens, Then Plucks Them Down Into Icey [sic] Waters," *TAGline*, February 1995, 1, 3, 5.

137. Stephen D. Moore, "Wellcome Advises Shareholders to Accept $15.15 Billion Takeover Offer from Glaxo," *Wall Street Journal*, 8 March 1995, A-3.

138. Rick Loftus and David Gold, "Protease Inhibitors: Where Are They Now?" *GMHC Treatment Issues,* January 1995.

139. "AIDS Activists Seek Speedy Access to Protease Drugs," *Nature* 374 (2 March 1995): 4.

140. Diane Naughton, "Drug Lotteries Raise Questions: Some Experts Say System of Distribution May Be Unfair," *Washington Post,* 26 September 1995, Z-14.

141. Loftus and Gold, "Protease Inhibitors."

142. Claire O'Brien, "HIV Integrase Structure Catalyzes Drug Search," *Science* 266 (23 December 1994): 1946.

143. Warren E. Leary, "Experts Press for Fast Action on AIDS Drug," *New York Times,* 8 November 1995.

144. Philip J. Hilts, "Acting with Unusual Speed, Drug Agency Approves New AIDS Treatment," *New York Times,* 2 March 1996, 7; Philip J. Hilts, "With Record Speed, F.D.A. Approves a New AIDS Drug," *New York Times,* 15 March 1996, A-9.

145. Lawrence K. Altman, "A New AIDS Drug Yielding Optimism as Well as Caution," *New York Times,* 2 February 1996, A-1.

146. Daniel Hoth, interview by author, tape recording, Foster City, Calif., 11 July and 19 October 1994.

147. Jon Cohen, "Bringing AZT to Poor Countries," *Science* 269 (4 August 1995): 624–625.

148. Mark Barnes, "Treatment's High Cost," *New York Times,* 28 November 1995, A-14 (letter to the editor).

149. Richard Preston, *The Hot Zone* (New York: Anchor Books, 1994). For a more sober treatment, see Laurie Garrett, *The Coming Plague: Newly Emerging Diseases in a World Out of Balance* (New York: Farrar, Straus and Giroux, 1994).

150. Lawrence K. Altman, "AIDS Is Now the Leading Killer of Americans from 25 to 44," *New York Times,* 31 January 1995, B-8; "First 500,000 AIDS Cases—United States, 1995," *Morbidity and Mortality Weekly Report* 44 (24 November 1995): 849–853.

151. See Elizabeth Fee and Daniel M. Fox, eds., *AIDS: The Making of a Chronic Disease* (Berkeley: Univ. of California Press, 1992).

152. See H. P. Kitschelt, "Political Opportunity Structures and Political Protest: Anti-Nuclear Movements in Four Democracies," *British Journal of Political Science* 16 (January 1986): 57–85.

153. "Clinton Administration Names AIDS Panel to Speed Drug Search," *New York Times,* 7 February 1994, A-9.

154. Hoth, interview.

155. Jon Cohen, "AIDS Task Force Fizzles Out," *Science* 271 (26 January 1996): 438.

156. "15 Drug Firms Announce Alliance on AIDS Research," *Los Angeles Times,* 20 April 1993, D-2.

157. David R. Olmos, "The Cost of a Cure," *Los Angeles Times,* 2 March 1994, B-5.

158. Garance Franke-Ruta, interview by author, tape recording, New York City, 29 April 1994.

159. Braverman, interview.

160. Moisés Agosto, interview by author, tape recording, New York City, 26 April 1994.

161. Link, interview.

162. See Eric L. Hirsch, "Sacrifice for the Cause: Group Processes, Recruitment, and Commitment in a Student Social Movement," *American Sociological Review* 55 (April 1990): 243–254.

163. Sarah Schulman, *My American History: Lesbian and Gay Life During the Reagan/Bush Years* (New York: Routledge, 1994), 12.

164. Mark Harrington, interview by author, tape recording, New York City, 29 April 1994.

165. See Scott A. Hunt, Robert D. Benford, and David A. Snow, "Identity Fields: Framing Processes and the Social Construction of Movement Identities," in *New Social Movements: From Ideology to Identity*, ed. Enrique Laraña, Hank Johnston, and Joseph R. Gusfield (Philadelphia: Temple Univ. Press, 1994), 185–208.

166. Chris Bull, "No News Is Bad News," *The Advocate*, 13 July 1993, 24–27.

167. Franke-Ruta, interview.

168. Kolata, "Scientists Say U.S. Research on AIDS Needs Redirection."

Conclusion

1. As Bourdieu has argued more generally, "the question of the limits of the field is a very difficult one, if only because it is *always a stake in the field itself* and therefore admits of no *a priori* answer. . . . Thus the boundaries of the field can only be determined by an empirical investigation" (Pierre Bourdieu and Loïc J. D. Wacquant, *An Invitation to Reflexive Sociology* [Chicago: Univ. of Chicago Press, 1992], 100 [emphasis in the original]).

2. Exceptions are discussed in the introduction.

3. See Steven Shapin and Simon Schaffer, *Leviathan and the Air-Pump: Hobbes, Boyle, and the Experimental Life* (Princeton, N.J.: Princeton Univ. Press, 1985); Harry Collins, *Changing Order: Replication and Induction in Scientific Practice*, 2d ed. (Chicago: Univ. of Chicago Press, 1992); Harry Collins and Trevor Pinch, *The Golem: What Everyone Should Know about Science* (Cambridge: Cambridge Univ. Press, 1993). For an analysis of such debates in the interpretation of clinical trials, see Evelleen Richards, *Vitamin C and Cancer: Medicine or Politics?* (New York: St. Martin's, 1991).

4. Douglas Richman, interview by author, tape recording, San Diego, 1 June 1994.

5. Rae Goodell, "The Role of the Mass Media in Scientific Controversies," in *Scientific Controversies: Case Studies in the Resolution and Closure of Disputes in Science and Technology*, ed. H. Tristram Engelhardt Jr. and Arthur L. Caplan (Cambridge, England: Cambridge Univ. Press, 1987), 585–597, quote from 590. This echoes Anthony Fauci's criticism of media coverage of Peter Duesberg (see chapter 4).

6. Todd Gitlin, *The Whole World Is Watching: Mass Media in the Making*

and Unmaking of the New Left (Berkeley: Univ. of California Press, 1980), chapter 5.

7. See Alvin Gouldner's discussion of the "culture of critical discourse" in *The Future of Intellectuals and the Rise of the New Class* (New York: Oxford Univ. Press, 1979), 27–47. For a similar argument about researchers' felt need to take AIDS activists' scientific arguments seriously, see William Francis Patrick Crowley III, "Gaining Access: The Politics of AIDS Clinical Drug Trials in Boston" (undergraduate thesis, Harvard College, 1991), 76–77.

8. On obligatory passage points in science, see Bruno Latour, *Science in Action* (Cambridge, Mass.: Harvard Univ. Press, 1987).

9. For an analysis of how debates within expert circles can expand outward to incorporate activists, see Brian Balogh, *Chain Reaction: Expert Debate and Public Participation in American Commercial Nuclear Power, 1945–1975* (Cambridge, England: Cambridge Univ. Press, 1991).

10. Latour, *Science in Action.*

11. Cf. Bourdieu and Wacquant, *Invitation to Reflexive Sociology,* 99.

12. Donna J. Haraway, *Simians, Cyborgs, and Women: The Reinvention of Nature* (New York: Routledge, 1991), chapter 9.

13. Giovanna Di Chiro, "Defining Environmental Justice: Women's Voices and Grassroots Politics," *Socialist Review,* October-December 1992, 93–130, esp. 120.

14. Anthony Fauci, interview by author, tape recording, Bethesda, Md., 31 October 1994.

15. Jonathan Kwitny, *Acceptable Risks* (New York: Poseidon Press, 1992), 461.

16. Robert Gallo, interview by author, tape recording, Bethesda, Md., 3 November 1994.

17. Douglas Richman, interview by author, tape recording, San Diego, 1 June 1994.

18. John Phair, interview by author, tape recording, Chicago, 15 November 1994.

19. Andrew Abbott, *The System of Professions: An Essay on the Division of Expert Labor* (Chicago: Univ. of Chicago Press, 1988), 75–76.

20. Gina Kolata, "F.D.A. Urges Special Access to Rejected Alzheimer Drug," *New York Times,* 23 March 1991, A-7; David Feigal, interview by author, tape recording, Rockville, Md., 1 November 1994.

21. Peter S. Arno and Karyn L. Feiden, *Against the Odds: The Story of AIDS Drug Development, Politics and Profits* (New York: HarperCollins, 1992); Jonathan Kwitny, *Acceptable Risks* (New York: Poseidon Press, 1992).

22. Figures from a handout prepared by Division of AIDS, NIAID, labeled "Adult ACTG Accrual." In general, subject populations in community-based research initiatives have been more demographically diverse than those in ACTG trials.

23. Minutes of the ACTG Executive Committee meeting (Joint Session with the Principal Investigators), Division of AIDS, NIAID, 7 March 1989; Minutes of the ACTG Executive Committee Meeting, Division of AIDS, NIAID, 6 October 1988.

24. Philip J. Hilts, "F.D.A. Ends Ban on Women in Drug Testing," *New York Times,* 25 March 1993, B-8.

25. Fauci, interview.

26. Susan Ellenberg, interview by author, tape recording, Rockville, Md., 25 April 1994.

27. Donald Abrams, interview by author, tape recording, San Francisco, 16 December 1993.

28. Paula Treichler has made a similar point about community-based AIDS research projects. See "How to Have Theory in an Epidemic: The Evolution of AIDS Treatment Activism," in *Technoculture,* ed. Constance Penley and Andrew Ross (Minneapolis: Univ. of Minnesota Press, 1991), 57–106, esp. 79.

29. Michelle Roland, interview by author, tape recording, Davis, Calif., 18 December 1993.

30. Phair, interview.

31. For the terminology of "lay expert" and "lay lay" activists, I am indebted to Gilbert Elbaz, "The Sociology of AIDS Activism, the Case of ACT UP/New York, 1987–1992" (Ph.D. diss., City University of New York, 1992), 488.

32. Roland, interview.

33. Some activists who criticize groups like TAG, such as Maxine Wolfe of the Women's Caucus of ACT UP/New York (interview by author, tape recording, New York City, 27 April 1994), do take a more radical stance in objecting to the randomized clinical trial. But this is a minority position.

34. Richards, *Vitamin C and Cancer,* 204, 232–234, 5.

35. Quoted in Paul Cotton, "HIV Surrogate Markers Weighed," *Journal of the American Medical Association* 265 (20 March 1991): 1357, 1361, 1362, quote from 1362.

36. Mark Harrington, "The Crisis in Clinical AIDS Research" (Treatment Action Group, New York, 1 December 1993, photocopy), 7.

37. Conveying to the public a deeper sense of the uncertainty endemic to the process of scientific investigation is similar to the mission expressed by Collins and Pinch in *Golem.* See also Sheila Jasanoff, *The Fifth Branch: Science Advisers as Policymakers* (Cambridge, Mass.: Harvard Univ. Press, 1990).

38. "Public Hearings at FDA Juxtapose Old Cries of Access with Those of Integrity, Accountability," *TAGline,* October 1994, 2.

39. Brian Wynne, "Unruly Technology: Practical Rules, Impractical Discourses and Public Understanding," *Social Studies of Science* 18 (February 1988): 147–167; Collins and Pinch, *Golem.*

40. Alberto Melucci, *Nomads of the Present: Social Movements and Individual Needs in Contemporary Society* (Philadelphia: Temple Univ. Press, 1989), 73–76.

41. Thomas Merigan, interview by author, tape recording, Palo Alto, Calif., 29 June 1994.

42. Gina Kolata, "Their Treatment, Their Lives, Their Decisions," *New York Times Magazine,* 24 April 1994, 66, 100, 105.

43. Andrew Feenberg, "On Being a Human Subject: Interest and Obligation in the Experimental Treatment of Incurable Disease," *The Philosophical Forum* 23 (spring 1992): 213–230; Carol Levine, Nancy Neveloff Dubler, and Robert J. Levine, "Building a New Consensus: Ethical Principles and Policies for Clinical Research on HIV/AIDS," *AIDS Patient Care*, April 1992, 67–85.

44. Robert M. Wachter, *The Fragile Coalition: Scientists, Activists, and AIDS* (New York: St. Martin's, 1991), xiii.

45. Roland, interview.

46. Rebecca Smith, interview by author, tape recording, Providence, R.I., 26 October 1994.

47. See Mark A. Chesler, "Mobilizing Consumer Activism in Health Care: The Role of Self-Help Groups," *Research in Social Movements, Conflicts and Change* 13 (1991): 275–305; Miriam J. Stewart, "Expanding Theoretical Conceptualizations of Self-Help Groups," *Social Science and Medicine* 31 (May 1990): 1057–1066; and the special issue of the *American Journal of Community Psychology* 19 (October 1991).

48. David S. Meyer and Nancy Whittier, "Social Movement Spillover," *Social Problems* 41 (May 1994): 277–298; David A. Snow and Robert D. Benford, "Master Frames and Cycles of Protest," in *Frontiers in Social Movement Theory*, ed. Aldon D. Morris and Carol McClurg Mueller (New Haven: Yale Univ. Press, 1992), 133–155.

49. Marian Uhlman, "Revolt by Patients Threatens Test of Lou Gehrig Drug," *Philadelphia Inquirer*, 21 March 1994, A-1; Tim Kingston, "The 'White Rats' Rebel: Chronic Fatigue Patients Sue Drug Manufacturer for Breaking Contract to Supply Promising CFIDS Drug," *San Francisco Bay Times*, 7 November 1991, 8, 44; Marcia Barinaga, "Furor at Lyme Disease Conference," *Science* 256 (5 June 1992): 1384–1385; "Marching for Alzheimer's," *Wall Street Journal*, 24 September 1992 (editorial); Lisa W. Foderaro, "Mentally Ill Gaining New Rights with the Ill as Their Own Lobby," *New York Times*, 14 October 1995, A-1; Christina Smith, "Living with Environmental Illness," *San Francisco Bay Times*, December 1990.

50. See Robert M. Wachter, "AIDS, Activism, and the Politics of Health," *New England Journal of Medicine* 326 (9 January 1992): 128–133.

51. "MD Telethon Boycott Urged," *San Francisco Examiner*, 2 September 1991, B-1.

52. Malcolm Gladwell, "Beyond HIV: The Legacies of Health Activism," *Washington Post*, 15 October 1992, A-29.

53. Susan Ferraro, "The Anguished Politics of Breast Cancer," *New York Times Magazine*, 15 August 1993, 26. See also Jackie Winnow, "Lesbians Evolving Health Care: Cancer and AIDS," *Feminist Review*, summer 1992, 68–77; Judy Brady, ed., *1 in 3: Women with Cancer Confront an Epidemic* (Pittsburgh and San Francisco: Cleis Press, 1991); Alisa Solomon, "The Politics of Breast Cancer," *Camera Obscura* 28 (January 1992): 157–177.

54. Ferraro, "Anguished Politics of Breast Cancer," 27. See also Gina Kolata, "Weighing Spending on Breast Cancer Research," *New York Times*, 20 October 1993, B-9.

55. Jane Gross, "Turning Disease into Political Cause: First AIDS, and Now Breast Cancer," *New York Times*, 7 January 1991, A-12. See also Lisa

M. Krieger, "Breast Cancer Activists Look to AIDS Forces," *San Francisco Examiner,* 5 May 1991, A-1, A-16.

56. Gross, "Turning Disease into Political Cause."

57. "ACT UP Fights for Breast Cancer Drug," *AIDS Treatment News,* 23 December 1994.

58. Bruce Mirken, "Quiet Collaboration between AIDS and Breast Cancer Activists Is Beginning to Pay Off," *San Francisco Bay Times,* 10 March 1994, 8–9.

59. Brenda Lein, interview by author, tape recording, San Francisco, 18–19 December 1993.

60. Lein, interview; Mirken, "Quiet Collaboration."

61. Mark Harrington, interview by author, tape recording, New York City, 29 April 1994.

62. Richard E. Sclove, *Democracy and Technology* (New York: Guilford, 1995), 26–27.

63. Sheldon Krimsky, "Beyond Technocracy: New Routes for Citizen Involvement in Social Risk Assessment," in *Citizen Participation in Science Policy,* ed. James C. Petersen (Amherst: Univ. of Massachusetts Press, 1984), 43–61; James C. Petersen, "Citizen Participation in Science Policy," in *Citizen Participation in Science Policy* (above), 1–17; Loet Leydesdorff and Peter Van den Besselaar, "What We Have Learned from the Amsterdam Science Shop," in *The Social Direction of the Public Sciences,* ed. Stuart Blume et al. (Dordrecht, Holland: D. Reidel, 1987), 135–160. For general perspectives on the democratization of science, technology, and research practices, see John Gaventa, "The Powerful, the Powerless, and the Experts: Knowledge Struggles in an Information Age," in *Voices of Change: Participatory Research in the United States and Canada,* ed. Peter Park et al. (Westport, Conn.: Bergin & Garvey, 1993), 21–40; Andrew Feenberg, *Critical Theory of Technology* (New York: Oxford Univ. Press, 1991); Joseph Turner, "Democratizing Science: A Humble Proposal," *Science, Technology & Human Values* 15 (summer 1990): 336–359; Michael Goldhaber, *Reinventing Technology: Policies for Democratic Values* (New York: Routledge, 1986); Brian Martin, "The Goal of Self-Managed Science: Implications for Action," *Radical Science Journal* 10 (1980): 3–16.

64. See Robert Kleidman, "Volunteer Activism and Professionalism in Social Movement Organizations," *Social Problems* 41 (May 1994): 257–276; Barbara Epstein, *Political Protest and Cultural Revolution: Nonviolent Direct Action in the 1970s and 1980s* (Berkeley: Univ. of California Press, 1991), 271; Ronald J. Troyer, "From Prohibition to Regulation: Comparing Two Antismoking Movements," *Research in Social Movements, Conflicts and Change* 7 (1984): 53–69.

65. Robert W. Rycroft, "Environmentalism and Science: Politics and the Pursuit of Knowledge," *Knowledge: Creation, Diffusion, Utilization* 13 (December 1991): 150–169, esp. 163–164.

66. Franke-Ruta, interview.

67. Moisés Agosto, interview by author, tape recording, New York City, 26 April 1994.

68. A fully adequate consideration of these issues would include an

analysis of relations of power, knowledge, and expertise in a global context—
for example, an examination of the ways in which, at times, "the concerns of
the developing world pale beside the new alliance of medical smocks and ACT
UP t-shirts" (Dennis Altman, *Power and Community: Organizational and
Cultural Responses to AIDS* [London: Taylor & Francis, 1994], 133).

69. Gregg Gonsalves and Mark Harrington, "AIDS Research at the NIH:
A Critical Review. Part I: Summary" (Treatment Action Group, New York,
1992, photocopy), 1-2.

Methodological Appendix

1. See Eugene Garfield, "Which Medical Journals Have the Greatest Impact?" *Annals of Internal Medicine* 105 (August 1986): 313-320.

2. David Bloor, *Knowledge and Social Imagery,* 2d ed. (Chicago: Univ. of
Chicago Press, 1991), 7, 175-179.

3. Pam Scott, Evelleen Richards, and Brian Martin, "Captives of Controversy: The Myth of the Neutral Social Researcher in Contemporary Scientific
Controversies," *Science, Technology, & Human Values* 15 (fall 1990): 475.

4. For debates about "symmetry" and "neutrality," see Scott, Richards,
and Martin, "Captives of Controversy"; H. M. Collins, "Captives and Victims: Comments on Scott, Richards, and Martin," *Science, Technology, &
Human Values* 16 (spring 1991): 249-251.

5. Michel Foucault, *The Order of Things: An Archaeology of the Human
Sciences* (New York: Vintage Books, 1973); Michel Foucault, *The Archaeology of Knowledge* (New York: Pantheon, 1972).

6. Michel Foucault, *Power/Knowledge* (New York: Pantheon, 1980), 83-
85.

7. On "situated knowledges," see Donna J. Haraway, *Simians, Cyborgs,
and Women: The Reinvention of Nature* (New York: Routledge, 1991), chapter 9.

8. For general procedures in performing content analysis, see Klaus Krip-
pendorff, *Content Analysis: An Introduction to Its Methodology* (Beverly
Hills, Calif.: Sage, 1980); Richard W. Budd, Robert K. Thorp, and Lewis Don-
ohew, *Content Analysis of Communication* (New York: Macmillan, 1967).

9. Eugene Garfield, ed., *Science Citation Index Journal Citation Reports*
(Philadelphia: Institute for Scientific Information), 1985, 1986, 1987.

10. Other specialty journals, such as the *Journal of Biological Chemistry*
and the *Journal of the American Chemical Society* also ranked high on this
list. But a check of the articles citing Gallo's paper revealed that practically no
authors who wrote for these journals cited Gallo. Therefore, these journals
were not included.

11. Other medical journals, such as the *WHO Technical Report Series,*
also ranked high on this list. But again, authors who wrote for these more
specialized publications were not among those citing Gallo's paper. On medical publications, see also Garfield, "Which Medical Journals Have the Greatest Impact?"

12. See C. Self, W. Filardo, and W. Lancaster, "Acquired Immunodeficiency Syndrome (AIDS) and the Epidemic Growth of Its Literature," *Scientometrics* 17 (July 1989): 49–60; I. N. Sengupta and Lalita Kumari, "Bibliometric Analysis of AIDS Literature," *Scientometrics* 20 (January 1991): 297–315.

13. I consulted the 1987 issue because the *SCI* does not report some citations until the year after their publication date.

14. Garfield, "Which Medical Journals Have the Greatest Impact?" 313, 315.

15. There were thirty-four such articles in the *Annals of Internal Medicine*, twenty-seven in *JAMA*, thirty-one in *Lancet*, nineteen in *Nature*, thirty-four in the *New England Journal*, thirty-three in the *Proceedings*, and sixty-six in *Science*.

16. I looked at the citing sentence only, unless that sentence did not permit a determination. In that case, I looked at the three preceding and three subsequent sentences to see if they provided additional context.

17. My original coding was more elaborate, differentiating between Gallo and the other coauthors and examining whether or not Gallo was the first author. In the end, there proved to be too few cases in most of these categories, so I combined the data, to distinguish simply between articles with an author from the Gallo group and articles without such an author.

18. A comparison of the four medical journals as an aggregate versus the three general science journals as an aggregate did not reveal any interesting differences. Therefore, I do not report these data.

INDEX

Abbott (pharmaceutical company), 323, 324

Abbott, Andrew, 366n.61, 371n.108, 384n.56, 413n.22, 438n.19; on academic researchers, 215; on advisory jurisdictions, 339; on the germ theory, 58; on the professions, 23, 372n.113

Aboulker, Jean-Pierre, 245, 301

Abraham, John, 375n.155

Abrams, Donald: on activism, 252, 319, 341; on clinical trials, 248; on ddI licensing, 277; forms the County Community Consortium, 216, 217

Abrams, Garry, 140

academic freedom, 176

accelerated approval program, 278–79, 280, 315–16. *See also* conditional approval program

Acker, Caroline Jean, 375n.147

Acquired Immunodeficiency Syndrome. *See* AIDS

ACTG (AIDS Clinical Trials Group), 211, 259, 281, 340; activist involvement in, 284–87, 290–91

ACTG 016 trial, 213–14, 237

ACTG 019 trial, 213–14, 237–40

ACTG 076 trial, 291, 311–12, 325

ACTG 155 trial, 266–67, 307–9, 312–15, 318

activism: cancer movement, 9, 20, 223, 348–49; environmental movement, 351; of Haitians, 66; of people with hemophilia, 289–90; against paternalism,

190, 206, 222. *See also* ACT UP; AIDS movement; feminist health movement; gay movement; social movements; treatment activism

actor-network theory of scientific knowledge, 18

ACT UP (AIDS Coalition to Unleash Power), 116, 117, 173, 219–21; accused of racism, 291; chapters worldwide, 219; demonstration at NIH headquarters, 285, 287; identity politics of, 21; involvement in the ACTG, 284–87; meetings by consensus, 220; negotiations with the FDA, 226; people of color in, 289, 291; rifts within, 291–94; street theater of, 220, 226, 247; Western *vs.* alternative medicine, 293–94. *See also specific chapters*

ACT UP/Boston, 1–2, 220

ACT UP/Chicago, 219, 292

ACT UP/Golden Gate, 292, 294, 299, 317–18, 349

ACT UP/Houston, 219

ACT UP/Los Angeles, 220

ACT UP/New Orleans, 219

ACT UP/New York: "AIDS Treatment Research Agenda," 246–47, 281; dominance of, 220; "FDA Action Handbook," 224–25; Media Committee, 225; Treatment & Data Committee, 281, 286, 288, 291, 292, 293; Women's Action Committee, 292; Women's Caucus, 288, 291, 292. *See also* TAG

maintaining legitimacy, 16–17; manufacture of, 2, 337; patients as, 9; power
of, 4; *vs.* laypeople, 3, 12, 292–93,
350; within social movements, 8–10,
13, 285, 292–93, 332, 342
Eyerman, Ron, 368n.80
Ezrahi, Yaron, 362n.20, 407n.132

Factor VIII (blood product), 56
Fain, Nathan, 76, 98
Farber, Celia, 112, 116, 176
Farmer, Paul, 378n.168, 385n.87
Fauci, Anthony: on AIDS vaccine, 182;
assumption of AIDS/gay link, 56; on
AZT, 210–11, 240; on the CCG, 290;
on community-based research, 219; on
covert infection of lymphoid cells, 164;
criticized by activists for incompetence,
196, 236; on drug testing, 212, 218,
261; on Duesberg, 119, 120, 170; on
HIV hypothesis, 115; on the media,
175; and National Conference on
Women and HIV Infection, 289; supports activists, 235–36, 249, 286–87,
321, 328, 338; supports parallel track
program, 236–37; on surrogate markers, 271, 316
FDA (Food and Drug Administration):
accelerated approval of drugs, 278–79,
280, 315–16; Anti-Infective Advisory
Committee, 199, 200; Antiviral Advisory Committee, 239, 275–80, 316;
AZT approved by, 199; blood screening test licensed by, 182; and buyers
clubs, 223–24; clinical trials required
for drug licensing, 185–86, 250–51,
270, 408n.12; compassionate-use approval of drugs, 188, 222; conditional
approval of drugs, 273–74; criticized
by activists, 222–26; criticized by conservatives, 223; d4T approved by, 315;
on HIV hypothesis, 83; ignores buyers
clubs, 267, 269; pentamidine approved
by, 218; on surrogate markers, 275–
76; Treatment Investigational New
Drugs, 222; women in clinical trials,
attitude toward, 260, 340
"FDA Action Handbook," 224–25
Fee, Elizabeth, 362n.12, 364n.30
Feenberg, Andrew, 440n.43, 441n.63
Feiden, Karyn, 40, 410n.46, 414n.32,
415n.51, 417n.93, 427n.83, 438n.21

Feigal, David, 274, 278
Feinberg, Mark, 283
Feinstein, Alvan, 255
feminist health movement, 7, 9–10, 12,
205
Feorino, Paul, 89, 90, 390n.28, 391n.37
Fettner, Ann, 122
fever, 147
field, definition of, 18–19, 367n.75,
437n.1
Fields, Bernard, 320
Figert, Anne E., 371n.101
Filardo, W., 376n.159, 388n.2, 443n.12
Financial Times, 151
Fineman, Norman, 412n.84
Fischl, Margaret, 193, 198, 201, 214,
266, 284; ACTG 155 trial, 266–67,
307–9, 312–15, 318
flu (influenza A), 182
fluoridation controversy, 172–73, 174
Food and Drug Administration. *See* FDA
Food, Drug, and Cosmetic Act (1938),
185
Fortin, Alfred J., 377n.165, 394n.84
Foucault, Michel, 371n.99, 380n.14,
382n.26; on genealogical research,
357; on the microphysics of power, 4;
on the power of professionals, 23; on
sexuality, 20
Foundation for Alternative AIDS Re-
search (Netherlands), 154
"Founding Statement of People with
AIDS/ARC," 206
Fox, Daniel M., 362n.12, 378n.170
Fox, Rene C., 432n.65
Frader, Joel, 40, 412n.97
framing, 24–25, 77–78, 221, 264, 285
Francis, Donald, 28, 89
Frankel, Henry, 374n.140
Franke-Ruta, Garance, 326–27, 328,
347, 352
Franks, Pat, 383n.42
freedom of thought, 176
Friedland, Gerald, 239
Friedman, Samuel R., 377n.167,
378n.168
Friedman-Kien, Alvin, 46–47, 160–61
Freidson, Eliot, 23, 49, 372n.108,
372n.111, 381n.17; on professional au-
thority, 205
Fujimura, Joan, 68, 366n.49, 367n.73,
391n.41; on the causation controversy,

Markle, Gerald, 363n.29, 369n.81,
 415n.56; on resource mobilization,
 20
Marks, Harry, 374–75n.147, 408n.11,
 424n.14; on clinical trials, 197; on doctors *vs.* researchers, 255; on drug evaluation, 185, 408n.12
Martin, Brian, 361n.2, 392n.60,
 441n.63, 442n.3; on fluoridation
 controversy, 172–73, 174
Martin, Emily, 39
Marx, Jean, 193
Mason, James, 72, 101
Mass, Lawrence, 54; on epidemiology,
 61–62; on gay men's promiscuity as
 cause of AIDS, 46; on medical advice,
 65; on virus as cause of AIDS, 56
Masur, Henry, 47
Matthews, J. Rosser, 375n.147
Mausner, Judith S., 76
Maver, Robert, 143
media: credibility and, 22–23, 174–76,
 335; gay/alternative press, 174; journal-
 ists' dependence on sources, 175–76;
 journalists' professional orientation,
 372n.113. *See also specific publica-
 tions*
medicine, field of. *See* biomedicine; doc-
 tors
Meditel Productions, 112, 130, 174
Medline database, 106, 394n.2
Mehan, Hugh, 369n.84
Meier, Paul, 278
Meldrum, Marcia Lynn, 375n.147
Meltzer, Monte S., 209
Melucci, Alberto, 21, 369n.83, 370n.87;
 on social movements, 346
Merck, 323, 324
Merigan, Thomas, 263, 284, 346
Merton, Robert K., 363n.24
"Methodological Issues in AIDS Clinical
 Trials" (symposium), 251, 253
Meyer, David S., 365n.40, 440n.48
microbes. *See* monocausal/microbial
 model of illness
Mildvan, Donna, 46
Mineshaft (New York City bath house),
 134
Mitsuya, Hiroaki, 192
Monette, Paul, 207
monocausal/microbial model of illness:
 criticism of, 57; dominance of, 57, 58;

vs. immune overload hypothesis, 57;
 left-wing rejection of, 158. *See also* viral hypothesis
monogamy, 63, 97. *See also* promiscuity
 of gay men
mononucleosis, 108
Montagnier, Luc: alleged defection of,
 154–55; on autoimmune mechanisms,
 103, 184; cited by others, 388–89n.8;
 on cofactors, 84, 129, 140, 150, 155,
 284; discovers HIV-2, 80, 208; discovers LAV, 69–71; on Duesberg, 152;
 LAV antibodies study, 88–89; on mycoplasma, 129, 140, 155; publishes LAV
 research in *Science,* 70; sends LAV sample to Gallo, 71
Montini, Theresa, 367n.70, 432n.65
Moore, Kelly, 368n.79, 369n.81
Morris, Aldon D., 370n.87
movements: cancer movement, 9, 20,
 223, 348–49; environmental movement, 351; Haitian movement, 66; hemophiliac movement, 289–90. *See also*
 AIDS movement; feminist health movement; gay movement; social movements
Mueller, Carol McClurg, 370n.87
Mueller, Mary-Rose, 40, 379n.174; on
 community-based research, 216
Mukerji, Chandra, 366n.59
Mulkay, Michael, 366n.49
Mullis, Kary, 151, 153, 156, 169
multiple chemical sensitivity, 348
Murbach, Ruth, 411n.74
Murdoch, Rupert, 150. *See also specific
 newspapers*
Murray, Stephen, 40, 362n.19, 381n.19,
 382n.31, 415n.42
muscular dystrophy, 348
mycoplasmas, 92, 129, 140

Names Project AIDS Quilt, 225
National Academy of Sciences (NAS):
 Confronting AIDS, 102–3, 109, 126–
 27. *See also Proceedings of the National Academy of Sciences*
National Breast Cancer Coalition, 348–
 49
National Cancer Institute (NCI), 184,
 210, 298
National Commission for the Protection
 of Human Subjects, 189–90

Palca, Joseph, 145
Panem, Sandra, 378n.170
parallel track program, 236–37, 340
Pasteur Institute (Paris): on HIV hypothesis, 84; LAV antibodies study, 88–89; LAV discovered at, 69–72 (see also Montagnier, Luc); patent dispute with U.S. government over blood screening test, 77
paternalism, activism against, 190, 206, 222
pathogenesis, 145, 283; vs. etiology, 123–24, 157; and viral load, 316–17
patients: activism of, 348–50; education of, 9, 10; noncompliance of, 204–5, 206–7, 238, 249; self-help groups, 9. See also activism; treatment activism
"Patient's Bill of Rights," 206
Patton, Cindy, 39, 373n.126, 377n.168, 380n.13, 381n.18, 383n.42, 393n.63, 427n.89; on AIDS activism, 408n.18
Paul, William, 320
Pauling, Linus, 127–128
Payne, Kenneth, 40, 362n.19, 381n.19, 382n.31
PCP (Pneumocystis carinii pneumonia), 45–46, 49, 132, 133, 199, 218; among hemophiliacs, 56
PCR (polymerase chain reaction), 120, 151, 156, 163, 272, 306
pentamidine, aerosolized, 218
Penthouse, 27
Perrow, Charles, 378n.170
Petersen, James, 363n.29, 369n.80, 415n.56, 441n.63; on resource mobilization, 20
Petrow, Steven, 383n.42
Phair, John, 338
pharmaceutical companies, 326. See also specific companies
Philadelphia, incidence of AIDS in, 259
Phillips, David, 22
physicians. See doctors
Physicians for Human Rights, 54
Pickering, Andrew, 366n.49
Pierret, Janine, 377n.166, 378n.170
Pinch, Trevor, 362n.11, 366n.49, 367n.68, 375n.153, 437n.3, 439n.37; on scientific controversy, 171; on value of experiments, 167
Pinching, Anthony, 244, 309–10
Pinn-Wiggins, Vivian, 262

placebos in clinical trials: activists' criticism of, 190, 202–4, 214; activists' support of, 251; function/effectiveness of, 193, 203, 209–10, 214, 250; vs. historical controls, 203, 251; and noncompliance, 204; as unethical, 202–3, 214, 245
PNAS. See Proceedings of the National Academy of Sciences
Pneumocystis carinii pneumonia. See PCP
pneumonia, 147. See also PCP
Poirier, Richard, 378n.171
Policy Review (Heritage Foundation publication), 141; publishes Duesberg and Ellison article on risk-AIDS hypothesis, 131–37, 138
polio vaccine, 201
Pollak, Michaël, 378n.170
polymerase chain reaction. See PCR
poppers. See nitrite inhalants
Popular Health Movement, 205
Porter, Theodore M., 375n.155, 410n.53
power, microphysics of, 4
President's Commission on the HIV Epidemic, 119–20, 127, 218–19
Preston, Richard, 436n.149
prevention guidelines, 63, 96–97
Proceedings of the National Academy of Sciences (PNAS), 358; refuses to publish Duesberg, 146; publishes Duesberg, 127–29, 146
Proctor, Robert N., 362n.9
professions: authority of, 205, 268–69; autonomy of, 255, 269; logic of practice, 372n.113; and the medical field, 23–24; sociology of, 5, 23–24
programmed cell death, 155
Project AIDS International, 302
Project Inform (San Francisco), 117, 155, 223, 233, 275, 299; on accelerated approval, 316; advocates early intervention, 213, 242, 243; criticizes AZT dissenters, 243; criticizes HIV dissenters, 156–58, 159; on ddI licensing, 277; founding/goals of, 189, 233–34; Immune Restoration Think Tank, 318–19, 320–21; PI Perspectives, 233–34, 243; receives funds from Burroughs Wellcome, 299–300; researches Compound Q, 257–58; on surrogate markers, 271–72

thalidomide, 185, 408n.12
Third World, treatment in, 325
Thomas, Stephen B., 423n.102
Thomas Jr., Charles, 143, 144, 158–59
Thorp, Robert K., 442n.8
3TC, 322–23
TIBO, 295
Time, 162, 200, 315, 356
Times (London), 150, 151, 152; coverage of Duesberg, 27
Toronto Star (Canada), 154
Touraine, Alain, 370n.87
toxoplasmosis, 132
transfusion. *See* blood transfusion
Trauner, Joan, 383n.37
treatment: AIDS/cancer therapies similarities, 324; antiviral drugs, 183–85, 191; drug trials/licensing, length of time for, 186, 194, 210, 270; early intervention, 213, 239–40, 243–46, 309–10, 322; hit-and-miss approach to research, 183, 212; logical approach to research, 183, 212; NIH recommendations, 310; politics of, 31–38, 182; in poorer countries, 325. *See also* clinical trials; combination therapy; FDA; treatment activism; *specific drugs*
Treatment Action Group. *See* TAG
Treatment & Data Committee (of ACT UP/New York), 281, 286, 288, 291, 292, 293
treatment activism, 32–33, 177–78; basic research, involvement in, 298–99, 318–22; biostatisticians as allies, 247–48, 250, 254, 262–63; buyers clubs, 223–24, 229; and clinical-trial design, 227–28, 246–64, 340–46, 439n.33; community-based trials, 216–19, 438n.22; and conservatives, 223; constituencies within, 290–94; credibility of activists, 252–53, 335–39; criticism of the FDA, 222–26; decline of, 326–28; demonstration in Rockville, Md., against FDA, 225, 227; diversification of, 288–90; donations from Burroughs Wellcome, 299–300; drug development, discouragement over pace/failures of, 295–97, 429n.4; and drug-development bottleneck, 281–84; drug smuggling/bootlegging, 188; East Coast *vs.* West Coast, 317–18; education of communities, 35; effectiveness

of, 34, 35, 253–56, 338–40; effects on doctor-patient relationship, 346–47; expertification of activists, 13–14, 195–96, 207, 229–32, 285–86, 287–88, 293, 350–53; expertise about the community, 249–50; genesis of, 186–89; grassroots publications, 195 (see also *ATN*); hemophilia activists, 289–90; insider/outsider status of, 232–34, 287–88, 342, 351–52; at International Conference on AIDS, 236, 246–47; involvement in the ACTG, 284–87; and need for knowledge, 343–44; for patient autonomy/risk taking, 190, 206, 222; patient/research-subject roles, 202, 215–16; against placebos in clinical trials, 190, 202–4, 214; researchers' respect for, 337–39; respect for scientists, 328; situated knowledge of activists, 337; specialization within, 350–51; and surrogate markers, 270–76, 304, 341. *See also* ACT UP; AIDS movement; FDA; Project Inform
treatment controversy *vs.* causation controversy, 37–38, 177–78
Treatment Investigational New Drugs (Treatment INDs), 222
Treichler, Paula, 39, 80–81, 84, 379n.173, 387n.133, 398n.92, 419n.39; on community-based research, 439n.28
tricosanthin (Compound Q), 257–58
Troyer, Ronald J., 441n.64
Trueheart, Charles, 141
trust, 5–8, 14–17, 351. *See also* credibility
Tsiatis, Anastasios (Butch), 275
tuberculosis, 132–33, 147
Tuchman, Gaye, 392n.49
Turner, Bryan S., 370n.94
Turner, Joseph, 441n.63
Turner, Stephen P., 366n.57
Tuskegee syphilis study, 189, 259

uncertainty, 62–66, 241–42, 246, 305–6, 309; and clinical trials, 343–46; and credibility, 331–34; and distance from research front, 411n.82, 432n.65
United States government: applies for patent for blood screening test, 72; National Commission for the Protection of Human Subjects, 189–90; patent